INTRODUCTION TO BIOMEDICAL IMAGING

IEEE Press Series in Biomedical Engineering

The focus of our series is to introduce current and emerging technologies to biomedical and electrical engineering practitioners, researchers, and students. This series seeks to foster interdisciplinary biomedica engineering education to satisfy the needs of the industrial and academic areas. This requires an innovativ approach that overcomes the difficulties associated with the traditional textbook and edited collections.

Books in the IEEE Press Series in Biomedical Engineering

Webb, A., *Introduction to Biomedical Imaging*
Baura, G., *System Theory and Practical Applications of Biomedical Signals*
Rangayyan, R. M., *Biomedical Signal Analysis*
Akay, M., *Time Frequency and Wavelets in Biomedical Signal Processing*
Hudson, D. L. and Cohen, M. E., *Neural Networks and Artificial Intelligence for Biomedical Engineering*
Khoo, M. C. K., *Physiological Control Systems: Analysis, Simulation, and Estimation*
Liang, Z-P. and Lauterbur, P. C., *Principles of Magnetic Resonance Imaging: A Signal Processing Perspective*
Akay, M., *Nonlinear Biomedical Signal Processing: Volume I, Fuzzy Logic, Neural Networks and New Algorithms*
Akay, M., *Nonlinear Biomedical Signal Processing: Volume II, Dynamic Analysis and Modeling*
Ying, H., *Fuzzy Control and Modeling: Analytical Foundations and Applications*

INTRODUCTION TO BIOMEDICAL IMAGING

Andrew Webb

University of Illinois
Urbana, IL

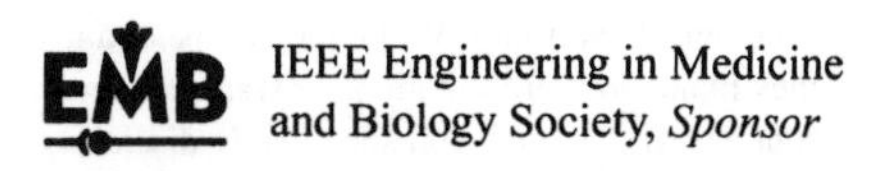

IEEE Engineering in Medicine
and Biology Society, *Sponsor*

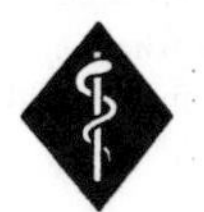

IEEE Press Series on Biomedical Engineering
Metin Akay, *Series Editor*

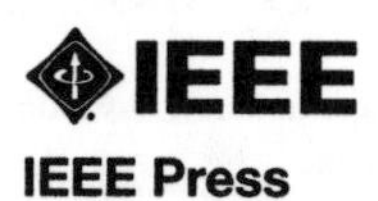

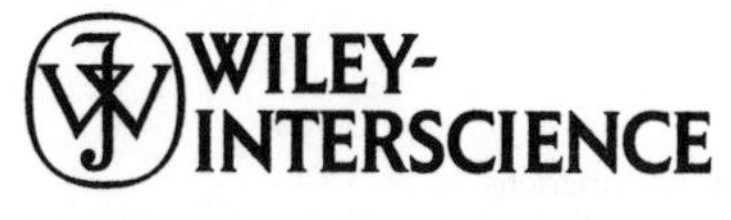

JOHN WILEY & SONS, INC.

Published by John Wiley & Sons, Inc., Hoboken, New Jersey.

For general information on our other products and services please contact our Customer Care Department within the U.S. at 877-762-2974, outside the U.S. at 317-572-3993 or fax 317-572-4002.

Wiley also publishes its books in a variety of electronic formats. Some content that appears in print, however, may not be available in electronic format.

Library of Congress Cataloging-in-Publication Data is available.

ISBN 0-471-23766-3

Printed in the United States of America

10 9 8 7 6 5 4 3

CONTENTS

PREFACE

This book grew out of notes developed for a course in biomedical imaging in the Electrical and Computer Engineering Department at the University of Illinois at Urbana-Champaign. As part of the IEEE Press Series in Biomedical Engineering, the approach and level of the material are aimed at junior- to senior-level undergraduates in bioengineering and/or other engineering disciplines. The content, however, should also be suitable for practitioners in more clinically related professions in which imaging plays an important role. One of the major goals was to prepare a textbook that would be suitable for a one-semester course, with an integrated and consistent description of each imaging modality. This involved choosing areas to discuss in detail, survey, or ignore. Sources of additional material not included in this book are suggested at the end of this preface.

The approach of this book is to cover physical principles, instrumental design, data acquisition strategies, image reconstruction techniques, and clinical applications of the four imaging techniques most commonly used in clinical medicine as well as in academic and commercial research. The first four chapters cover, respectively, X-ray and computed tomography, nuclear medicine, ultrasonic imaging, and magnetic resonance imaging. In each chapter, particular emphasis is placed on the basic science and engineering design involved in each imaging modality. Recent developments, such as multislice spiral computed tomography, harmonic and subharmonic ultrasonic imaging, multislice positron emission tomography, and functional magnetic resonance imaging, are also highlighted. The sections on clinical applications are relatively brief, comprising a few examples illustrative of the types of images that provide useful diagnostic information. Many hundreds of specialized diagnostic clinical imaging books exist, written by authors far more expert in these areas. The fifth chapter deals with general image characteristics, such as spatial resolution and signal-to-noise ratio, common to all of the imaging modalities. Finally, two appendices cover basic mathematics and transform methods, again common to many of the modalities. Suggestions are made at the end of each chapter for further reading. These lists comprise a selection of original "classic" papers in each field, recent books and review articles covering specific aspects of an area in considerably more detail than possible here, and a list of journals specific to the particular imaging modality. These selections are by necessity somewhat subjective and certainly not comprehensive. Those readers interested in historical aspects of the development of medical imaging should consult the elegant and succinct description in Chapter 1 of the book by S. Webb or the expansively detailed account in the book by B. H. Kevles, both listed in the Further Reading section below.

FURTHER READING

General

B. H. Kevles, *Naked to the Bone,* Rutgers University Press, New Brunswick, New Jersey (1997).

A. B. Wolbarst, *Looking Within: How X-Ray, CT, MRI, Ultrasound, and Other Medical Images Are Created, and How They Help Physicians Save Lives,* University of California Press, Berkeley (1999).

Introductory Imaging Texts

E. Krestel, ed. *Imaging Systems for Medical Diagnosis: Fundamentals and Technical Solutions—X-Ray Diagnostics-Computed Tomography-Nuclear Medical Diagnostics-Magnetic Resonance Imaging-Ultrasound Technology,* Wiley, New York (1990).

K. K. Shung, M. B. Smith, and B. Tsui, *Principles of Medical Imaging,* Academic Press, San Diego, California (1992).

D. J. Dowsett, P. A. Kenney, and R. E. Johnston, *The Physics of Diagnostic Imaging,* Chapman and Hall Medical, London (1998).

J. T. Bushberg, J. A. Seibert, E. M. Leidholdt, Jr., and J. M. Boone, *The Essential Physics of Medical Imaging,* Lippincott, Williams and Wilkins, Philadelphia (2001).

Advanced Texts Covering Many Imaging Modalities

S. Webb, *The Physics of Medical Imaging,* Adam Hilger, Bristol, England (1988).

Z.-H. Cho, J. P. Jones, and M. Singh, *Foundations of Medical Imaging,* Wiley, New York (1993).

W. R. Hendee and E. R. Ritenour, *Medical Imaging Physics,* 4th ed., Wiley, New York (2002).

Image Visualization

R. A. Robb, *Biomedical Imaging, Visualization, and Analysis,* Wiley-Liss, New York (1999).

Journals Containing Articles on a Wide Range of Imaging Modalities

Diagnostic Imaging

IEEE Transactions on Biomedical Engineering

IEEE Transactions on Medical Imaging

Investigative Radiology

Medical Physics

Physics in Medicine and Biology

Radiology

ACKNOWLEDGMENTS

The suggestion for this book came originally from the IEEE Series Editor, Metin Akay, and was supported enthusiastically by Zhi-Pei Liang. I would like to thank several people for their input, suggestions, and corrections including Nadine Smith (Penn State University), Mark Griswold and Robin Heidemann (University of W¨urzburg), Vikas Gulani (University of Michigan), and Xiaozhong Zhang (University of Illinois at Urbana-Champaign). The assistance and patience of Christina Kuhnen, Associate Acquisitions Editor at IEEE Press, has been invaluable in the preparation of this book. ATL Ultrasound was kind enough to provide many of the images in Chapter 3. Finally, this project was aided considerably by research support from the National Institutes of Health, the National Science Foundation, and the Alexander von Humboldt Foundation.

University of Illinois at Urbana-Champaign ANDREW WEBB

1

X-Ray Imaging and Computed Tomography

1.1. GENERAL PRINCIPLES OF IMAGING WITH X-RAYS

X-ray imaging is a transmission-based technique in which X-rays from a source pass through the patient and are detected either by film or an ionization chamber on the opposite side of the body, as shown in Figure 1.1. Contrast in the image between different tissues arises from differential attenuation of X-rays in the body. For example, X-ray attenuation is particularly efficient in bone, but less so in soft tissues. In planar X-ray radiography, the image produced is a simple two-dimensional projection of the tissues lying between the X-ray source and the film. Planar X-ray radiography is used for a number of different purposes: intravenous pyelography (IVP) to detect diseases of the genitourinary tract including kidney stones; abdominal radiography to study the liver, bladder, abdomen, and pelvis; chest radiography for diseases of the lung and broken ribs; and X-ray fluoroscopy (in which images are acquired continuously over a period of several minutes) for a number of different genitourinary and gastrointestinal diseases.

Planar X-ray radiography of overlapping layers of soft tissue or complex bone structures can often be difficult to interpret, even for a skilled radiologist. In these cases, X-ray computed tomography (CT) is used. The basic principles of CT are shown in Figure 1.2. The X-ray source is tightly collimated to interrogate a thin "slice" through the patient. The source and detectors rotate together around the patient, producing a series of one-dimensional projections at a number of different angles. These data are reconstructed to give a two-dimensional image, as shown on the right of Figure 1.2. CT images have a very high spatial resolution ($\sim$1 mm) and provide reasonable contrast between soft tissues. In addition to anatomical imaging, CT is the imaging method that can produce the highest resolution angiographic images, that is,

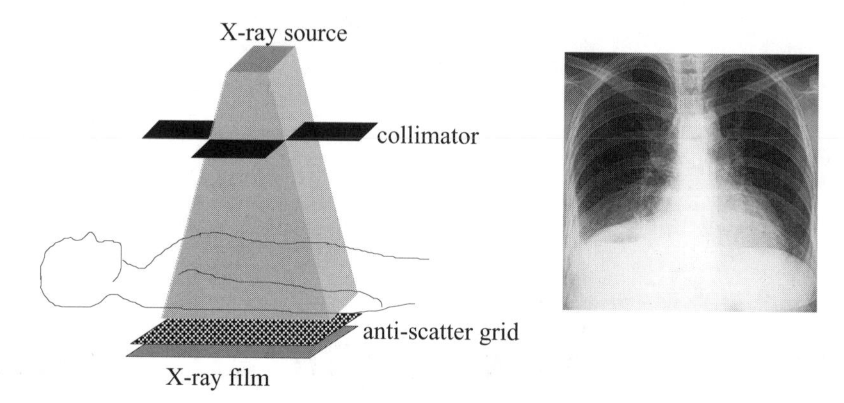

FIGURE 1.1. *(Left) The basic setup for X-ray imaging. The collimator restricts the beam of X-rays so as to irradiate only the region of interest. The antiscatter grid increases tissue contrast by reducing the number of detected X-rays that have been scattered by tissue. (Right) A typical planar X-ray radiograph of the chest, in which the highly attenuating regions of bone appear white.*

images that show blood flow in vessels. Recent developments in spiral and multislice CT have enabled the acquisition of full three-dimensional images in a single patient breath-hold.

The major disadvantage of both X-ray and CT imaging is the fact that the technique uses ionizing radiation. Because ionizing radiation can cause tissue damage, there is a limit on the total radiation dose per year to which a patient can be subjected. Radiation dose is of particular concern in pediatric and obstetric radiology.

1.2. X-RAY PRODUCTION

The X-ray source is the most important system component in determining the overall image quality. Although the basic design has changed little since the mid-1900s, there have been considerable advances in the past two decades in designing more

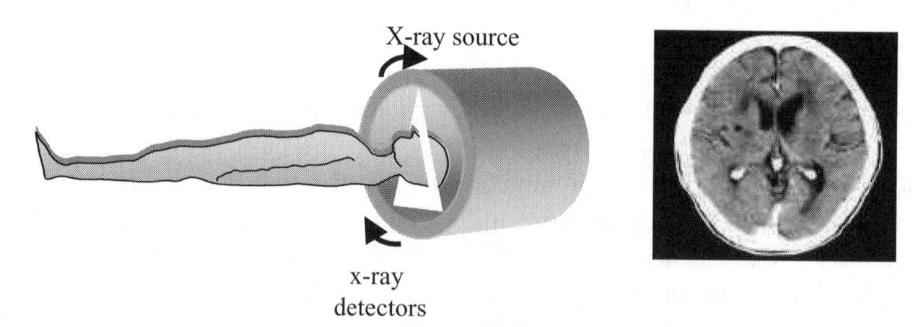

FIGURE 1.2. *(Left) The principle of computed tomography with an X-ray source and detector unit rotating synchronously around the patient. Data are essentially acquired continuously during rotation. (Right) An example of a single-slice CT image of the brain.*

efficient X-ray sources, which are capable of delivering the much higher output levels necessary for techniques such as CT and X-ray fluoroscopy.

1.2.1. The X-Ray Source

The basic components of the X-ray source, also referred to as the X-ray tube, used for clinical diagnoses are shown in Figure 1.3. The production of X-rays involves accelerating a beam of electrons to strike the surface of a metal target. The X-ray tube has two electrodes, a negatively charged cathode, which acts as the electron source, and a positively charged anode, which contains the metal target. A potential difference of between 15 and 150 kV is applied between the cathode and the anode; the exact value depends upon the particular application. This potential difference is in the form of a rectified alternating voltage, which is characterized by its maximum value, the kilovolts peak (kV_p). The maximum value of the voltage is also referred to as the accelerating voltage. The cathode consists of a filament of tungsten wire ($\sim$200 μm in diameter) coiled to form a spiral $\sim$2 mm in diameter and less than 1 cm in height. An electric current from a power source passes through the cathode, causing it to heat up. When the cathode temperature reaches $\sim$2200°C the thermal energy absorbed by the tungsten atoms allows a small number of electrons to move away from the metallic surface, a process termed thermionic emission. A dynamic equilibrium is set

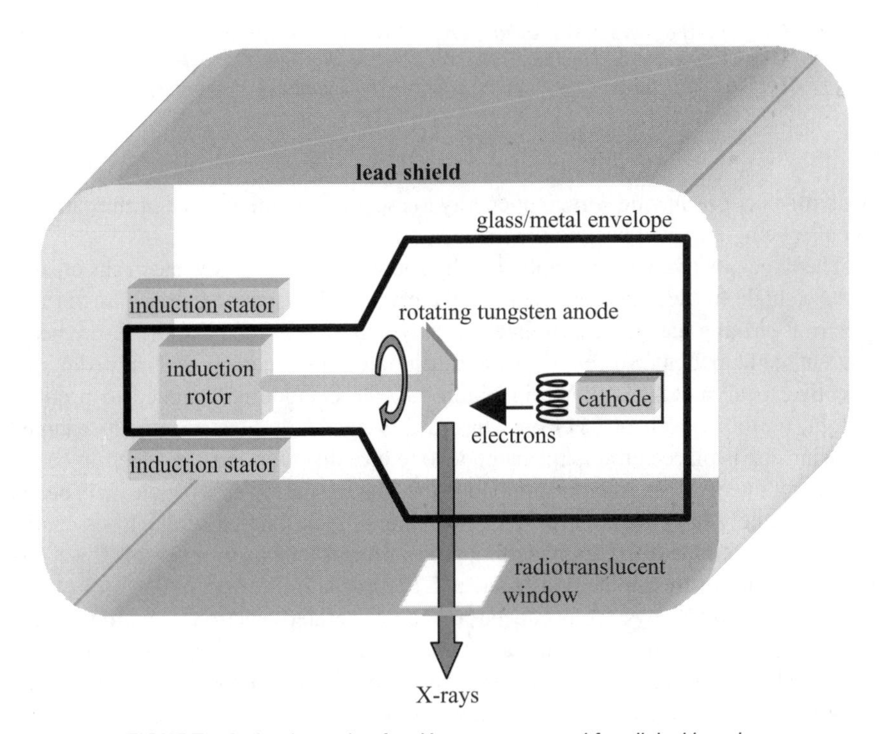

FIGURE 1.3. *A schematic of an X-ray source used for clinical imaging.*

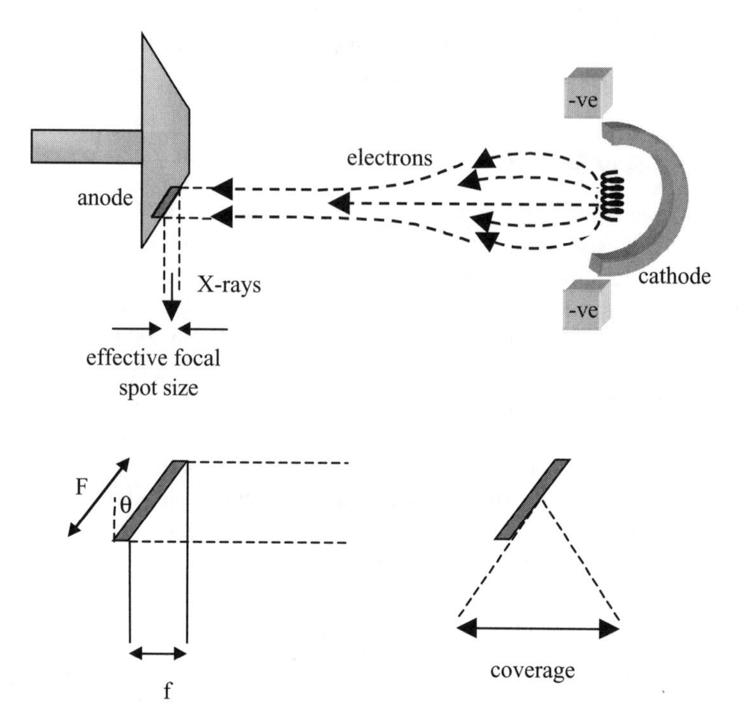

FIGURE 1.4. *(Top) A negatively charged focusing cup within the X-ray cathode produces a tightly focused beam of electrons and increases the electron flux striking the tungsten anode. (Bottom) The effect of the anode bevel angle θ on the effective focal spot size f and the X-ray coverage.*

up, with electrons having sufficient energy to escape from the surface of the cathode, but also being attracted back to the metal surface.

The large positive voltage applied to the anode causes these free electrons created at the cathode surface to accelerate toward the anode. The spatial distribution of these electrons striking the anode correlates directly with the geometry of the X-ray beam that enters the patient. Since the spatial resolution of the image is determined by the effective focal spot size, shown in Figure 1.4, the cathode is designed to produce a tight, uniform beam of electrons. In order to achieve this, a negatively charged focusing cup is placed around the cathode to reduce divergence of the electron beam. The larger the negative potential applied to the cup, the narrower is the electron beam. If an extremely large potential ($\sim$2 kV) is applied, then the flux of electrons can be switched off completely. This switching process forms the basis for pulsing the X-ray source on and off for applications such as CT, covered in Section 1.10.

At the anode, X-rays are produced as the accelerated electrons penetrate a few tens of micrometers into the metal target and lose their kinetic energy. This energy is converted into X-rays by mechanisms covered in detail in Section 1.2.3. The anode must be made of a metal with a high melting point, good thermal conductivity, and low vapor pressure (to enable a vacuum of less than 10^{-7} bar to be established within the vessel). The higher the atomic number of the metal in the target, the higher is the efficiency of X-ray production, or radiation yield. The most commonly used anode metal is tungsten, which has a high atomic number of 74, a high melting point of 3370°C, and the lowest vapor pressure, 10^{-7} bar at 2250°C, of all metals. Elements with higher atomic number, such as platinum (78) and gold (79), have much lower melting points and so are not practical as anode materials. For mammography, in which the X-rays required are of much lower energy, the anode usually consists of molybdenum rather than tungsten. Even with the high radiation yield of tungsten, most of the energy absorbed by the anode is converted into heat, with only ~1% of the energy being converted into X-rays. If pure tungsten is used, then cracks form in the metal, and so a tungsten–rhenium alloy with between 2% and 10% rhenium has been developed to overcome this problem. The target is about 700 μm thick and is mounted on the same thickness of pure tungsten. The main body of the anode is made from an alloy of molybdenum, titanium, and zirconium and is shaped into a disk.

As shown in Figure 1.4, the anode is beveled, typically at an angle of 5–20°, in order to produce a small effective focal spot size, which in turn reduces the geometric "unsharpness" of the X-ray image (Section 1.6.2). The relationship between the actual focal spot size F and the effective focal spot size f is given by

$$f = F \sin\theta \tag{1.1}$$

where θ is the bevel angle. Values of the effective focal spot size range from 0.3 mm for mammography to between 0.6 and 1.2 mm for planar radiography. In practice, most X-ray tubes contain two cathode filaments of different sizes to give the option of using a smaller or larger effective focal spot size. The effective focal spot size can also be controlled by increasing or decreasing the value of the negative charge applied to the focusing cup of the cathode.

The bevel angle θ also affects the coverage of the X-ray beam, as shown in Figure 1.4. The approximate value of the coverage is given by

$$\text{coverage} = 2(\text{source-to-patient distance}) \tan\theta \tag{1.2}$$

All of the components of the X-ray system are contained within an evacuated vessel. In the past, this was constructed from glass, but more recently glass has been replaced by a combination of metal and ceramic. The major disadvantage with glass is that vapor deposits, from both the cathode filament and the anode target, form on the inner surface of the vessel, causing electrical arcing and reducing the life span of the tube. The evacuated vessel is surrounded by oil for both cooling and electrical isolation. The whole assembly is surrounded by a lead shield with a glass window, through which the X-ray beam is emitted.

1.2.2. X-Ray Tube Current, Tube Output, and Beam Intensity

The tube current (mA) of an X-ray source is defined in terms of the number of electrons per second that travel from the tungsten cathode filament to the anode. Typical values of the tube current are between 50 and 400 milliamps for planar radiography and up to 1000 mA for CT. Much lower tube currents are used in continuous imaging techniques such as fluoroscopy. If the value of kV_p is increased, the tube current also increases, until a saturation level is reached. This level is determined by the maximum temperature in, or current through, the cathode filament. X-ray tubes are generally characterized in terms of either the tube output or tube power rating. The tube output, measured in watts, is defined as the product of the tube current and the applied potential difference between the anode and cathode. In addition to the kV_p value, the tube output also depends upon the strength of the vacuum inside the tube. A stronger vacuum enables a higher electron velocity to be established, and also a greater number of electrons to reach the anode, due to reduced interactions with gas molecules. A high tube output is desirable in diagnostic X-ray imaging because it means that a shorter exposure time can be used, which in turn decreases the possibility of motion-induced image artifacts in moving structures such as the heart.

The tube power rating is defined as the maximum power dissipated in an exposure time of 0.1 s. For example, a tube with a power rating of 10 kW can operate at a kV_p of 80 kV with a tube current of 1.25 A for 0.1 s. The ability of the X-ray source to achieve a high tube output is ultimately limited by anode heating. The anode rotates at roughly 3000 rpm, thus increasing the effective surface area of the anode and reducing the amount of power deposited per unit area per unit time. The maximum tube output is, to a first approximation, proportional to the square root of the rotation speed. Anode rotation is accomplished using two stator coils placed close to the neck of the X-ray tube, as shown in Figure 1.3. The magnetic field produced by these stator coils induces a current in the copper rotor of the induction motor which rotates the anode. A molybdenum stem joins the main body of the anode to the rotor assembly. Because molybdenum has a high melting point and low thermal conductivity, heat loss from the anode is primarily via radiation through the vacuum to the vessel walls.

The intensity I of the X-ray beam is defined to be the power incident per unit area and has units of joules/square meter. The power of the beam depends upon two factors, the total number of X-rays and the energy of these X-rays. The number of X-rays produced by the source is proportional to the tube current, and the energy of the X-ray beam is proportional to the square of the accelerating voltage. Therefore, the intensity of the X-ray beam can be expressed as

$$I \propto (kV_p)^2(mA) \tag{1.3}$$

In practice, the intensity is not uniform across the X-ray beam, a phenomenon known as the heel effect. This phenomenon is due to differences in the distances that X-rays created in the anode target have to travel through the target in order to be emitted. This distance is longer for X-rays produced at the "anode end" of the target than at the "cathode end." The greater distance at the anode end results in greater absorption of the X-rays within the target and a lower intensity emitted from the source. An increase in the bevel angle can be used to reduce the magnitude of the heel effect, but this also increases the effective focal spot size.

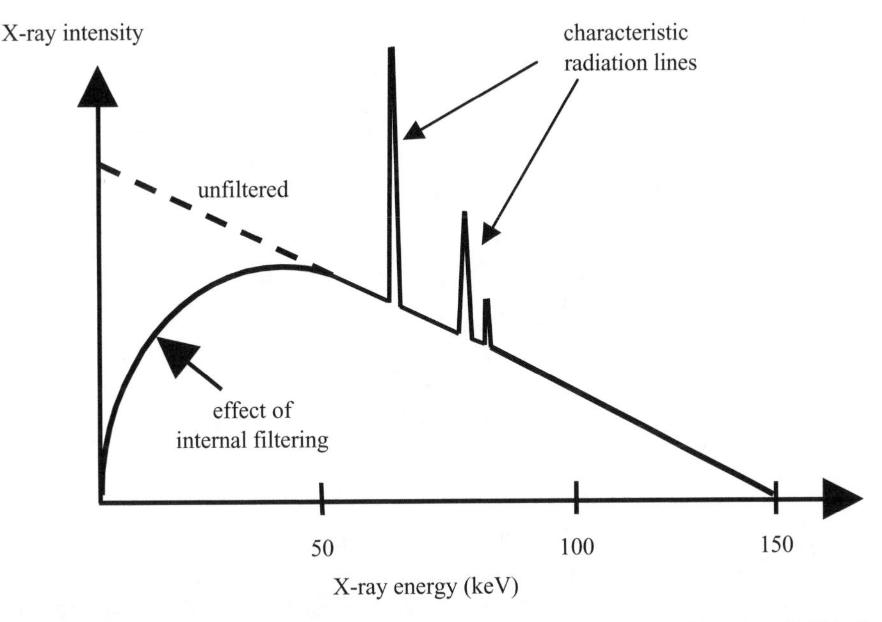

FIGURE 1.5. *A typical X-ray energy spectrum produced from a tube with a kV_p value of 150 keV, using a tungsten anode. Low-energy X-rays (dashed line) are absorbed by the components of the X-ray tube itself. Characteristic radiation lines from the anode occur at approximately 60 and 70 keV.*

1.2.3. The X-Ray Energy Spectrum

The output of the source consists of X-rays with a broad range of energies, as shown in Figure 1.5. High-energy electrons striking the anode generate X-rays via two mechanisms: bremsstrahlung, also called general, radiation and characteristic radiation. Bremsstrahlung radiation occurs when an electron passes close to a tungsten nucleus and is deflected by the attractive force of the positively charged nucleus. The kinetic energy lost by the deflected electron is emitted as an X-ray. Many such encounters occur for each electron, with each encounter producing a partial loss of the total kinetic energy of the electron. These interactions result in X-rays with a wide range of energies being emitted from the anode. The maximum energy E_{max} of an X-ray created by this process corresponds to a situation in which the entire kinetic energy of the electron is transformed into a single X-ray. The value of E_{max} (in units of keV) therefore corresponds to the value of the accelerating voltage $\mathrm{kV_p}$. The efficiency η of bremsstrahlung radiation production is given by

$$\eta = k(\mathrm{kV_p})Z \tag{1.4}$$

where k is a constant (with a value of 1.1×10^{-9} for tungsten) and Z is the atomic number of the target metal. Bremsstrahlung radiation is characterized by a linear decrease in X-ray intensity with increasing X-ray energy. However, many X-rays

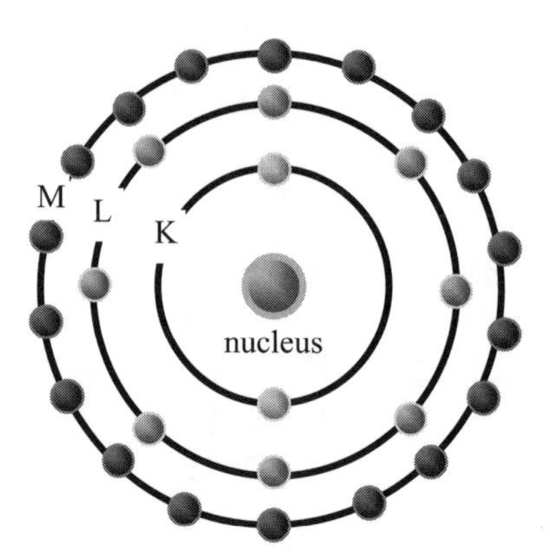

FIGURE 1.6. *The atomic structure of a model element showing the maximum number of electrons that can occupy the K, the L, and the M shells.*

with low energies are absorbed within the X-ray tube and its housing, resulting in the "internally filtered" spectrum shown in Figure 1.5. Additional filters external to the tube are used in order to reduce further the number of X-rays with low energies that are emitted from the tube because such X-rays do not have sufficient energy to pass through the patient and reach the detector, and therefore add to the patient dose, but are not useful for imaging. For values of kV_p up to 50 kV, 0.5-mm-thick aluminum is used; between 50 and 70 kV, 1.5-mm-thick aluminum is used; and above 70 kV, 2.5-mm-thick aluminum is used. These filters can reduce skin dose by up to a factor of 80. For mammography studies, where the kV_p value is less than 30 kV, a 30-μm-thick molybdenum filter is typically used.

Sharp peaks are also present in the X-ray energy spectrum, and these arise from the second mechanism, characteristic radiation. Surrounding the nucleus of any atom are a number of electron "shells" as shown in Figure 1.6. The innermost shell is termed the *K* shell (with a maximum occupancy of 2 electrons), and outside this are the *L* shell (maximum 8 electrons), *M* shell (maximum 18 electrons), etc. The electrons in the *K* shell have the highest binding energy, that is, they are bound the tightest of all electrons. When electrons accelerated from the cathode collide with a tightly bound electron in the *K* shell of the tungsten anode, a bound electron is ejected, and the resulting "hole" is filled by an electron from an outer shell. The loss in potential energy due to the different binding energies of the electrons in the inner and the outer shells is radiated as a single X-ray. This X-ray corresponds to a characteristic radiation line, such as shown in Figure 1.5.

An electron from the cathode must have an energy greater than 70 keV to eject a *K*-shell electron from the tungsten anode. An electron that falls from the *L* shell to fill the hole in the *K* shell has a binding energy of ~11 keV, and therefore the characteristic X-ray emitted from the anode has an energy of ~59 keV. The actual situation is more complicated, because electrons within the *L* shell can occupy three different sublevels, each having slightly different binding energies. There are also additional characteristic lines in the energy spectrum corresponding to electron transitions from the M to the K shell, and from the N to the K shell. There is no characteristic radiation below a kV_p value of 70 kV, but between kV_p values of 80 and 150 kV characteristic radiation makes up between 10% and 30% of the intensity of the X-ray spectrum.

Although the X-ray energy spectrum is inherently polychromatic, it can be characterized in terms of an effective, or average, X-ray energy, the value of which usually lies between one-third and one-half of E_{max}. For example, an X-ray source with a tungsten anode operating at a kV_p of 150 kV has an effective X-ray energy of approximately 68 keV.

1.3. INTERACTIONS OF X-RAYS WITH TISSUE

Contrast between tissues in X-ray images arises from differential attenuation of the X-rays as they pass from the source through the body to the film or detector. A certain fraction of X-rays pass straight through the body and undergo no interactions with tissue: these X-rays are referred to as primary radiation. Alternatively, X-rays can be scattered, an interaction that alters their trajectory between source and detector: such X-rays are described as secondary radiation. Finally, X-rays can be absorbed completely in tissue and not reach the detector at all: these constitute absorbed radiation. In the X-ray energy range (25–150 keV) used for diagnostic radiology, three dominant mechanisms describe the interaction of X-rays with tissue: coherent scatter and Compton scatter are both involved in the production of secondary radiation, whereas photoelectric interactions result in X-ray absorption.

1.3.1. Coherent Scattering

Coherent, also called Rayleigh, scattering represents a nonionizing interaction between X-rays and tissue. The X-ray energy is converted into harmonic motions of the electrons in the atoms in tissue. The atom then reradiates this energy in a random direction as a secondary X-ray with the same wavelength as the incident X-ray. Therefore, coherent scatter not only reduces the number of X-rays reaching the detector, but also alters the X-ray trajectory between source and detector. The probability $P_{coherent}$ of a coherent scattering event is given by

$$P_{coherent} \propto \frac{Z_{eff}^{8/3}}{E^2} \tag{1.5}$$

where E is the energy of the incident X-rays and Z_{eff} is the effective atomic number of the tissue. Muscle has a Z_{eff} of 7.4, whereas bone, containing calcium, has a value close to 20. For X-rays with energies in the diagnostic range, coherent scattering typically only accounts for between 5% and 10% of the interactions with tissue.

1.3.2. Compton Scattering

Compton scattering refers to the interaction between an incident X-ray and a loosely bound electron in an outer shell of an atom in tissue. A fraction of the X-ray energy is

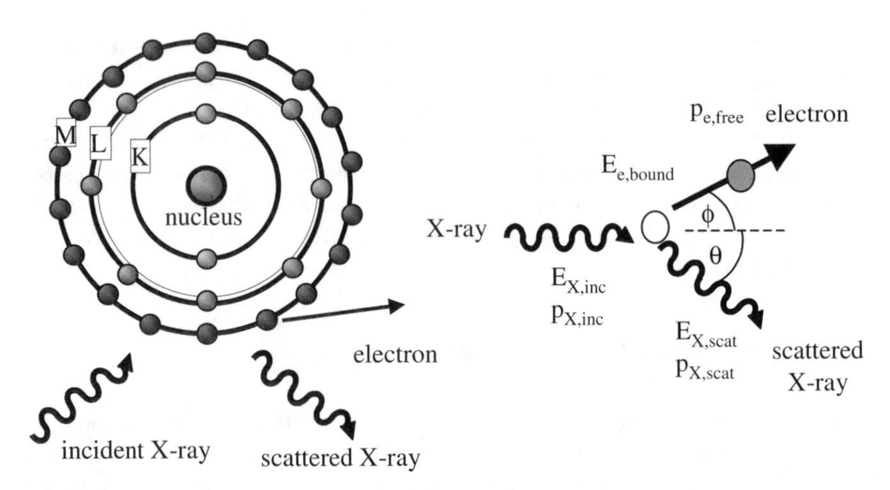

FIGURE 1.7. *(Left). A schematic of Compton scattering of an incident X-ray by an atom in tissue. (Right) Compton scattering of the incident X-ray with energy $E_{X,inc}$ and momentum $p_{X,inc}$ by a loosely bound electron with energy $E_{e,bound}$ produces a scattered X-ray with energy $E_{X,scat}$ and momentum $p_{X,scat}$ and a free electron with energy $E_{e,free}$ and momentum $p_{e,free}$.*

transferred to the electron, the electron is ejected, and the X-ray is deflected from its original path as shown in Figure 1.7. If the angle of deflection θ is relatively small, then the scattered X-ray has a similar energy to that of the incident X-ray and has sufficient energy to pass through the body and be detected by the film.

The energy of the scattered X-ray can be calculated by applying the laws of conservation of momentum and energy. In this case, conservation of momentum can be expressed as

$$\mathbf{p}_{e,\text{free}} = \mathbf{p}_{\text{X,inc}} - \mathbf{p}_{\text{X,scat}} \tag{1.6}$$

where **p** represents momentum. The equation for the conservation of energy is

$$E_{\text{X,inc}} + E_{e,\text{bound}} = E_{\text{X,scat}} + E_{e,\text{free}} \tag{1.7}$$

After some algebraic manipulation, the energy of the Compton-scattered X-ray is given by

$$E_{\text{X,scat}} = \frac{E_{\text{X,inc}}}{1 + (E_{\text{X,inc}}/\text{mc}^2)(1 - \cos\theta)} \tag{1.8}$$

where m is the mass of the ejected electron and c is the speed of light. Table 1.1 shows the energy of Compton-scattered X-rays as a function of the incident X-ray energy and scattering angle. The relatively small difference in energy between incident and scattered X-rays means that secondary radiation is detected with approximately the same efficiency as primary radiation.

The probability of an X-ray undergoing Compton scattering is essentially independent of the effective atomic number of the tissue, is linearly proportional to the tissue electron density, and is weakly dependent on the energy of the incident X-ray.

TABLE 1.1. The Energies of Compton-Scattered X-Rays as a Function of Scattering Angle for Various Energies of Incident X-Rays

Scattering angle (deg)	Energy of Compton-scattered X-rays (keV) $E_{X,inc} = 25$	$E_{X,inc} = 50$	$E_{X,inc} = 100$	$E_{X,inc} = 150$
30	24.8	49.4	97.5	144.4
60	24.4	47.7	91.2	131.0
90	23.8	41.9	72.1	94.6

Considering these factors in turn, the independence with respect to atomic number means that scattered X-rays contain little contrast between, for example, soft tissue, fat, and bone. A small degree of contrast does arise from the differences in electron density, which have values of 3.36×10^{23} electrons per gram for muscle, 3.16×10^{23} electrons per gram for fat, and 5.55×10^{23} electrons per gram for bone. As described in the next section, photoelectric interactions (which produce excellent tissue contrast) are highly unlikely to occur at high incident X-ray energies. The weak dependence of the probability of Compton scattering on the incident X-ray energy means that Compton scattering is the dominant interaction at high energies and results in poor image contrast at these energies.

1.3.3. The Photoelectric Effect

Photoelectric interactions in the body involve the energy of an incident X-ray being absorbed by an atom in tissue, with a tightly bound electron being emitted from the *K* or *L* shell as a "photoelectron," as shown in Figure 1.8. The kinetic energy of the

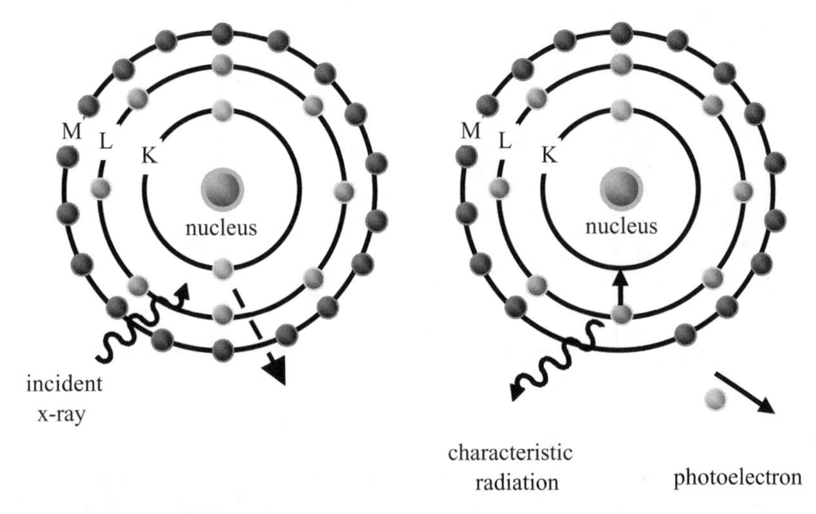

FIGURE 1.8. A schematic of the first two stages of absorption of an X-ray in tissue via a photoelectric interaction. Almost all of the energy of the incident X-ray is transferred to the ejected photoelectron.

photoelectron is equal to the difference between the energy of the incident X-ray and the binding energy of the electron. A second electron from a higher energy level then fills the "hole" created by the ejection of the photoelectron, a process accompanied by the emission of a "characteristic" X-ray with an energy equal to the difference in the binding energies of the outer electron and the photoelectron. If the energy of the incident X-ray is lower than the K-shell binding energy, then the photoelectron is ejected from the L shell. If the incident X-ray has sufficient energy, then a K-shell electron is emitted and an L- or M-shell electron fills the hole. The characteristic X-ray has a very low energy and is absorbed within a short distance. For example, the 4-keV characteristic radiation from a photoelectric interaction with a calcium atom in bone only travels about 0.1 mm in tissue. The net result of the photoelectric effect in tissue is that the incident X-ray is completely absorbed and does not reach the detector.

There is also a second, less common form of the photoelectric interaction, in which the difference between the inner and the outer electron binding energies is transferred to an outer shell electron (Auger electron), which then escapes, leaving a nucleus with a double-positive charge. The two electron-shell vacancies are filled by other outer electrons, producing very low energy characteristic X-rays or further Auger electrons. Again, no radiation, neither photoelectrons nor characteristic radiation, reaches the detector.

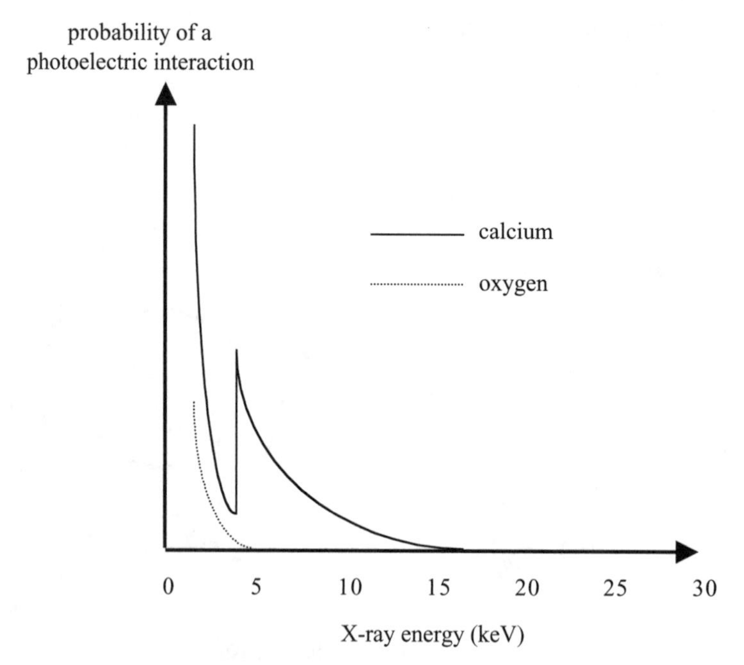

FIGURE 1.9. *A plot of the probability of a photoelectric interaction as a function of the incident X-ray energy for oxygen (water, tissue) and calcium (bone). The K-edge at 4 keV for calcium results in much higher attenuation of X-rays for bone at low X-ray energies.*

For energies of the incident X-rays less than the binding energy of the inner K electrons, photoelectric interactions are limited to the ejection of L- and M-shell electrons. However, at an energy just higher than the K-shell binding energy, the probability of photoelectric interactions increases dramatically, typically by a factor of five to eight. This phenomenon is known as the "K-edge." Above this energy, the photoelectric interaction probability P_{pe} is given by

$$P_{\text{pe}} \propto \frac{Z_{\text{eff}}^3}{E^3} \tag{1.9}$$

Figure 1.9 shows the probability of photoelectric interactions for ^{8}O and ^{20}Ca, illustrating both the higher attenuation for ^{20}Ca, due to its higher atomic number, and also its K-edge at 4 keV. At low energies of the incident X-rays there is, therefore, excellent contrast between bone and tissue. However, equation (1.9) also shows that photoelectric attenuation of X-rays drops off very rapidly as a function of the incident X-ray energy.

1.4. LINEAR AND MASS ATTENUATION COEFFICIENTS OF X-RAYS IN TISSUE

Attenuation of the intensity of the X-ray beam as it travels through tissue can be expressed mathematically by

$$I_{\text{x}} = I_0 e^{-\mu x} \tag{1.10}$$

where I_0 is the intensity of the incident X-ray beam, I_{x} is the X-ray intensity at a distance x from the source, and μ is the linear attenuation coefficient of tissue measured in cm^{-1}. A high value of the constant μ corresponds to efficient absorption of X-rays by tissue, with only a small number of X-rays reaching the detector. The value of μ can be represented by the sum of individual contributions from each of the interactions between X-rays and tissue described in the previous section:

$$\mu = \mu_{\text{photoelectric}} + \mu_{\text{Compton}} + \mu_{\text{coherent}} \tag{1.11}$$

Figure 1.10 shows the contributions of the photoelectric interactions and Compton scattering (coherent scattering is usually ignored due to its small effect) to the linear attenuation coefficient of tissue as a function of the incident X-ray energy. The contribution from photoelectric interactions dominates at lower energies, whereas Compton scattering is more important at higher energies. X-ray attenuation is often characterized in terms of a mass attenuation coefficient, equal to the linear attenuation coefficient divided by the density of the tissue. Figure 1.10 also plots the mass attenuation coefficient of fat, bone, and muscle as a function of the incident X-ray energy. At low incident X-ray energies bone has much the highest mass attenuation coefficient. The probability of photoelectric interactions is much higher in bone than tissue because bone contains calcium, which has a relatively high atomic number.

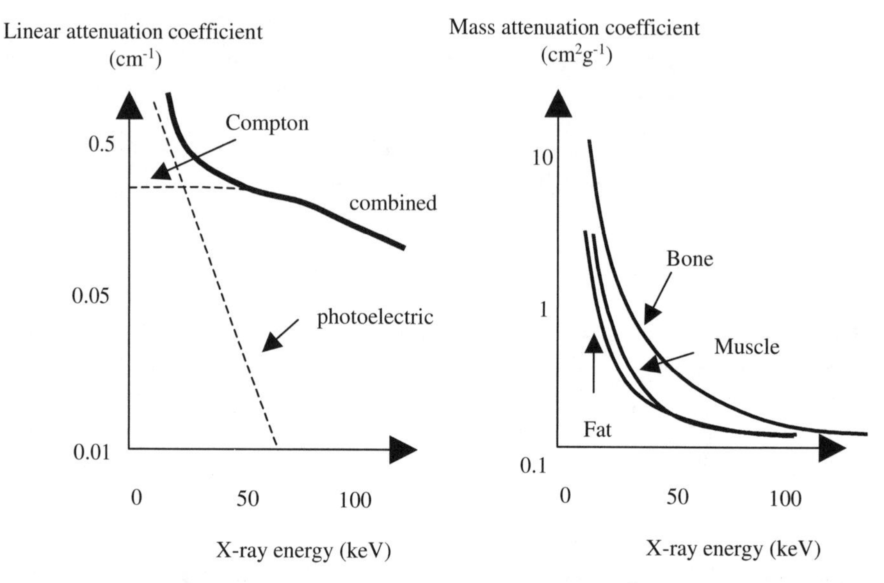

FIGURE 1.10. *(Left) The relative contributions from Compton scattering and photoelectric interactions to the linear attenuation coefficient in soft tissue as a function of the incident X-ray energy. The dashed lines represent straight-line approximations to the relative contributions, with the solid line representing actual experimental data corresponding to the sum of the contributions. (Right) The mass attenuation coefficient in bone, muscle, and fat as a function of X-ray energy.*

As the incident X-ray energy increases, the probability of photoelectric interactions decreases and the value of the mass attenuation coefficient becomes much lower. At X-ray energies greater than about 80 keV, Compton scattering is the dominant mechanism, and the difference in the mass attenuation coefficients of bone and soft tissue is less than a factor of two. At incident X-ray energies greater than around 120 keV, the mass attenuation coefficients for bone and soft tissue are very similar. Figure 1.10 also shows that differentiation between soft tissues, such as fat and muscle, is relatively difficult using X-rays. This is because the effective atomic number of muscle (7.4) is only slightly higher than that of fat (5.9). Low-energy X-rays produce a reasonable amount of contrast, but at higher energies little differentiation is possible because the electron density of both species is very similar.

A parameter used commonly to characterize X-ray attenuation in tissue is the half-value layer (HVL), which is defined as the thickness of tissue that attenuates the intensity of the X-ray beam by a factor of one-half. From equation (1.10) the value of the HVL is given by $(\ln 2)/\mu$. Table 1.2 lists values of the HVL for muscle and bone at four different values of the energy of the incident X-rays. The data in Table 1.2 indicate that the vast majority of the X-rays from the source are actually absorbed in the patient. For chest radiographs only about 10% of the incident X-rays are detected, that is, 90% are attenuated in the body. Other examinations result in even higher X-ray absorption: 95% for mammograms and 99.5% for abdominal scans.

As described at the end of Section 1.2.3, the effective X-ray energy from a source using a tungsten anode is around 68 keV. However, in calculating the HVL and

TABLE 1.2. The Half-Value Layer (HVL) for Muscle and Bone as a Function of the Energy of the Incident X-Rays

X-ray energy (keV)	HVL, muscle (cm)	HVL, bone (cm)
30	1.8	0.4
50	3.0	1.2
100	3.9	2.3
150	4.5	2.8

attenuation characteristics of tissue, the phenomenon of "beam hardening" must be considered. From Figure 1.10 it is clear that the lower energy X-rays in the beam are attenuated preferentially in tissue, and so the average energy of the X-ray beam increases as it passes through tissue. If the X-rays have to pass through a large amount of tissue, such as in abdominal imaging, then beam hardening reduces image contrast by increasing the proportion of Compton-scattered X-rays due to the higher effective energy of the X-ray beam. Beam hardening must be corrected for in CT scanning, otherwise significant image artifacts can result, as outlined in Section 1.11.1.

1.5. INSTRUMENTATION FOR PLANAR X-RAY IMAGING

This section covers the remaining components of an X-ray imaging system. A typical system comprises a variable field-of-view (FOV) collimator, which restricts the X-ray beam to the desired imaging dimensions, an antiscatter grid to reduce the contribution of scattered X-rays to the image, and a combined intensifying screen/X-ray film to record the image.

1.5.1. Collimators

The geometry of the X-ray beam emanating from the source, as indicated in Figure 1.1, is a divergent beam. Often, the dimensions of the beam when it reaches the patient are larger than the desired FOV of the image. This has two undesirable effects, the first of which is that the patient dose is increased unnecessarily. The second effect is that the number of Compton-scattered X-rays contributing to the image is greater than if the extent of the beam had been matched to the image FOV. In order to restrict the dimensions of the beam, a collimator, also called a beam restrictor, is placed between the X-ray source and the patient. The collimator consists of sheets of lead, which can be slid over one another to restrict the beam in either one or two dimensions.

1.5.2. Antiscatter Grids

Ideally, all of the X-rays reaching the detector would be primary radiation, with no contribution from Compton-scattered X-rays. In this case, image contrast would be affected only by differences in attenuation from photoelectric interactions in the various tissues. However, in practice, a large number of X-rays that have undergone

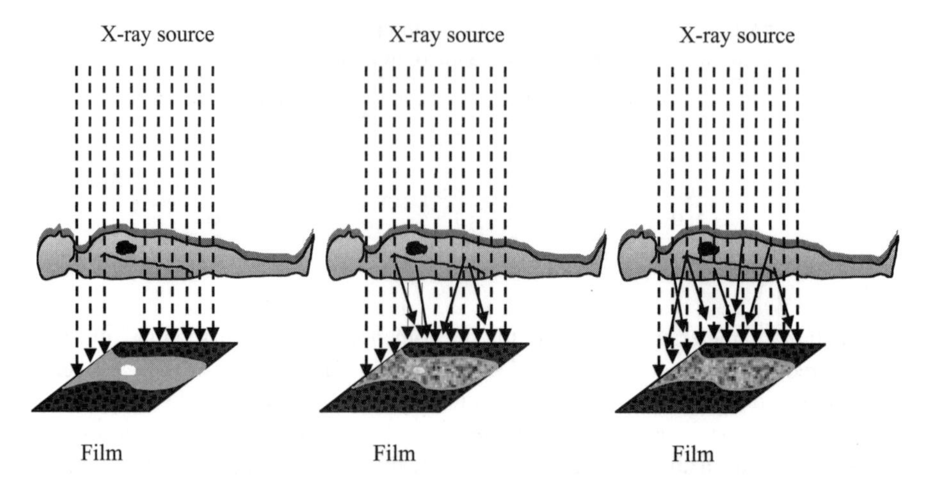

FIGURE 1.11. The effect of Compton scattering on the X-ray image. A highly attenuating pathology is represented as a black object within the body. (Left) The ideal situation in which only photoelectric interactions occur leading to complete X-ray attenuation in the pathology. (Center) As the contribution of Compton-scattered X-rays to the image increases, the image contrast is reduced. (Right) In the case where only Compton-scattered X-rays are detected, image contrast is almost zero.

Compton scattering reach the detector. As mentioned previously, the contrast between tissues from Compton-scattered X-rays is inherently low. In addition, secondary radiation contains no useful spatial information and is distributed randomly over the film, thus reducing image contrast further. The effect of scattered radiation on the X-ray image is shown schematically in Figure 1.11. If the assumption is made that scattered radiation is uniformly distributed on the X-ray film, then the image contrast is reduced by a factor of $(1 + R)$, where R is the ratio of secondary to primary radiation. The value of R depends upon the FOV of the image. For a small FOV, below about 10 cm, the contribution of scattered radiation is proportional to the FOV. This relationship levels off, reaching a constant value at a FOV of roughly 30 cm.

As described in the previous section, collimators can be used to restrict the beam dimensions to the image FOV and therefore decrease the number of scattered X-rays contributing to the image, but even with a collimator in place secondary radiation can represent between 50% and 90% of the X-rays reaching the detector. Additional measures, therefore, are necessary to reduce the contribution of Compton-scattered X-rays.

One method is to place an antiscatter grid between the patient and the X-ray detector. This grid consists of strips of lead foil interspersed with aluminum as a support, with the strips oriented parallel to the direction of the primary radiation, as shown in Figure 1.12. The properties of the grid are defined in terms of the grid ratio and strip line density:

$$\text{grid ratio} = \frac{h}{d}, \qquad \text{strip line density} = \frac{1}{d+t} \tag{1.12}$$

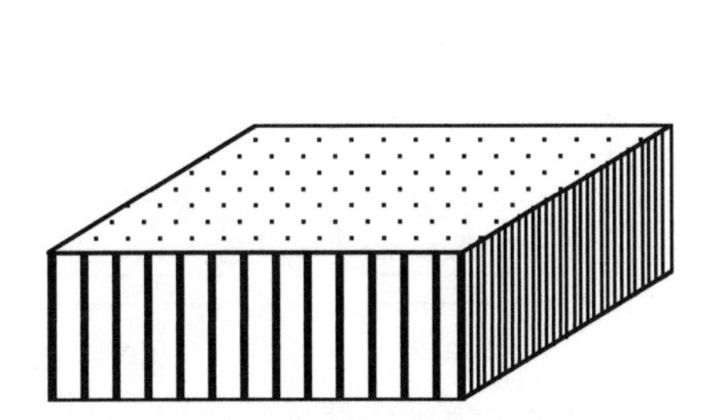

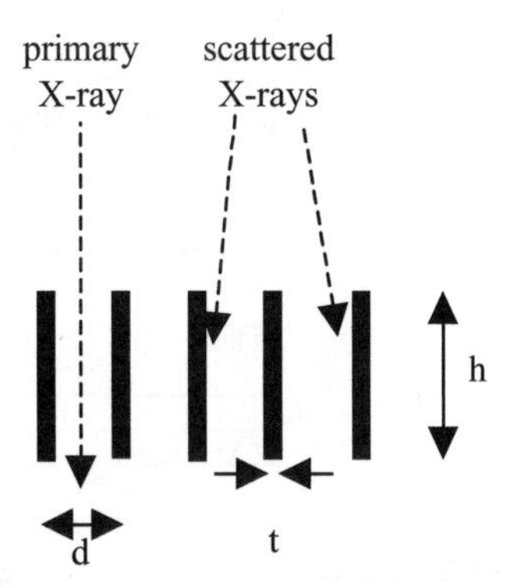

FIGURE 1.12. *(Left) A two-dimensional schematic of an antiscatter grid, which is placed on top of the X-ray detector. The black areas represent thin lead septa, separated by the aluminum support. (Right) A one-dimensional representation of the antiscatter grid. Primary X-rays pass between the lead septa, whereas those X-rays that have undergone a significant deviation in trajectory from Compton scattering are absorbed by the septa.*

where h, t, and d are the length and the thickness of the lead strips and the distance between the centers of the strips, respectively. Typical values of the grid ratio range from 4:1 to 16:1 and the strip line density varies from 25 to 60 per cm. If the lead strips are sufficiently narrow, no degradation of image quality is apparent from the shadowing effects of the grid. However, if this is not the case, then the grid can be moved in a reciprocating motion during the exposure. There is, of course, a tradeoff between the reduction of scattered radiation (and hence improvement in image contrast) and the patient dose that must be delivered to give the same number of detected X-rays. This tradeoff can be characterized using a parameter known as the Bucky factor F of a grid, which is defined as

$$F = \frac{\text{X-ray exposure with the grid in place}}{\text{X-ray exposure with no grid}} \tag{1.13}$$

1.5.3. Intensifying Screens

The intrinsic sensitivity of photographic film to X-rays is very low, meaning that its use would require high patient doses of radiation to produce high-quality images. In order to circumvent this problem, intensifying screens are used to convert X-rays into light, to which film is much more sensitive. A schematic of such an intensifying screen/film combination is shown in Figure 1.13. An outer plastic protective layer ($\sim$15 μm thick), transparent to X-rays, lies above the phosphor layer (100–500 μm thick), which converts the X-rays into light. The polyester base ($\sim$200 μm thick) gives mechanical stability to the entire intensifying screen. Because the light produced in the phosphor layer travels in all directions, a reflective layer (20 μm thick) containing titanium oxide is placed between the phosphor and plastic base to reflect light, which would otherwise be lost through the base, back toward the film. The screen is generally double-sided, as shown in Figure 1.13, except for X-ray mammography studies,

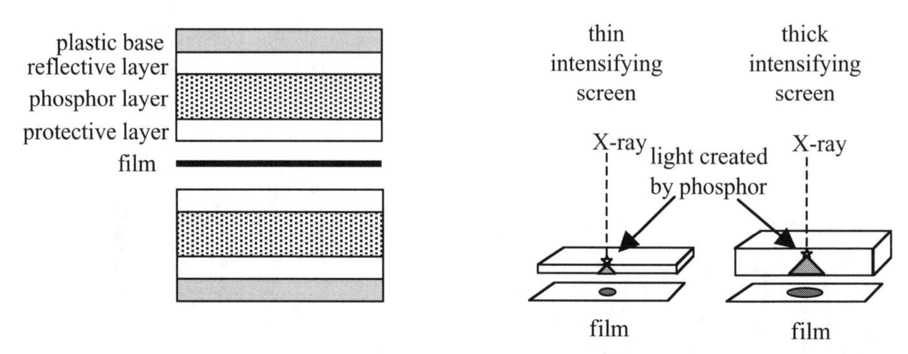

FIGURE 1.13. *(Left) A schematic of a double-layer intensifying screen/X-ray film, which is placed in a "cassette" for imaging. (Right). The effect of the thickness of the intensifying screen on the spatial resolution of the image. A thin screen means that light formed in the screen travels a relatively short distance before striking the X-ray film, and so diffusion within the screen results in a relatively sharp image. In contrast, a thicker screen results in a greater degree of light diffusion and therefore a lower spatial resolution.*

described in Section 1.9.1. Compared to direct detection of X-rays by film alone, the intensifying screen/film combination results in a greater than 50-fold increase in sensitivity. The more sensitive the film, the lower is the necessary tube current and patient dose. Alternatively, the same tube current could be used, but with a shorter exposure time, which can reduce image blurring due to patient motion.

The phosphor layer in the screen contains a rare earth element such as gadolinium (Gd) or lanthanum (La) suspended in a polymer matrix. The two most common screens contain terbium-doped gadolinium oxysulfide (Gd_2O_2S:Tb) or terbium-doped lanthanum oxybromide (LaOBr:Tb). Gd_2O_2S:Tb emits light in the green part of the spectrum at 540 nm, and since Gd has a K-edge at 50 keV, absorption of X-rays via photoelectric interactions is very efficient. The compound has a high energy-conversion efficiency of 20%, that is, one-fifth of the energy of the X-rays striking the phosphor layer is converted into light photons. LaOBr:Tb emits light in the blue part of the spectrum at 475 nm (with a second peak at 360 nm), has a K-edge at 39 keV, and an energy conversion efficiency of 18%. This compound has the advantage of using film technology that had been developed for a previously widely used phosphor, cadmium tungstate.

The thickness of the phosphor layer contributes to both the signal-to-noise ratio (SNR) and the spatial resolution of the X-ray image. The attenuation of X-rays by the intensifying screen can be characterized by a linear attenuation coefficient μ_{screen}. A thicker screen means that more X-rays are detected, that is, absorbed, and the SNR is higher. Double-layer intensifying screens, such as the one shown in Figure 1.13, effectively double the thickness of the phosphor layer. However, light created in the phosphor crystals must diffuse a certain distance through the phosphor layer before developing the film. The thicker the phosphor layer, the more uncertainty there is in the position of the original X-ray, and therefore the lower is the spatial resolution. The uncertainty can be described mathematically in terms of a "light-spread function," represented geometrically as a cone on the right of Figure 1.13.

1.5.4. X-Ray Film

Depending upon whether the intensifying screen is Gd- or La-based, the X-ray film should be maximally sensitive to either green or blue light. Two types of film, monochromatic and orthochromatic, are generally used. Monochromatic films are sensitive to ultraviolet and blue visible light, and are therefore spectroscopically matched to the output of intensifying screens based on La rare earths. Orthochromatic films have a sensitizer added to make the film more sensitive to green light for matching to the output of Gd-based intensifying screens. Most films are double emulsion ($\sim$10 μm thick) with one emulsion layer on either side of a central transparent plastic sheet ($\sim$150 μm thick). The emulsion contains silver halide particles with diameters between 0.2 and 1.5 μm. The majority of the particles are silver bromide bound in a gelatin matrix, with smaller amounts of a silver iodide sensitizer. When the particles are exposed to light, a "latent image" is formed. After exposure, the developing process involves chemical reduction of these exposed silver salts to metallic silver, which appears black. Developed films therefore consist of darker areas corresponding to tissues that attenuate relatively few X-rays and lighter regions corresponding to highly attenuating tissues. The degree of film "blackening" depends upon the product of the intensity of the light from the intensifying screen and the time for which the film is exposed to the light. Film blackening is quantified by a parameter known as the optical density (OD), which is defined as

$$\mathrm{OD} = \log\frac{I_{\mathrm{i}}}{I_{\mathrm{t}}} \tag{1.14}$$

where I_{i} is the intensity of light incident on, and I_t the intensity transmitted through, the X-ray film. The darker the film, therefore, the higher is the value of the OD of the film. A logarithmic scale of the OD is defined because the physiological response of the eye to light intensity is itself logarithmic.

The relationship between the OD and the exposure, is shown in Figure 1.14. The graph is referred to as the characteristic, or *D*/log *E*, curve. Several points should be noted. First, the OD without any X-ray exposure does not have a value of zero. This baseline, or "fog," level corresponds to the natural opacity of the X-ray film and the small amount of silver halide that is chemically reduced during the developing process. Typically, the fog level has an OD value between 0.1 and 0.3. Second, at both low and high values of exposure, termed the toe and shoulder regions, respectively, the plot of OD versus log exposure becomes highly nonlinear. Thus, too low or too high an exposure time or total radiation dose results in very poor image contrast. The ideal region of the curve in which to operate corresponds to a linear relationship between the OD and log exposure.

X-ray film, as for standard photographic film, can be characterized in terms of parameters such as contrast, speed, and latitude. The speed of the film is defined as the inverse of the exposure needed to produce a given OD above the fog level. For example, a fast film produces a given OD for a given exposure in a faster time than a slow film, as shown on the right of Figure 1.14. A measure of the film contrast is

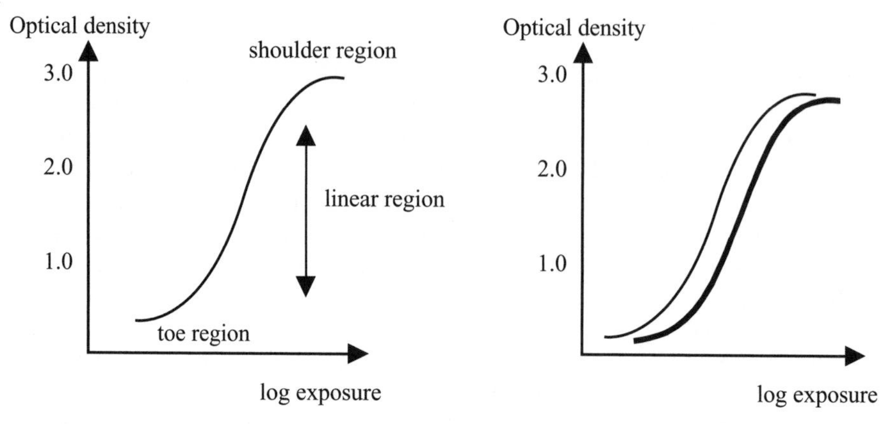

FIGURE 1.14. (Left) The characteristic curve for an X-ray film. (Right) A comparison of two characteristic curves for a fast film (thin line) and a slow film (thick line).

given by the value of the film gamma (γ), defined as the maximum slope of the linear region of the characteristic curve:

$$\gamma = \frac{\mathrm{OD}_2 - \mathrm{OD}_1}{\log E_2 - \log E_1} \tag{1.15}$$

A high value of gamma means that a given difference in exposures for two areas of the X-ray film results in high contrast between those regions in the developed film. The film latitude is defined as the range of exposure values (typically OD values between 0.5 and 2.0) for which useful contrast can be seen in the image. A large value of the film latitude corresponds to a low value of γ, and this means low image contrast. The latitude is also sometimes referred to as the dynamic range of the film.

In terms of the physical composition of the film, a large size of the silver halide particles corresponds to high film sensitivity, but poor spatial resolution, and vice-versa. A mixed-particle size film gives high image contrast, with a single particle size resulting in low image contrast.

In practice, a procedure called automatic exposure control (AEC) is used to optimize the exposure time of the X-ray film to produce an image with the highest possible contrast. AEC uses a flat ionization chamber, covered in Section 1.10.2, usually filled with xenon gas, which can be placed in front of the film cassette without interfering with the image. This chamber provides a separate measure of the intensity of the X-ray beam reaching the film, and once the value has reached the desired level, the X-ray source is shut off.

1.5.5. Instrumentation for Computed and Digital Radiography

Although X-ray film has the advantage of speed, simplicity, and a long history of radiological interpretation, the future of all imaging modalities undoubtedly lies in digital display and storage. Digital images can be archived and transferred rapidly between clinical centers and, where appropriate, the data can be postprocessed using different algorithms or filters. In order for digital imaging to become a medical standard, however, it is absolutely necessary for the quality of the images to be at least as good as those produced using film. Two techniques, computed radiography and digital radiography, are currently being used and evaluated for digital X-ray imaging.

Computed radiography (CR) uses a photostimulable, phosphor-based storage imaging plate to replace the standard intensifying screen/X-ray film combination. This imaging plate contains a phosphor layer of fine-grain barium fluorohalide crystals doped with divalent europium (Eu^{2+}). When the imaging plate is exposed to X-rays, electrons in the phosphor screen are excited to higher energy levels and are trapped in halide vacancies, forming "color centers." Holes created by the missing valence electrons cause Eu^{2+} to be oxidized to Eu^{3+}. This chemical oxidation persists for time periods of many hours to several days. At the appropriate time, the exposed imaging plate is read using a scanning laser system. When the phosphor crystals are irradiated by the laser, the color centers absorb energy, releasing the trapped electrons, which return to their equilibrium valence positions. As they do so, they release blue light at a wavelength of 390 nm. This light is captured by detector electronics in the image reader, and the signals are digitized and assembled into an image. After the image reading process, a bright light can be used to erase the imaging plate, which can be reused numerous times.

The second technique, digital radiography (DR), is based on large-area, flat-panel detectors (FPD) using thin-film transistor (TFT) arrays, the same technology as in, for example, the screens of laptop computers. The FPD is fabricated on a single monolithic glass substrate. A thin-film amorphous silicon transistor array is then layered onto the glass. Each pixel of the detector consists of a photodiode and associated TFT switch. On top of the array is a structured thallium-doped cesium iodide (CsI) scintillator, a reflective layer, and a graphite protective coating. The CsI layer consists of many thin, rod-shaped cesium iodide crystals (approximately 6–10 μm in diameter) aligned parallel to one another and extending from the top surface of the CsI layer to the substrate on which they are manufactured.

When an X-ray is absorbed in a CsI rod, the CsI scintillates and produces light. The light undergoes internal reflection within the fiber and is emitted from one end of the fiber onto the TFT array. The light is then converted into an electrical signal by the photodiodes in the TFT array. This signal is amplified and converted into a digital value for each pixel using an analog-to-digital (A/D) converter. Each pixel typically has dimensions of 200×200 μm. A typical commercial DR system has flat-panel dimensions of 41×41 cm, with an TFT array of 2048×2048 elements. An antiscatter grid with a grid ratio of $\sim$13:1 and a strip line density of $\sim$70 lines per centimeter is used for scatter rejection.

In terms of image quality, the advantages of DR include the wide dynamic range available from A/D converters and a higher detective quantum efficiency (DQE) and latitude than is possible with intensifying screen/film combinations. The DQE is defined as

$$\mathrm{DQE} = \left[\frac{\mathrm{SNR_{out}}}{\mathrm{SNR_{in}}}\right]^2 \tag{1.16}$$

FIGURE 1.15. *The appearance of noise in X-ray images, with the film being exposed to a "uniform" X-ray beam. (Left) The image with no quantum mottle, (Center) a low value of quantum mottle, and (Right) a higher value of quantum mottle.*

The value of the DQE is always less than one because the detector must introduce some noise into the system, but the higher the value, the larger is the SNR for a given number of photons entering the detector. The higher DQE of the flat panel compared to film arises from the X-ray absorption properties of CsI, the dense filling of the pixel matrix, and the low-noise readout electronics.

1.6. X-RAY IMAGE CHARACTERISTICS

The three most common parameters used to measure the "quality" of an image are the SNR, the spatial resolution, the and contrast-to-noise ratio (CNR). An image ideally has a high value of each of these parameters, but often there are tradeoffs among the parameters, and compromises have to be made. General concepts relating to SNR, spatial resolution, and CNR for all the imaging modalities in this book are covered in Chapter 5.

1.6.1. Signal-to-Noise Ratio

If an X-ray film is exposed to a beam of X-rays, with no attenuating medium between the source and the film, one would imagine that the image should have a spatially uniform OD. In fact, however, a nonuniform distribution of signal intensities is seen, as shown in Figure 1.15.

There are two sources for this nonuniformity: the first is the statistical distribution of X-rays from the source, and the second is the spatial nonuniformity in the response of the film. The first factor is typically the dominant source of noise, and can be defined in terms of "quantum mottle," that is, the statistical variance in the number of X-rays per unit area produced by the source. This statistical variance is characterized by a Poisson distribution, as covered in Section 5.3.1. If the total number of detected X-rays per unit area is denoted by N, then the image SNR is proportional to the square root of N. Therefore, the factors that affect the SNR include the following:

1. The exposure time and X-ray tube current: The SNR is proportional to the square root of the product of the exposure time and the X-ray tube current.

2. The kV_p value: The higher the kV_p value, the greater is the number of high-energy X-rays produced. This, in turn, increases the number of X-rays reaching the detector and results in a higher SNR.
3. The degree of X-ray filtration: The higher the degree of filtering, the smaller is the number of X-rays reaching the detector, and the lower is the SNR for a given kV_p and mA.
4. The size of the patient: The greater the thickness of tissue through which the X-rays have to travel, the greater is the attenuation and the lower is the SNR.
5. The thickness of the phosphor layer in the intensifying screen: The thicker the layer, the greater is the proportion of incident X-rays that produce light to develop the film and the higher is the SNR.
6. The geometry of the antiscatter grid: A grid with a higher ratio of septal height to separation attenuates a greater degree of Compton-scattered X-rays than one with a smaller ratio, and therefore reduces the image SNR.

One further factor affecting the SNR is:

7. The uniformity of the spatial response of the intensifying screen/film combination: A nonuniform response is due mainly to differences in the number of grains of silver halide per unit area across the film, and secondarily to the spatial variations in the density of phospors per unit area in the screen. The higher the nonuniformity, the lower is the SNR of the image.

1.6.2. Spatial Resolution

Several factors which affect the spatial resolution of the X-ray image have already been described:

1. The thickness of the intensifying screen: The thicker the screen, the broader is the light spread function and the coarser is the spatial resolution.
2. The speed of the X-ray film: A fast film consists of relatively large particles of silver halide, and therefore has a poorer spatial resolution than a slow film.

Two other important factors are as follows:

3. The effective size of the X-ray focal spot (Figure 1.4): The fact that the X-ray source has a finite size results in a phenomenon known as geometric unsharpness. This causes blurring in the image, which is most apparent at the edges of different tissues, in which case the effect is referred to as a penumbra. The degree of image blurring depends on the effective focal spot size f and the distances between the X-ray source and the patient S_0 and the X-ray source and the detector S_1, as shown in Figure 1.16.

Using simple trigonometry, we obtain the size of the penumbra region, denoted P, from

$$P = \frac{f(S_1 - S_0)}{S_0} \tag{1.17}$$

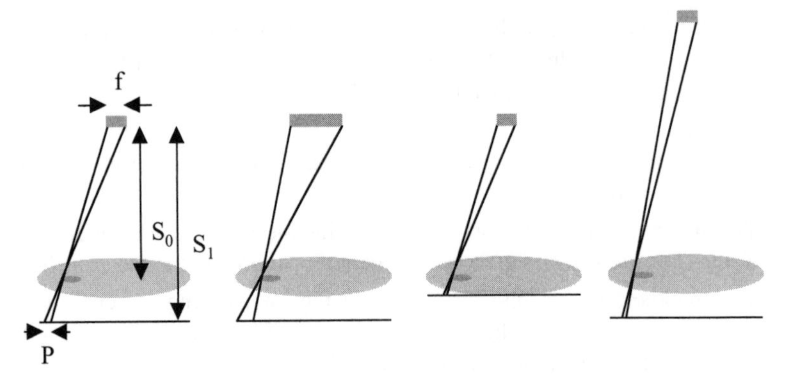

FIGURE 1.16. *(Left) A finite value of the effective focal spot size f of the source means that a penumbra P of geometric unsharpness exists in the image. (Left to right). Increasing the source diameter increases the unsharpness. Decreasing the object-to-detector distance decreases the unsharpness. Increasing the source-to-object distance, keeping the factor $S_1 - S_0$ constant, also decreases the unsharpness.*

In order to improve the image spatial resolution, therefore, the distance from the source to the detector should be as large, and the effective focal spot size as small, as possible.

4. The magnification factor associated with the imaging process: From Figure 1.16, the magnification factor m is given by

$$m = \frac{S_1}{S_0} \tag{1.18}$$

For standard imaging parameters with the size of the effective focal spot being between 0.6 and 1.2 mm, increasing the value of m increases the geometric unsharpness, and so the patient should be placed as close to the detector as possible. In procedures involving magnification radiography, where a special anode is used to produce an effective focal spot size of typically 0.1 mm, magnification factors of up to 1.5 are achieved by placing the detector some distance away from the patient.

Each part of the imaging system contributes a certain degree of blurring, and the spatial resolution R_{total} of the image represents the combination of all these contributions:

$$R_{\text{total}} = \sqrt{R_{\text{screen}}^2 + R_{\text{film}}^2 + R_{\text{spot size}}^2 + R_{\text{mag}}^2} \tag{1.19}$$

where R_{screen}, R_{film}, $R_{\text{spot size}}$, and R_{mag} refer to the contributions of the parameters described in detail above. The most useful measure of spatial resolution for X-ray radiography is the line spread function (LSF), described in detail in Section 5.2.2.

The LSF is most easily measured using a grid consisting of parallel lead septa. The wider is the LSF, the more blurring occurs in the image. It is also common to calculate the modulation transfer function (MTF) of the imaging system, which is covered in Section 5.2.3.

1.6.3. Contrast-to-Noise Ratio

Image contrast relates to the difference in signal intensity from various regions of the body. For example, in chest radiography, the contrast can be defined in terms of signal differences from areas of the X-ray film that correspond to bone and soft tissue. The ability of a physician to interpret an image depends upon the value of the CNR, that is, the difference in the SNR between bone and soft tissue, as discussed in Section 5.4. Therefore, all of the factors that affect the image SNR, for example, exposure time, tube current, kV_p value, X-ray filtration, patient size, detector efficiency, and film response uniformity, also affect the CNR. In addition, the spatial resolution also has an effect on CNR. A broad point spread function blurs the boundaries between different tissues and therefore reduces the image CNR. Parameters described in the previous section, such as the size of the X-ray focal spot, the thickness of the intensifying screen, the magnification factor, and the film speed, therefore affect the CNR.

In addition, the following parameters also affect the image CNR:

1. The energy of the X-rays produced by the source: If low-energy X-rays are used, the photoelectric effect dominates, and the values of μ_{bone} and $\mu_{\text{soft tissue}}$ are substantially different. If high-energy X-rays are used, then Compton scattering is the dominant interaction, and because the probability of this occurring is essentially independent of atomic number, the contrast is reduced considerably. There is still some contrast because the probability of Compton scattering depends upon electron density and bone has a slightly higher electron density than soft tissue, but the contrast is much reduced compared to that at low X-ray energies. However, as described previously, using very low energy X-rays also produces a relatively large noise level due to quantum mottle.
2. The FOV of the X-ray image: Between values of the FOV of 10 and 30 cm, the proportion of Compton-scattered radiation reaching the detector increases linearly with the FOV, and therefore the CNR is reduced with increasing FOV. Above a FOV of 30 cm, the proportion remains constant.
3. The thickness of the body part being imaged: The thicker the section, the larger is the contribution from Compton-scattered X-rays and the lower is the number of X-rays detected. Both factors reduce the CNR of the image.
4. The geometry of the antiscatter grid: As outlined in Section 1.5.2, there is a tradeoff between the SNR of the image and the contribution of Compton-scattered X-rays to the image. The factor by which contrast is improved by using an antiscatter grid is given by

$$\text{Contrast improvement} = \frac{1 + R}{1 + Rs/p} \tag{1.20}$$

where R, as defined previously, is the ratio of scattered to primary X-rays incident upon the grid, p is the primary radiation transmitted through the grid, and s is the scattered radiation transmitted through the grid.

5. The properties of the intensifying screen/film combination: Ideally, the detector amplifies the intrinsic contrast due to X-ray attenuation, such that differences in the OD of the developed film are larger than the differences in the incident X-ray intensities.

1.7. X-RAY CONTRAST AGENTS

X-ray contrast agents are chemicals that are introduced into the body to increase image contrast. For example, barium sulfate is used to investigate abnormalities such as ulcers, polyps, tumors, or hernias in the gastrointestinal (GI) tract. Because the element barium has a K-edge at 37.4 keV, X-ray attenuation is much higher in areas where the agent accumulates than in surrounding tissue. Barium sulfate, made up as a suspension in water, can be administered orally, rectally, or via a nasal gastric tube. Orally, barium sulfate is used to explore the upper GI tract, including the stomach and esophagus. As an enema, barium sulfate can be used either as a single or "double" contrast agent. As a single agent it fills the entire lumen of the GI tract and can detect large abnormalities. As a double contrast agent, barium sulfate is introduced first, followed usually by air: the barium sulfate coats the inner surface of the GI tract and the air distends the

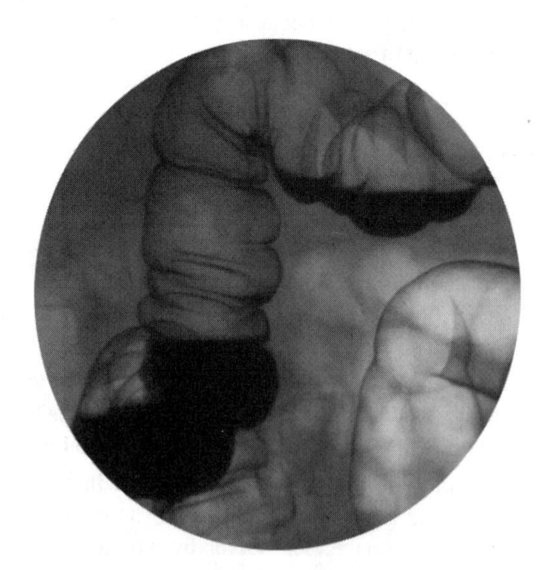

FIGURE 1.17. *An X-ray image showing the passage of barium sulfate through the GI tract. In this image, areas of high X-ray attenuation appear dark. The image corresponds to a double contrast (barium sulfate and air).*

lumen. This double-agent approach is used to characterize smaller disorders of the large intestine, colon, and rectum. An example image is shown in Figure 1.17.

Iodine-based X-ray contrast agents are used for a number of applications including intravenous urography, angiography, and intravenous and intraarterial digital subtraction angiography (covered in the next section). An iodine-based agent is injected into the bloodstream and because iodine has a *K*-edge at 33.2 keV, X-ray attenuation in blood vessels is enhanced compared to the surrounding soft tissue. This makes it possible to visualize arteries and veins within the body. Iodinated agents can also used in the detection of brain tumors and metastases, as covered in detail in Section 1.15.1. Iodine-containing X-ray contrast agents are usually based on triiodinated benzene rings, as shown in Figure 1.18. Important parameters in the design of a particular agent are the iodine load, that is, the amount of iodine in a given injected dose, and the osmolarity of the solution being injected. An increase in iodine load typically comes at the expense of an increased osmolarity, which can cause cells to shrink or swell, and can also result in adverse reactions, particularly in patients with kidney disease, asthma, or diabetes. Historically, the first contrast agents used were ionic, high-osmolarity contrast media (HOCM), such as sodium diatrizoate. Ionic, low-osmolarity contrast media (LOCM) subsequently became available in the form of compounds such as ioxaglate. The design of nonionic LOCM, such as iohexol, iopamidol, iopromol (shown in Figure 1.18), and iopental, reduced the adverse side effects of iodinated contrast agents considerably. The latest developments are nonionic isoosmotic contrast agents such as iodixanol (Visipaque), also shown in Figure 1.18.

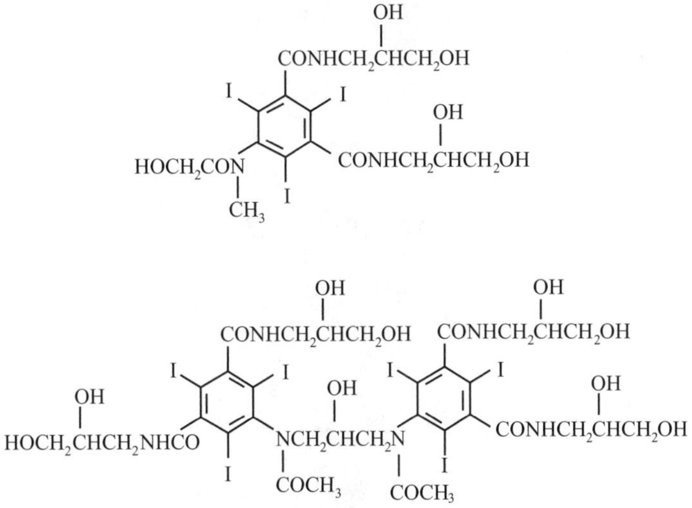

FIGURE 1.18. *(Top) The chemical structure of iopromol, a nonionic, low-osmolarity X-ray contrast agent. (Bottom) The chemical structure of iodixanol, a nonionic, isoosmotic X-ray contrast agent.*

1.8. X-RAY IMAGING METHODS

In addition to planar X-ray imaging, there are a number of different imaging techniques which use X-rays. These include angiography, which uses injected iodinated contrast agents; fluoroscopy, which is a real-time imaging method often used in conjunction with barium contrast agents; and dual-energy imaging, which can produce separate images corresponding to bone and soft tissue.

1.8.1. X-Ray Angiography

Angiographic techniques produce images that show selectively the blood vessels in the body. This type of imaging is used to investigate diseases such as stenoses and clotting of arteries and veins and irregularities in systemic and pulmonary blood flow. In X-ray angiography, a bolus of iodine-based contrast agent is injected into the bloodstream before imaging. The X-ray image shows increased attenuation from the blood vessels compared to the tissue surrounding them. A related imaging technique is called digital subtraction angiography (DSA), in which one image is taken before the contrast agent is administered, a second after injection of the agent, and the difference between the two images is computed. DSA gives very high contrast between the vessels and tissue, as shown in Figure 1.19. Both DSA and conventional X-ray angiography can

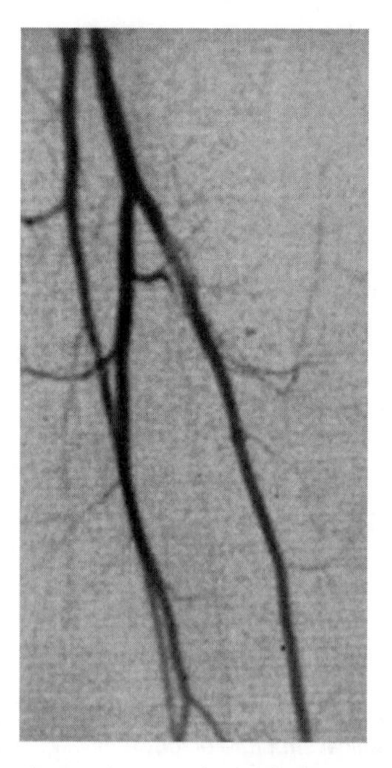

FIGURE 1.19. *A digital subtraction angiogram obtained after contrast agent injection, showing a portion of the arterial tree distal to the renal arteries.*

produce angiograms with extremely high spatial resolution, resolving vessels down to $\sim 100\,\mu m$ in diameter.

1.8.2. X-Ray Fluoroscopy

X-ray fluoroscopy is a continuous imaging technique using X-rays with very low energies, typically in the range 25–30 keV. This technique is used for placement of stents and catheters, patient positioning for interventional surgery, and many studies of the GI tract. The X-ray source is identical to that described previously, except that a lower tube current (1–5 mA) and accelerating voltage (70–90 kV) are used, and so a small number of low-energy X-rays are produced. The inherently low SNR of the technique, due to a high level of quantum mottle, requires the use of a fluoroscopic image intensifier, shown in Figure 1.20, in order to improve the SNR. A fluorescent screen is used to monitor continuously the area of interest within the body.

The image intensifier is surrounded by mu-metal to shield the electrostatic lenses from interference from external magnetic fields. The input window of the intensifier is constructed either of aluminum or titanium, both of which have a very low attenuation coefficient at low X-ray energies. The input fluorescent screen contains a thin, 0.2- to 0.4-mm thick, convex layer of sodium-doped cesium iodide (CsI:Na). This layer consists of columnar crystals, which are deposited directly onto the input window. Because both cesium and iodine have *K*-edges, 36 and 33 keV respectively, that are close to the energies of the X-rays being used, the probability of photoelectric

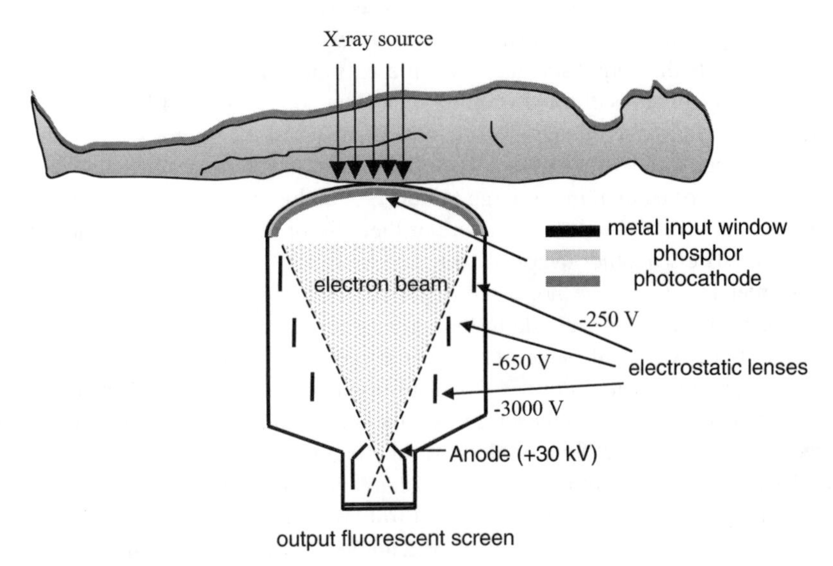

FIGURE 1.20. *A schematic of an image intensifier used for X-ray fluoroscopy. The intensifying screen can be above, below, or to the side of the patient, depending upon the particular clinical application.*

interactions between the incoming X-rays and the screen is very high, with approximately 60% of the incoming X-rays being absorbed. The photoelectrons produced from these photoelectric interactions in the screen are converted into light photons within the phosphor layer. Roughly 2000 low-energy (2-eV, 400-nm) light photons are produced for every incoming X-ray photon. The light photons produced from the screen are absorbed by the photocathode and converted into photoelectrons.

The photocathode, which contains antimony/cesium compounds, is in direct contact with the surface of the fluorescent screen. The maximum conversion efficiency of the photocathode occurs at 400 nm, matching the maximum output wavelength of the screen. The conversion efficiency at the photocathode is approximately 10%, that is, one photoelectron is produced for every 10 light photons striking the photocathode. These photoelectrons accelerate toward the positively charged anode, which has an applied potential difference of between 25 and 35 kV. They are focused onto the output screen, which is made from a layer, a few micrometers thick, of silver-activated zinc cadmium sulfide. Electrostatic "lenses," consisting of negatively charged electrodes, are used for this focusing. The exact voltage applied to the electrodes can be varied to change the area of the output screen onto which the photoelectrons are focused, giving a variable image magnification factor. The output phosphor screen converts the photoelectrons into photons, with wavelengths in the visible range of 500–600 nm. These photons can be visualized directly or recorded via a video recorder. Electron absorption at the output screen is 90% efficient, with the final step of light generation typically producing 1000 light photons for every photoelectron absorbed. The inner surface of the output screen is coated with a very thin layer of aluminum, which allows the electrons to reach the output screen, but prevents light created in the screen from returning to the photocathode and producing secondary electrons.

For every X-ray photon incident on the input screen, roughly 200,000 light photons are produced at the output screen. This represents an increase of a factor of 100 from the number of photons emitted from the input screen. The second factor in the high SNR gain of an image intensifier is that the diameter of the output screen is usually about 10 times smaller than that of the input screen, which ranges in size from small (23 cm) for cardiac imaging to large (57 cm) for abdominal studies. The increase in brightness is proportional to the square of the ratio of the respective diameters, that is, approximately another factor of 100.

In order for the image not to be distorted, each electron must travel the same distance from the photocathode to the output screen, and so a curved input screen must be used. A typical value of the spatial resolution at the center of the output screen is about 0.3 mm, with ~3–5% distortion due to differential electron paths at the edges of a 2.3-cm-diameter screen. Another important property of the intensifying screen is the signal retention, or "lag," from one image to the next. The value of the lag determines the maximum frame rate, that is, the highest number of images that can be acquired per second without signal from one image appearing in the next.

X-ray fluoroscopy can be carried out in a number of modes. The simplest is continuous visualization or video recording of the signal, often referred to as "cine mode." Cine-mode fluoroscopy is often used in cardiac studies with two X-ray source/image intensifiers situated at an angle of 90° to one other. By alternating data acquisition from each detector and pulsing the X-ray source, frame rates up to 150 per second are possible. Digital fluoroscopy can also be performed: in this case the video output of the camera is digitized and can be stored for subsequent data processing. Digital fluoroscopy is used for, among other applications, cardiac pacemaker implantation and orthopedic interventions.

1.8.3. Dual-Energy Imaging

Dual-energy X-ray imaging is a technique which produces two separate images corresponding to soft tissue and bone. The method is most commonly used clinically for imaging the chest region because both soft-tissue abnormalities and small calcifications can be visualized more clearly on these separate images than on a conventional planar X-ray scan. There are two ways of performing dual-energy imaging. The first method uses two X-ray exposures, one applied immediately after the other, with different kV_p values of the X-ray source. Because the X-rays in both scans contain a range of energies, some manipulation of the data is necessary to produce the final images. The second method uses a single exposure with the setup shown in Figure 1.21. The detector, usually made from Y_2O_2S or BaFBr, which is placed directly beneath the patient, preferentially absorbs lower energy X-rays. This detector effectively hardens the X-ray beam incident on the second detector, which is typically made from Gd_2O_2S. Therefore, the image from the first detector corresponds to a low-X-ray-energy, high-contrast image, and that from the second detector to a high-X-ray-energy, low-contrast image. As for the first method of dual-energy imaging, postacquisition data processing is performed to produce the final set of images. If extra beam hardening is required,

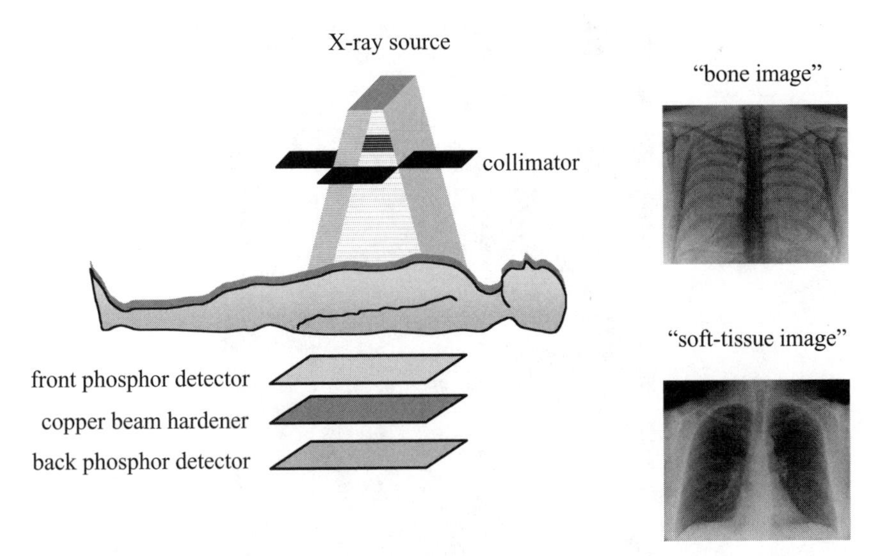

FIGURE 1.21. *A schematic of an instrumental setup used for dual-energy X-ray imaging. The front detector records an image primarily from lower-energy X-rays and the back detector primarily from higher-energy X-rays. Nonlinear combination of the two datasets results in images, shown on the right, corresponding to soft tissue and bone.*

a copper filter can be placed in front of the second detector. The detectors can either be in the form of storage phosphor screens, as used in computed radiography, or be coupled directly to a photodiode array to produce a digital output.

1.9. CLINICAL APPLICATIONS OF X-RAY IMAGING

A number of clinical applications of X-ray imaging have already been described. Plain film radiography is used for determining the presence and severity of fractures or cracks in the bone structure in the brain, chest, pelvis, arms, legs, hands, and feet. Dual-energy scanning is used for diagnosing lung disease and detecting other masses within the chest wall. Vascular imaging, using injected iodine-based contrast agents, is performed to study compromised blood flow, mainly in the brain and heart, but also in the peripheral venous and arterial systems. Diseases of the GI tract can be diagnosed using barium sulfate as a contrast agent, usually with continuous monitoring via X-ray fluoroscopic techniques. The following sections highlight two additional important applications of X-ray imaging.

1.9.1. Mammography

X-ray mammography is used to detect small lesions in the breast. Very high spatial resolution and CNR are needed to detect microcalcifications, which may be considerably smaller than 1 mm in diameter, as shown in Figure 1.22. A low radiation dose

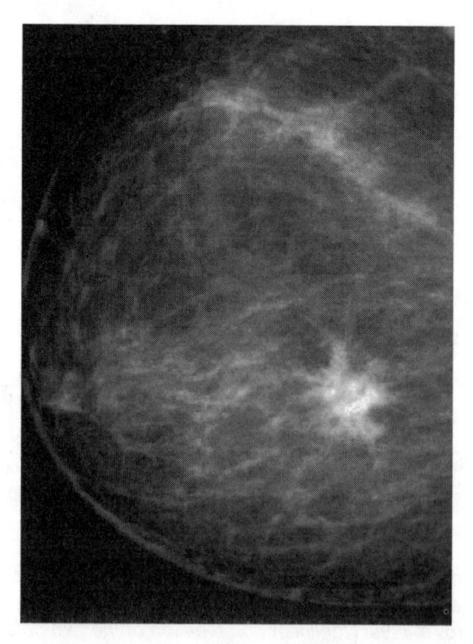

FIGURE 1.22. *An X-ray mammogram showing a calcification as a bright area in the image.*

is also important to avoid tissue damage. Fast intensifying screen/film combinations are necessary to allow the use of low kV_p values (generally 25–30 kV) to optimize contrast by maximizing the contribution of photoelectric interactions. Several modifications are also made to the conventional X-ray tube. The X-ray source uses an anode target made from molybdenum, which has K-edges at 17.9 and 19.6 keV. The cathode filament is flat in shape, rather than a spiral, in order to produce a more focused electron beam. The glass window in the X-ray tube is replaced by one fabricated from beryllium to reduce the degree of filtering of the low-energy X-rays. A molybdenum filter (30 μm thick) is used to reduce the amount of high-energy X-rays ($>$20 keV), which would otherwise give increased patient dose without improving image quality. Occasionally, with a radiopaque breast, in which attenuation of X-rays is particularly high, an aluminum filter can be used instead of molybdenum.

In order to reduce the effects of geometric unsharpness, large focal-spot-to-film distances (45–80 cm) and small focal spot sizes (0.1–0.3 mm) are used. A 4:1 or 5:1 grid ratio is used for the antiscatter grid, with septa density typically between 25 and 50 lines per cm, a septal thickness less than 20 μm, and a septal height less than 1 mm. Compression of the breast is necessary, normally to about 4 cm in thickness, in order to improve X-ray transmission and reduce the contribution from Compton scatter.

A relatively new technique, called digital mammography, is becoming increasingly important in the clinical setting. In this technique, the conventional intensifying screen/film combination is replaced by a phosphor screen, which is coupled through fiber-optic cables to a charge coupled device (CCD) detector with, typically, 1024 $\times$ 1024 elements. The CCD converts the light into an analog signal, which is digitized, stored, and displayed. CCDs typically have greater sensitivity and lower overall system noise, which translates into a lower patient dose, than the intensifying screen/film combination.

1.9.2. Abdominal X-Ray Scans

Investigations of the urinary tract are among the most common applications of planar X-ray imaging, and are carried out in the form of kidney, ureter, and bladder (KUB) scans and intravenous pyelograms (IVPs). The KUB scan is carried out without contrast agent, and can detect abnormal distributions of gas within the intestines, indicative of various conditions of the GI tract, and also large kidney stones. The KUB is usually the precursor to a follow-up imaging procedure, which would entail a GI scan with barium sulfate, or an IVP if problems with the urinary system are suspected. An IVP is performed using an injected iodinated contrast agent in order to visualize the filling and emptying of the urinary system, that is, the kidneys, the bladder, and the ureters. An example of an IVP is shown in Figure 1.23. Obstruction to normal flow through the system is usually caused by kidney stones, but can result from infections of the urinary system. An IVP is carried out as a series of images acquired at different times after injection of the contrast agent. Normal excretion of the agent from the bloodstream via the kidneys takes about 30 min, but obstructions can be detected or inferred from delayed passage of the contrast agent through the affected part of the urinary system.

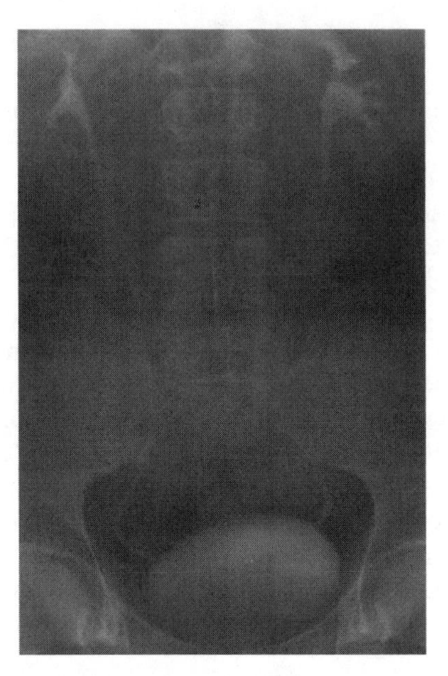

FIGURE 1.23. *An intravenous pyelogram, showing enhanced signal from the ureters and bladder, which contain iodinated contrast agent.*

1.10. COMPUTED TOMOGRAPHY

The technique of X-ray CT was invented by Godfrey Hounsfield in 1972, for which he, jointly with Allan Cormack, who had independently done earlier work on the mathematics of the technique, were awarded jointly the Nobel Prize in Medicine in 1979. CT enables the acquisition of two-dimensional X-ray images of thin "slices" through the body. Multiple images from adjacent slices can be obtained in order to reconstruct a three-dimensional volume. CT images show reasonable contrast between soft tissues such as kidney, liver, and muscle because the X-rays transmitted through each organ are no longer superimposed on one another at the detector, as is the case in planar X-ray radiography. The basic principle behind CT is that the two-dimensional internal structure of an object can be reconstructed from a series of one-dimensional "projections" of the object acquired at different angles. In order to obtain an image from a thin slice of tissue, the X-ray beam is collimated to give a thin beam. The detectors, which are situated opposite the X-ray source, record the total number of X-rays that are transmitted through the patient, producing a one-dimensional projection. The signal intensities in this projection are dictated by the two-dimensional distribution of tissue attenuation coefficients within the slice. The X-ray source and the detectors are then rotated by a certain angle and the measurements repeated. This process continues until sufficient data have been collected to reconstruct an image with high spatial resolution. Reconstruction of the image involves a process termed backprojection, which is covered in Section 1.11.2 and Appendix B.

The reconstructed image is displayed as a two-dimensional matrix, with each pixel corresponding to the CT number of the tissue at that spatial location.

1.10.1. Scanner Instrumentation

Several components of the CT system such as the X-ray source, collimator, and antiscatter grid are very similar to the instrumentation described previously for planar X-ray radiography. Over the past 30 years single-slice CT scanners have developed from systems with a single source and single detector, which took many minutes to acquire an image, to single-source, multiple-detector instruments, which can acquire an image in 1 s or less. Multislice systems have also been developed, and are described in Section 1.13. The principles of data acquisition and processing for CT can be appreciated by considering the development from the earliest, so-called "first-generation scanners" to the third- and fourth-generation systems found in most hospitals today. A schematic of the basic operation of a first-generation scanner is shown in Figure 1.24.

Motion of the X-ray source and the detector occurred in two ways, linear and rotational. In Figure 1.24, M linear steps were taken with the intensity of the transmitted X-rays being detected at each step. This produced a single projection with M data points. Then both the source and detector were rotated by $(180/N)$ degrees, where N is the number of rotations in the complete scan, and a further M translational lines were acquired at this angle. The total data matrix acquired was therefore $M \times N$ points. The spatial resolution could be increased by using finer translational steps and angular increments, up to a limiting value dictated by the effective X-ray focal spot size, but this resulted in a longer imaging time. Collimation of the X-ray beam gave a certain beam width in the axis perpendicular to the axis of rotation, and

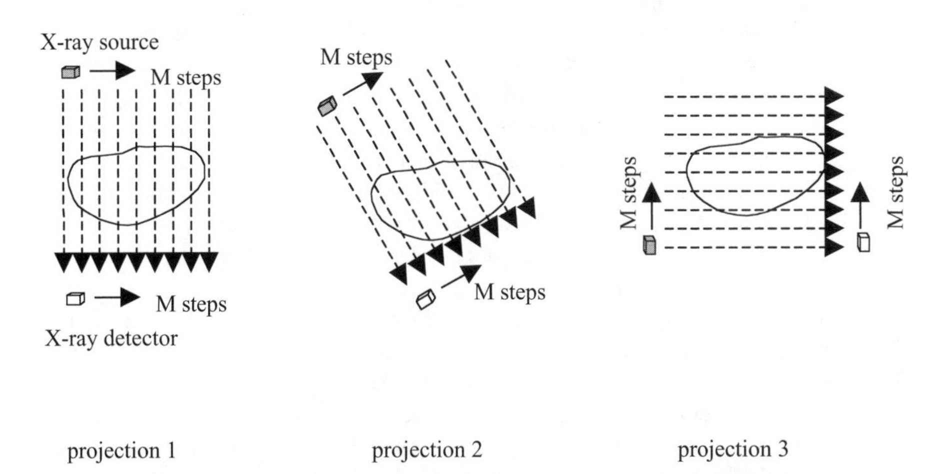

FIGURE 1.24. *The mode of operation of a first-generation CT scanner. The source and the detector move in a series of linear steps, and then both are rotated and the process repeated. Typically, the number of projections and the number M of steps in each projection are equal in value.*

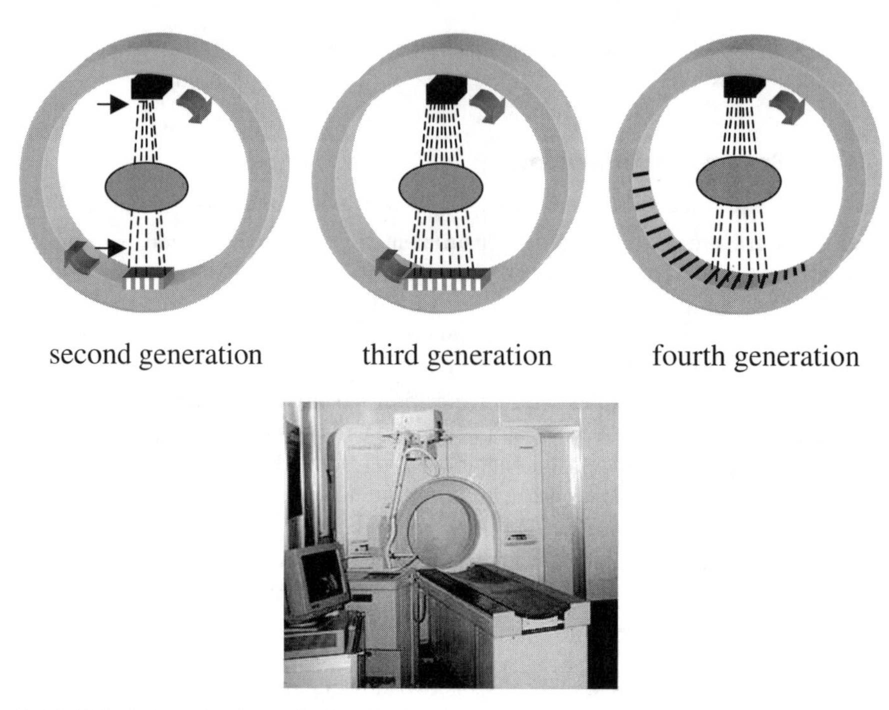

FIGURE 1.25. (Top) A schematic showing the development of second-, third-, and fourth- generation CT scanners. (Bottom) A photograph of a typical third-generation scanner with patient bed.

this determined the thickness of the slice. Typical data matrix sizes were 180 × 180 and scanning times were 4–5 min. Image reconstruction algorithms were based upon backprojection, discussed in Section 1.11.2 and Appendix B.

In second-generation scanners, instead of the single beam used in the first-generation scanners, a thin "fan beam" of X-rays was produced from the source and multiple X-ray detectors were used rather than a single one. The major advantage of the second-generation scanner, shown in Figure 1.25, was the reduction in total scanning time, which, for example, made abdominal imaging feasible within a single breath-hold. Image reconstruction required the development of "fan-beam" backprojection reconstruction algorithms, discussed in Section 1.11.3.

Third-generation scanners, also shown in Figure 1.25, use a much wider X-ray fan beam and a sharply increased number of detectors, typically between 512 and 768, compared to the second-generation systems. Two separate collimators are used in front of the source. The first collimator restricts the beam to an angular width of roughly 45°. The second collimator, placed perpendicular to the first, restricts the beam to the desired slice thickness, which is typically 1–5 mm. An intense pulse of X-rays is produced for a time period of 2 to 4 ms for each projection, and the X-ray tube/detector unit rotates through 360°. The scanner usually operates at a kV_p of 140 kV, with filtration giving an effective X-ray energy of 70–80 keV and a tube current between 70 and 320 mA. The focal spot size is between 0.6 and 1.6 mm. Typical operating conditions are a rotation speed of once per second, a data matrix of either 512×512 or 1024×1024, and a spatial resolution of $\sim$0.35 mm.

In the fourth-generation scanner a complete ring of detectors surrounds the patient. The X-ray tube rotates through 360° with a wide fan beam. There is no intrinsic decrease in scan time for fourth-generation with respect to third-generation scanners. In fact, the vast majority of scanners in hospitals are third generation.

1.10.2. Detectors for Computed Tomography

The most common detectors for CT scanners are xenon-filled ionization chambers, shown in Figure 1.26. Because xenon has a high atomic number of 66, there is a high probability of photoelectric interactions between the gas and the incoming X-rays. The xenon is kept under pressure at $\sim$20 atm to increase further the number of interactions between the X-rays and the gas molecules. An array of interlinked ionization chambers, typically 768 in number (although some commercial scanners have up to 1000), is filled with gas, with metal electrodes separating the individual chambers. X-rays transmitted through the body ionize the gas in the detector, producing electron–ion pairs. These are attracted to the electrodes by an applied voltage difference between the electrodes, and produce a current which is proportional to the number of incident X-rays. Each detector electrode is connected to a separate amplifier, and the outputs of the amplifiers are multiplexed through a switch to a single A/D converter. The digitized signals are logarithmically amplified and stored for subsequent image reconstruction. In this design of the ionization chamber, the metal

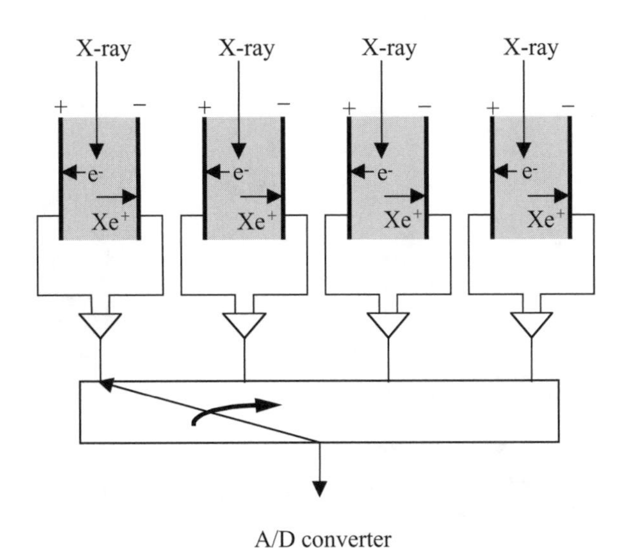

FIGURE 1.26. *A schematic of the Xe-filled detectors used in computed tomography, and the switched connections between multiple detectors and a single analog-to-digital converter.*

electrode plates also perform the role of an antiscatter grid, with the plates being angled to align with the focal spot of the X-ray tube. The plates are typically 10 cm in length, with a gap of 1 mm between adjacent plates.

1.11. IMAGE PROCESSING FOR COMPUTED TOMOGRAPHY

Image reconstruction takes place in parallel with data acquisition in order to minimize the delay between the end of data acquisition and the display of the images on the operator's console. As the signals corresponding to one projection are being acquired, those from the previous projection are being amplified and digitized, and those from the projection previous to that are being filtered and processed.

In order to illustrate the issues involved in image reconstruction, consider the raw projection data that would be acquired from a simple object such as an ellipse with a uniform attenuation coefficient, as shown in Figure 1.27. The reconstruction goal is illustrated on the right of Figure 1.27 for a simple 2×2 matrix of tissue attenuation coefficients: given a series of intensities I_1, I_2, I_3, I_4, what are the values of the attenuation coefficients μ_1, μ_2, μ_3, μ_4?

For each projection, the signal intensity recorded by each detector depends upon the attenuation coefficient and the thickness of each tissue that lies between the X-ray source and that particular detector. For the simple case shown on the right of Figure 1.27, two projections are acquired, each consisting of two data points: projection 1 (I_1 and I_2) and projection 2 (I_3 and I_4). If the image to be reconstructed is also a two-by-two matrix, then the intensities of the projections can be expressed in terms of the linear attenuation coefficients by

$$
\begin{aligned}
I_1 &= I_0 e^{-(\mu_1+\mu_2)x} \\
I_2 &= I_0 e^{-(\mu_3+\mu_4)x} \\
I_3 &= I_0 e^{-(\mu_1+\mu_3)x} \\
I_4 &= I_0 e^{-(\mu_2+\mu_4)x}
\end{aligned}
\tag{1.21}
$$

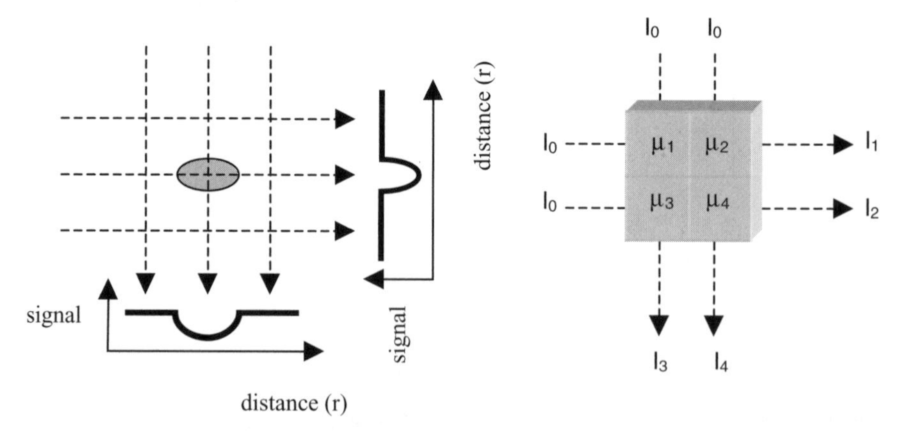

FIGURE 1.27. *(Left) Two projections acquired from an elliptical test object. (Right) Two projections acquired from an object consisting of a simple 2 × 2 matrix of tissue attenuation coefficients.*

where x is the dimension of each pixel. It might seem that this problem could be solved by matrix inversion or similar techniques. These approaches are not feasible, however, first due to the presence of noise in the projections (high noise levels can cause direct inversion techniques to become unstable), and second because of the large amount of data collected. If the data matrix size is, for example, 1024×1024, then matrix inversion techniques become very slow. Image reconstruction, in practice, is carried out using either backprojection algorithms or iterative techniques, both of which are covered in the following sections.

1.11.1. Preprocessing Data Corrections

Image reconstruction is preceded by a series of corrections to the acquired projections. The first corrections are made for the effects of beam hardening, in which the effective energy of the X-ray beam increases as it passes through the patient due to greater attenuation of lower X-ray energies. This means that the effective linear attenuation coefficient of tissue decreases with distance from the X-ray source. If not corrected, beam hardening results in significant artifacts in the reconstructed images (see Exercise 1.12). Correction algorithms typically assume a uniform tissue attenuation coefficient and estimate the thickness of the tissue through which the X-rays have traveled for each projection. These algorithms work well for images containing mainly soft tissue, but can give problems in the presence of bone.

The second type of correction is for imbalances in the sensitivities of individual detectors and detector channels. If these variations are not corrected, then a ring or halo artifact can appear in the reconstructed images. Imbalances in the detectors are usually measured using an object with a spatially uniform attenuation coefficent before the actual patient study. The results from this calibration scan can then be used to correct the clinical data.

1.11.2. The Radon Transform and Backprojection Techniques

The mathematical basis for reconstruction of an image from a series of projections is the Radon transform. For an arbitrary function $f(x, y)$, its Radon transform $\mathbb{R}$ is defined as the integral of $\rho(x, y)$ along a line L, as shown in Figure 1.28:

$$\mathbb{R}\{f(x, y)\} = \int_L f(x, y)\, dl \tag{1.22}$$

Each X-ray projection $p(r, \phi)$ can therefore be expressed in terms of the Radon transform of the object being studied:

$$p(r, \phi) = \mathbb{R}\{f(x, y)\} \tag{1.23}$$

where $p(r, \phi)$ refers to the projection data acquired as a function of r, the distance along the projection, and ϕ, the rotation angle of the X-ray source and detector.

Reconstruction of the image therefore requires computation of the inverse Radon transform of the acquired projection data. The most common methods of implementating the inverse Radon transform use backprojection or filtered backprojection

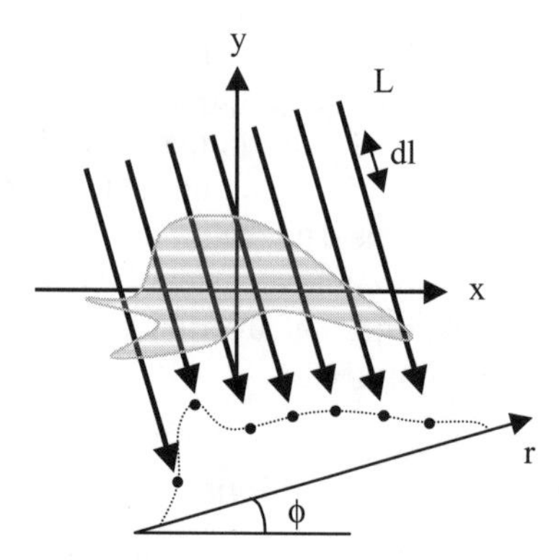

FIGURE 1.28. A representation of the X-ray line integrals defining the Radon transform of an object.

algorithms. These types of mathematical reconstructions are common to many imaging modalities, and the basic principles are covered in Appendix B.

After reconstruction, the image is displayed as a map of the tissue CT number, which is defined by

$$\mathrm{CT}_0 = 1000\frac{\mu_0 - \mu_{\mathrm{H_2O}}}{\mu_{\mathrm{H_2O}}} \tag{1.24}$$

where CT_0 is the CT number and μ_0 is the linear attenuation coefficient of the tissue. The reconstructed image consists of CT numbers varying in value from +3000 to −1000. The image display screen typically has only 256 gray levels and thus some form of nonlinear image windowing is used to display the image. Standard sets of contrast and window parameters exist for different types of scan.

1.11.3. Fan-Beam Reconstructions

The backprojection reconstruction methods outlined in Appendix B assume that each line integral corresponds to a parallel X-ray path from the source to detector. In third- and fourth-generation scanners, the geometry of the X-rays is a fan beam, as shown previously in Figure 1.25. Since the X-ray beams are no longer parallel to one another, image reconstruction requires modification of the backprojection algorithms to avoid introducing image artifacts.

The simplest modification is to "rebin" the acquired data to produce a series of parallel projections, which can then be processed as described previously. For example, in Figure 1.29, the X-ray beam from source position S_1 to detector D_3 is clearly not parallel to the beam from S_1 to detector D_1. However, when the source is rotated to position S_2, for example, the X-ray beam from S_2 to D_3 is parallel to that from S_1 to D_1. By resorting the data into a series of composite datasets consisting of parallel X-ray paths, for example, S_1D_1, S_2D_3, etc., one can reconstruct the image using standard

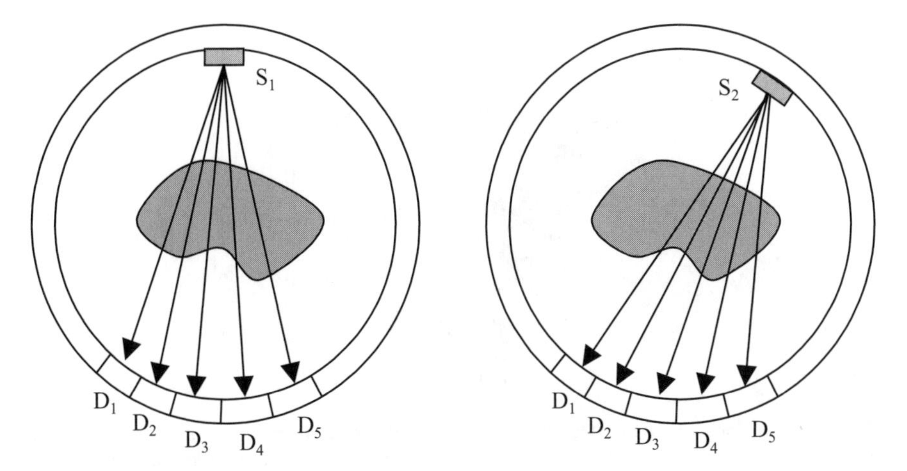

FIGURE 1.29. *Fan-beam projection data corresponding to two positions S_1 and S_2 of the X-ray source. By re-sorting the data from different positions of the source to produce composite data sets consisting of parallel X-ray beams, standard backprojection algorithms can be applied for image reconstruction.*

backprojection algorithms. Alternatively, filtered backprojection can be used directly on the fan-beam data, but each projection must be multiplied by the cosine of the fan-beam angle, and this angle is also incorporated into the convolution kernel for the filter.

1.11.4. Iterative Algorithms

An alternative approach to image reconstruction involves the use of iterative reconstruction algorithms. These algorithms start with an initial estimate of the two-dimensional matrix of attenuation coefficients. By comparing the projections predicted from this initial estimate with those that are actually acquired, changes are made to the estimated matrix. This process is repeated for each projection, and then a number of times for the whole dataset until the residual error between the measured data and those from the estimated matrix falls below a predesignated value. Iterative schemes are used relatively sparingly in standard CT scanning, where the SNR is sufficiently high for filtered backprojection algorithms to give good results. They are, however, used extensively in nuclear medicine tomographic techniques, which are covered in Chapter 2. There is a large number of methods for iterative reconstruction, most of which are based on highly complicated mathematical algorithms. One very simple illustrative method, called a ray-by-ray iteration method, is shown here.

Figure 1.30 shows two four-point projections from a two-dimensional matrix of tissue attenuation coefficients, μ_1–μ_{16}. In generating an initial estimate, the components of the horizontal projection, $0.2I_0$, $0.4I_0$, $0.3I_0$, and $0.1I_0$, are considered first (this choice is arbitrary). In the absence of prior knowledge, an initial estimate is formed by assuming that each pixel has the same X-ray attenuation coefficient. If the pixel dimensions are assumed to be square with height = length = 1 for simplicity,

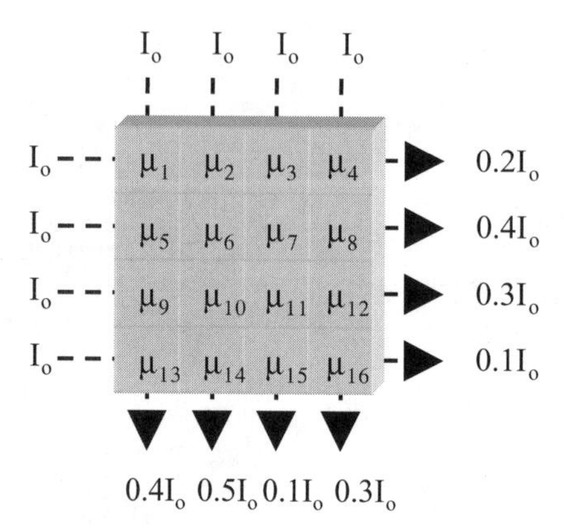

FIGURE 1.30. *The starting point for a ray-by-ray iterative reconstruction method. Two measured projections, each containing four data points, are shown. The aim is to use these data to estimate the values of* μ_1*–*μ_{16}*.*

then the following equations can be written:

$$
\begin{aligned}
0.2I_0 &= I_0 e^{-4\mu_A}, & \mu_A &= \mu_1 = \mu_2 = \mu_3 = \mu_4 \\
0.4I_0 &= I_0 e^{-4\mu_B}, & \mu_B &= \mu_5 = \mu_6 = \mu_7 = \mu_8 \\
0.3I_0 &= I_0 e^{-4\mu_C}, & \mu_C &= \mu_9 = \mu_{10} = \mu_{11} = \mu_{12} \\
0.1I_0 &= I_0 e^{-4\mu_D}, & \mu_D &= \mu_{13} = \mu_{14} = \mu_{15} = \mu_{16}
\end{aligned}
\tag{1.25}
$$

This gives the first iteration of the estimated matrix, shown on the left of Figure 1.31. Clearly the individual data points of the vertical projection calculated from this iteration do not agree with the measured data, $0.4I_0$, $0.5I_0$, $0.1I_0$, and $0.3I_0$. The mean squared error (MSE) per pixel is calculated as

$$
\text{MSE/pixel} = \tfrac{1}{4}I_0[(0.4 - 0.22)^2 + (0.5 - 0.22)^2 + (0.1 - 0.22)^2 + (0.3 - 0.22)^2]
\tag{1.26}
$$

The value of the MSE per pixel after the first iteration is approximately $0.0325I_0$. The next iteration forces the estimated data to agree with the measured vertical projection. Consider the component that passes through pixels μ_1, μ_5, μ_9, and μ_{13}. The measured data is $0.4I_0$, but the calculated data using the first iteration is $0.22I_0$. The values of the attenuation coefficients have been overestimated and must be reduced. The exact amount by which the attenuation coefficients μ_1, μ_5, μ_9, and μ_{13} should be reduced is unknown, and again the simple assumption is made that each value should be reduced by an equal amount. Applying this procedure to all four components of the horizontal projection gives the estimated matrix shown on the right of Figure 1.31. Now, of course, the estimated projection data do not agree with the measured data of the horizontal projection but the MSE per pixel has been reduced to $0.005I_0$. In a practical realization of a full ray-by-ray iterative reconstruction, many more projections would be acquired and processed. After a full iteration of all of the projections, the process can be repeated a number of times until the desired accuracy is reached or further iterations produce no significant improvements in the value of the MSE.

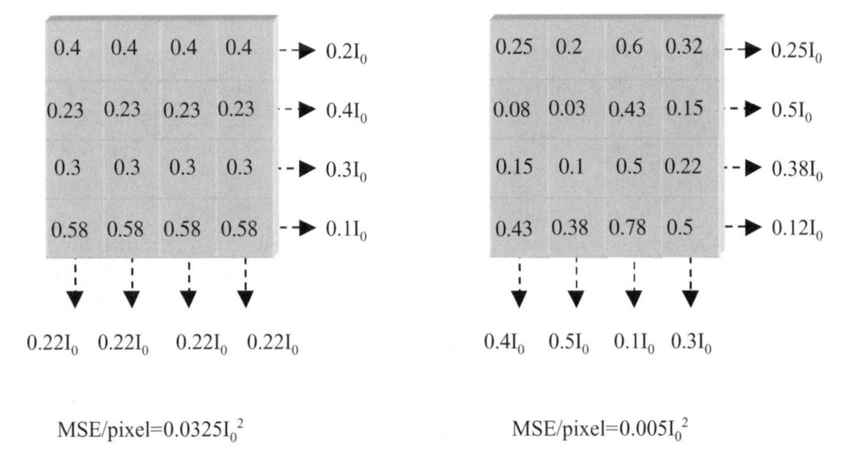

FIGURE 1.31. *(Left) The results from the first-pass iterative reconstruction based on the horizontal projection. (Right) The second-pass iteration incorporating the measured data from the vertical projection.*

1.12. SPIRAL/HELICAL COMPUTED TOMOGRAPHY

In the conventional CT systems described thus far, only a single slice can be acquired at one time. If multiple slices are required to cover a larger volume of the body, the entire thorax, for example, then the patient table is moved in discrete steps through the plane of the X-ray source and detector. A single slice is acquired at each discrete table position, with an inevitable time delay between obtaining each image. This process is both time-inefficient and can result in spatial misregistrations between slices if the patient moves. In the early 1990s a technique called spiral, or helical, CT was developed to overcome these problems by acquiring data as the table position is moved continuously through the scanner, as shown in Figure 1.32. The trajectory of the X-ray beam through the patient traces out a spiral, or helix: hence the name. This technique

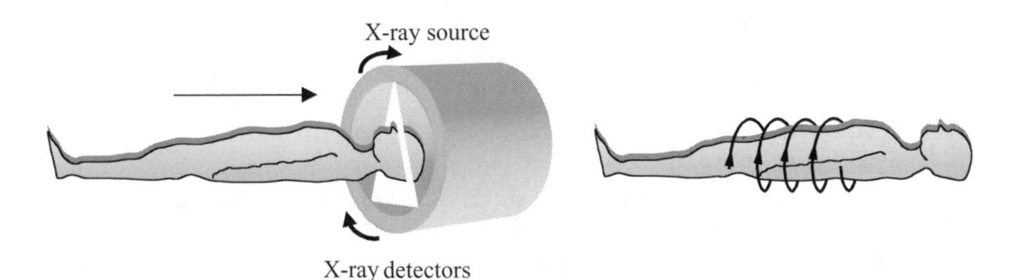

FIGURE 1.32. *The principle of spiral CT acquisition. Simultaneous motion of the patient bed and rotation of the X-ray source and detectors (left) results in a spiral trajectory (right) of the X-rays transmitted through the patient. The spiral can either be loose (a high value of the spiral pitch) or tight (a low value of the spiral pitch).*

represented a very significant advance in CT because it allowed scan times for a complete chest and abdominal study to be reduced from ~10 min to ~1 min. In addition, a full three-dimensional vascular imaging dataset could be acquired very shortly after injection of an iodinated contrast agent, resulting in a significant increase in the SNR of the angiograms. Incorporation of this new technology has resulted in three-dimensional CT angiography becoming the method of choice for diagnosing disease in the renal and the pulmonary arteries as well as the aorta.

The instrumentation for spiral CT is very similar to conventional third-generation CT scanners (some companies employ a fourth-generation design). However, because both the detectors and the X-ray source rotate continuously in spiral CT, it is not possible to use fixed cables to connect either the power supply to the X-ray source or the output of the photomultiplier tubes directly to the digitizer and computer. Instead, multiple slip-rings are used for power and signal transmission. Typical spiral CT scanners have dual-focal-spot X-ray tubes with three kV_p settings possible.

The main instrumental challenge in spiral CT scanning is that the X-rays must be produced continously, without the cooling period that exists between acquisition of successive slices in conventional CT. This requirement leads to very high temperatures being formed at the focus of the electron beam at the surface of the anode. Anode heating is particularly problematic in abdominal scanning, which requires higher values of tube currents and exposures than for imaging other regions of the body. Therefore, the X-ray source must be designed to have a high heat capacity and very efficient cooling. If anode heating is too high, then the tube current must be reduced, resulting in a lower number of X-rays and a degraded image SNR.

X-ray detector design is also critical in spiral CT because highly efficient detectors reduce the tube currents needed and help to alleviate issues of anode heating. The detectors used in spiral CT are either solid-state, ceramic scintillation crystals or pressurized xenon-filled ionization chambers, described previously. Scintillation crystals, usually made from bismuth germanate (BGO), have a high efficiency (75–85%) in converting X-rays to light and subsequently to electrical signals via coupled photomultiplier tubes. Gas-filled ionization chambers have a lower efficiency (40–60%), but are much easier and cheaper to construct. The total number of detectors is typically between 1000 (third-generation scanners) and 5000 (fourth-generation systems).

A number of data acquisition parameters are under operator control, the most important of which is the spiral pitch p. The spiral pitch is defined as the ratio of the table feed d per rotation of the X-ray source to the collimated slice thickness S:

$$p = \frac{d}{S} \tag{1.27}$$

The value of p lies between 0 and 2 for single-slice spiral CT systems. For p values less than 1, the X-ray beams of adjacent spirals overlap, resulting in a high tissue radiation dose. For p values greater than 2, gaps appear in the data sampled along the long axis of the patient. For large values of p, image blurring due to the continuous motion of the patient table during data acquisition is greater. A large value of p also increases the effective slice thickness to a value above the width of the collimated

X-ray beam: for example, at a spiral pitch value of 2, the increase is of the order of 25%. The value of p typically used in clinical scans lies between 1 and 2, which results in a reduction in tissue radiation dose compared to a single-slice scan by a factor equal to the value of p.

Due to the spiral trajectory of the X-rays throught the patient, modification of the backprojection reconstruction algorithm is necessary in order to form images that correspond to those acquired using a single-slice CT scanner. Reconstruction algorithms use linear interpolation of data points 180° apart on the spiral trajectory to estimate the data that would have been obtained at a particular position of a stationary patient table. Images with thicknesses greater than the collimation width can be produced by adding together adjacent reconstructed slices. Images are usually processed in a way which results in considerable overlap between adjacent slices. This has been shown to increase the accuracy of lesion detection, for example, because with overlapping slices there is less chance that a significant portion of the lesion lies between slices.

1.13. MULTISLICE SPIRAL COMPUTED TOMOGRAPHY

The efficiency of spiral CT can be increased further by incorporating an array of detectors in the z direction, that is, the direction of table motion. Such an array is shown in Figure 1.33. The increase in efficiency arises from the higher values of the

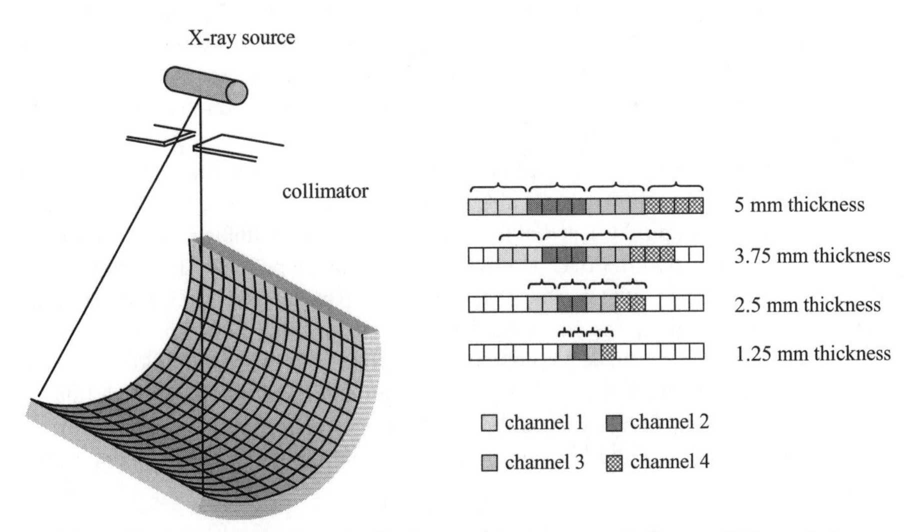

FIGURE 1.33. *(Left) A schematic of a fixed-array detector geometry for a multislice spiral scanner. (Right) Four configurations connecting the data acquisition channels to single or multiple elements of the arrayed detectors produce four different slice thicknesses. For 5-mm slices, the collimated beam shown on the left covers all 16 detectors. The degree of collimation can be increased progressively to cover only the central 12 (four 3.75-mm slices), the central 8 (four 2.5-mm slices), or the central 4 (four 1.25-mm slices) detectors.*

table feed per rotation that can be used. Multislice spiral CT can be used to image larger volumes in a given time, or to image a given volume in a shorter scan time, compared to single-slice spiral CT. The collimated X-ray beam can also be made thinner, giving higher quality three-dimensional scans. The spiral pitch p_{ms} for a multislice CT is defined slightly differently from that for a single-slice CT system:

$$p_{\mathrm{ms}} = \frac{d}{S_{\mathrm{single}}} \tag{1.28}$$

where S_{single} is the single-slice collimated beam width. For a four-slice spiral CT scanner, the upper limit of the effective spiral pitch is increased to a value of eight. In multislice spiral CT scanning the effective slice thickness is dictated by the dimensions of the individual detectors, rather than the collimated X-ray beam width.

In a multislice system the focal-spot-to-isocenter and the focal-spot-to-detector distances are shortened compared to those in a single-slice scanner, and the number of detectors in the longitudinal direction is increased from one long element to a number of shorter elements. There are two basic types of detector arrangements, called fixed and adaptive. The former consists of 16 elements, each of length 1.25 mm, giving a total length of 2 cm. The signals from sets of four individual elements are typically combined. With the setup shown in Figure 1.33, four slices can be acquired with thicknesses of 1.25, 2.5, 3.75, or 5 mm. These types of systems are typically run in either high-quality (HQ) mode with a spiral pitch of 3 or high-speed (HS) mode with a spiral pitch of 6. The second type of detector system is the adaptive array, which consists of eight detectors with lengths 5, 2.5, 1.5, 1, 1, 1.5, 2.5, and 5 mm, also giving a total length of 2 cm. As for the fixed detector system, four slices are usually acquired with 1, 2.5, or 5 mm thickness. Unlike the fixed detector system, in which only specific pitch values are possible, the pitch value in an adaptive array can be chosen to have any value between 1 and 8.

Fan-beam reconstruction techniques, in combination with linear interpolation methods, are used in multislice spiral CT. One important difference between single-slice and multislice spiral CT is that the slice thickness in multislice spiral CT can be chosen retrospectively after data acquisition, using an adaptive axial algorithm. The detector collimation is set to a value of 1, 2.5, or 5 mm before the scan is run. After the data have been acquired, the slices can be reconstructed with a thickness between 1 and 10 mm. Thin slices can be reconstructed to form a high-quality three-dimensional image, but the same dataset can also be used to produce a set of 5-mm-thick images with a high SNR. In Figure 1.34, the projections p_{z_R} acquired at every position z_R are averaged using a sliding filter $w(z)$ to give an interpolated set of projections $p_{z_R}^{\mathrm{int}}$ given by

$$p_{z_R}^{\mathrm{int}} = \frac{\sum_i w\left(z_i - z_R\right) p\left(z_i\right)}{\sum_i w\left(z_i - z_R\right)} \tag{1.29}$$

The width of the filter, which is usually trapezoidal in shape, determines the thickness of the reconstructed slice.

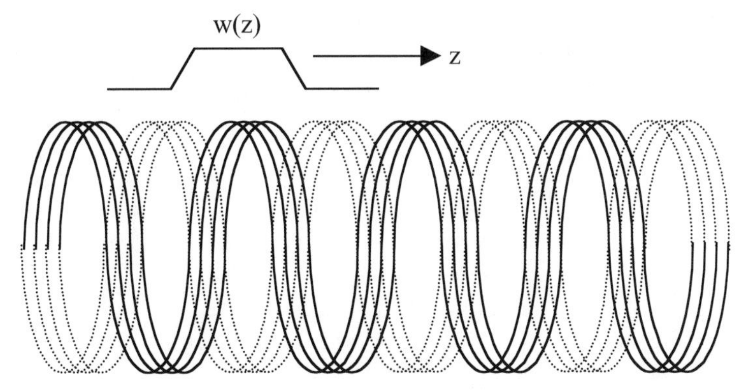

FIGURE 1.34. *The basic principle of data reconstruction using z-interpolation in multislice spiral CT. The solid lines show the acquired data, and the dotted lines represent the rebinned data from opposite rays. The projections are averaged at each z position by weighting the projections by the filter w(z).*

1.14. RADIATION DOSE

Ionizing radiation can cause damage to tissue in a number of ways. The largest risk is that of cancer arising from genetic mutations caused by chromosomal aberrations. The effects of radiation are both deterministic and stochastic. Deterministic effects are produced by high doses and are associated with cell death. These effects are characterized by a dose threshold below which cell death does not occur. In contrast, stochastic effects occur at lower radiation doses, but the actual radiation dose affects only the probability of damage occurring, that is, there is no absolute dose threshold.

The absorbed dose D is equal to the radiation energy E absorbed per unit mass. The value of D is given in units of grays (Gy), where 1 Gy equals 1 J/kg. Many publications still refer to absorbed dose in units of rads: 1 Gy is equal to 100 rads. The patient dose is often specified in terms of the entrance skin dose, with typical values of 0.1 mGy for a chest radiograph and 1.5 mGy for an abdominal radiograph. Such measurements, however, give little overall indication of the risk to the patient. The most useful measure of radiation dose is the effective dose equivalent H_{E}, which sums the dose delivered to each organ weighted by the radiation sensitivity w of that organ with respect to cancer and genetic risks:

$$H_{\mathrm{E}} = \sum_i w_i H_i \tag{1.30}$$

where i is the number of organs considered and H_i is the dose equivalent for each of the i organs. The value of H is given by the absorbed dose D multiplied by the quality factor (QF) of the radiation. The QF has a value of 1 for X-rays (and also for γ-rays), 10 for neutrons, and 20 for α-particles. The unit of H and H_{E} is the sievert (Sv). Older radiation literature quotes the units of dose equivalent and effective dose equivalent

TABLE 1.3. Effective Dose Equivalent H_E for Clinical X-Ray CT Exams

Clinical exam	H_E (mSv)
Breast	0.05
Chest X-ray	0.03
Skull X-ray	0.15
Abdominal X-ray	1.0
Barium fluoroscopy	5
Head CT	3
Body CT	10

in units of rems: 1 Sv equals 100 rems. Typical values of w for the calculation of H_E are: gonads, 0.2; lung, 0.12; breast, 0.1; stomach, 0.12; skin, 0.01; and thyroid, 0.05.

In CT, the radiation dose to the patient is calculated in a slightly different way because the X-ray beam profile across each slice is not uniform and adjacent slices receive some dose from one another. For example, in the United States, the Food and Drug Administration (FDA) defines the computed tomography dose index (CTDI) for a 14-slice exam to be

$$\text{CTDI} = \frac{1}{T} \int_{-7T}^{+7T} D_z \, dz \tag{1.31}$$

where D_z is the absorbed dose at position z and T is the thickness of the slice. In terms of assessing patient risk, again the value of H_E is a better measure. Table 1.3 lists typical values of H_E for standard clinical exams. The limit in annual radiation dose under federal law in the United States is 0.05 Sv (5000 mrem). This limit corresponds to over 1000 planar chest X-rays, 15 head CTs, or 5 full-body CTs.

1.15. CLINICAL APPLICATIONS OF COMPUTED TOMOGRAPHY

CT is used for a wide range of clinical conditions. The following list and series of images is by no means exhaustive. There are a large number of books devoted solely to the clinical applications of CT.

1.15.1. Cerebral Scans

One of the most important applications of CT is in head trauma, where it is used to investigate possible skull fractures, underlying brain damage, or hemorrhage. Hemorrhage shows up on CT scans as areas of increased signal intensity due to higher attenuation from the high levels of protein in hemoglobin. Edema, often associated with stroke, shows up as an area of reduced signal intensity on the image. For brain tumors, CT is excellent at showing calcification in lesions such as meningiomas or gliomas, and can be used to investigate changes in bone structure and volume in diseases of the sinus. Figure 1.35 shows an example of the sensitivity of CT, in this case able to detect a subacute infarct.

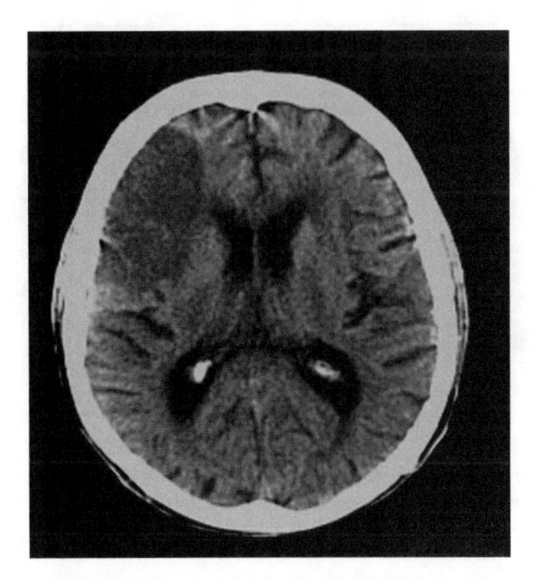

FIGURE 1.35. *CT image of a subacute infarct, which appears as a large area of low signal intensity on the left of the brain.*

In well-vascularized tumors such as meningiomas, iodinated contrast agents are often injected, and increase the signal intensity of the tumor. In healthy brain tissue, the blood brain barrier (BBB) selectively filters the blood supply to the brain, allowing only a limited number of naturally occurring substrates to enter brain tissue. If the brain is damaged, by a tumor, for example, the BBB is disrupted such that the injected contrast agent can now enter the brain tissue. As tumors grow, they develop their own blood supply, and blood flow is often higher in tumors, particularly in the periphery of the tumor, than in normal tissue. Abscesses, for example, often show a distinctive pattern in which the center of the pathology appears with a lower signal than surrounding tissue, but is encircled by an area of higher signal, a so-called "rim enhancement."

1.15.2. Pulmonary Disease

CT is particularly useful in the detection of pulmonary disease because lung imaging is extremely difficult using ultrasound and magnetic resonance imaging. CT can detect pulmonary malignancies as well as emboli, and is often used to diagnose diffuse diseases of the lung such as silicosis, fibrosis, and emphysema. Cystic fibrosis can also be diagnosed, as shown in Figure 1.36.

1.15.3. Abdominal Imaging

Compound fractures in organs such as the pelvis, which occur commonly in elderly patients, can be visualized in three dimensions using CT. CT is also very useful in the detection of abdominal tumors and ulcerations in the liver. Most of these latter studies use an iodinated contrast agent. Pathologies such as hepatic hemangiomas

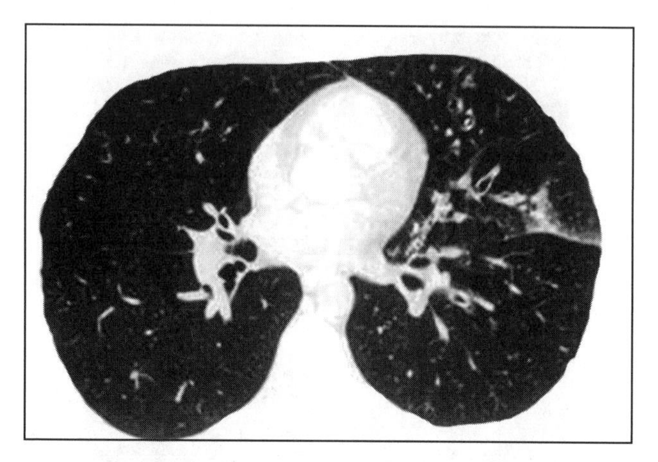

FIGURE 1.36. CT image of a patient with cystic fibrosis. The disease can be diagnosed by the thickening of the airways and the presence of small, opaque areas filled with mucus.

can be detected by acquiring a series of images after injection of the agent: the outside of the hemangioma increases in signal intensity very soon after injection, but within 30 min there is uniform enhancement of the whole tumor. Figure 1.37 shows an example of a hepatic meningioma detected in an abdominal CT scan.

EXERCISES

1.1. Figure 1.38 shows the intensity of X-rays produced from a source as a function of their energy. With respect to the reference graph shown on the left, one plot

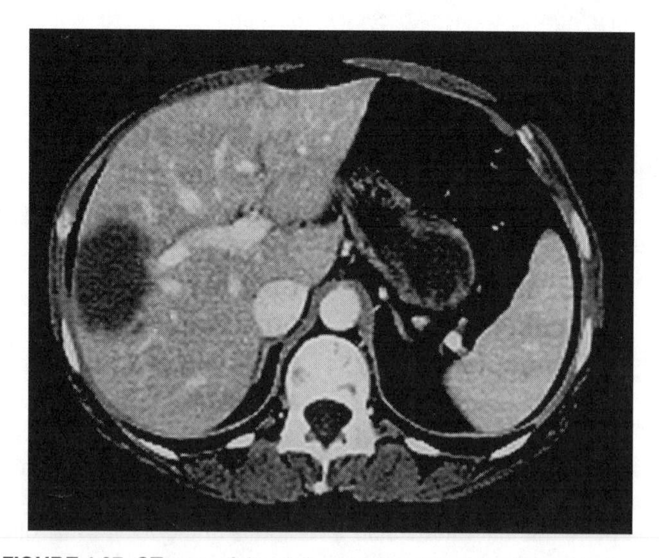

FIGURE 1.37. CT scan of the abdomen showing a hepatic meningioma.

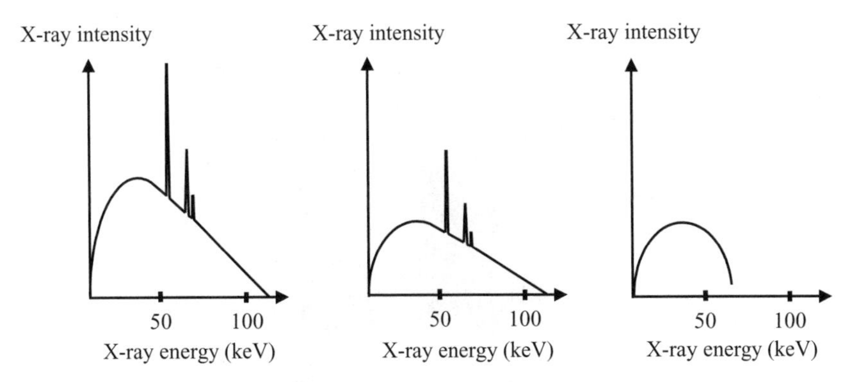

FIGURE 1.38. *Illustration for Exercise 1.1.*

corresponds to a decrease in tube current and the other to a decrease in the accelerating voltage (kV_p). Explain which plot corresponds to a decrease in which parameter.

1.2. The spectrum of X-ray energies changes as the X-rays pass through tissue due to the energy dependence of the linear attenuation coefficient: this is a phenomenon known as beam hardening. A typical energy distribution of the beam from the X-ray source is shown in Figure 1.39. Sketch the energy spectrum after the beam has passed through the body.

1.3. In Figure 1.40, calculate the X-ray intensity, as a function of the incident intensity I_0, that reaches the film for each of the three X-ray beams. The dark-shaded area represents bone and the light-shaded area represents tissue. The linear attenuation coefficients at the effective X-ray energy of 68 keV are 10 and 1 cm^{-1} for bone and tissue, respectively.

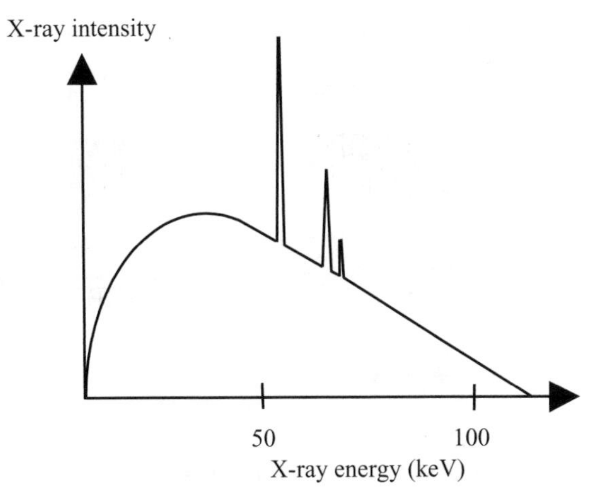

FIGURE 1.39. *Illustration for Exercise 1.2.*

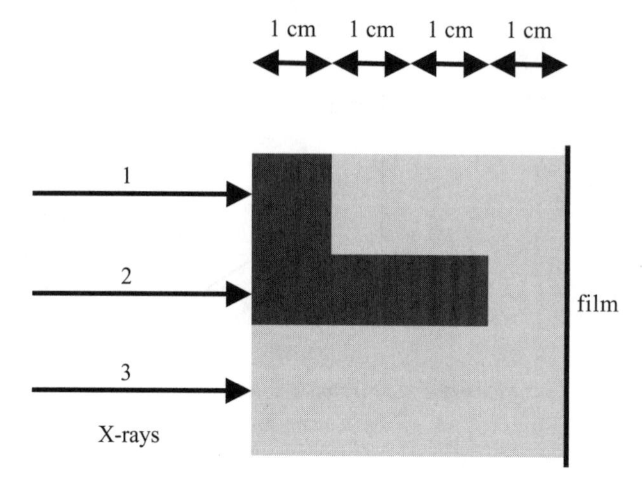

FIGURE 1.40. *Illustration for Exercise 1.3.*

1.4. Explain why $\mu_{\text{bone}} \gg \mu_{\text{tissue}}$ at low X-ray energies, but the two values of μ become closer as the X-ray energy increases.

1.5. The linear attenuation coefficient of a gadolinium-based phosphor used for detection of X-rays is 560 cm^{-1} at an X-ray energy of 150 keV. What percentage of X-rays are detected by phosphor layers of 100, 250 and 500 μm thickness? What are the tradeoffs in terms of spatial resolution?

1.6. In Figure 1.41, calculate the relative intensities of the signals S_1, S_2, and S_3 produced by each crystal. The value of μ_{tissue} is 0.5 cm^{-1}, μ_{bone} is 1 cm^{-1}, and μ_{crystal} is 2 cm^{-1}.

1.7. Intensifying screens (Section 1.5.3) can be placed on both sides of the X-ray film (double-sided) or on one side only (single-sided). Explain why

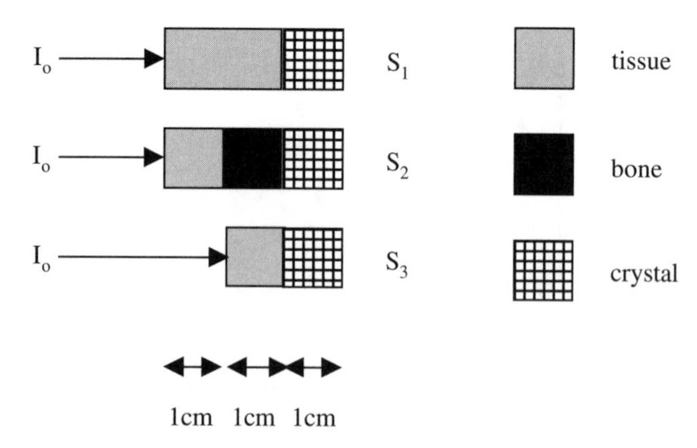

FIGURE 1.41. *Illustration for Exercise 1.6.*

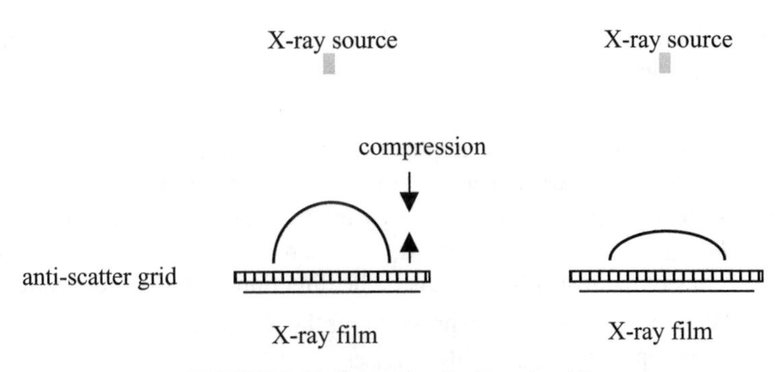

FIGURE 1.42. Illustration for Exercise 1.9.

double-sided screens give a higher image SNR, but single-sided screens have a better spatial resolution.

1.8. An X-ray with energy 60 keV strikes a gadolinium-based intensifying screen, producing photons at a wavelength of 415 nm. The energy conversion coefficient for this process is 20%. How many photons are produced for each incident X-ray? (Planck's constant = 6.63×10^{-34} J s, 1 eV = 1.602×10^{-19} J.)

1.9. In mammographic examinations, the breast is compressed between two plates, as shown in Figure 1.42. Answer the following with a brief explanation:

(a) Is the geometric unsharpness increased or decreased by compression?

(b) Why is the image contrast improved by this procedure?

(c) Is the required X-ray dose for a given image SNR higher or lower with compression?

1.10. For the two X-ray film characteristic curves shown in Figure 1.43:

(a) Which one corresponds to the film with the higher speed?

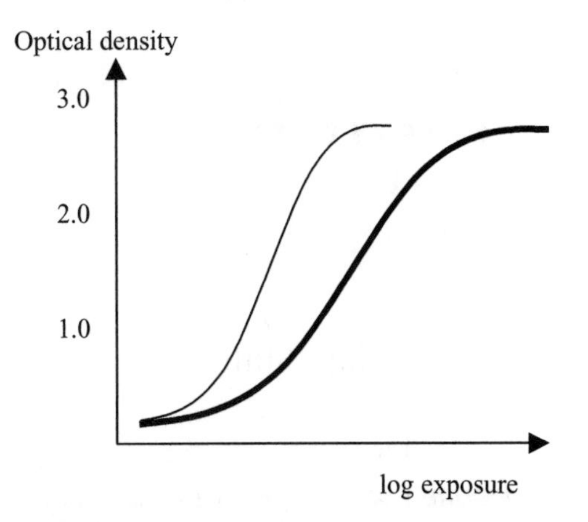

FIGURE 1.43. Illustration for Exercise 1.10.

(b) Which one corresponds to the film with the broader modulation transfer function?

1.11. In digital subtraction angiography, two images are acquired, the first before injection of the contrast agent and the other postinjection.

(a) Write an expression for the X-ray intensity I_1 in the first scan in terms of I_0, μ_{tissue}, x_{tissue}, μ_{blood}, and x_{vessel}, where x_{tissue} and x_{vessel} are the dimensions of the respective organs in the direction of X-ray propagation.

(b) Write a corresponding expression for the X-ray intensity I_2 for the second scan, replacing μ_{blood} with $\mu_{\text{constrast}}$.

(c) Is the image signal intensity from static tissue removed by subtracting the two images?

(d) Show that the signal from static tissue is removed by computing the quantity $\log(I_2) - \log(I_1)$.

1.12. In digital subtraction angiography, what is the effect of doubling the X-ray intensity on the SNR of the image? What would be the effect of doubling the dose of contrast agent on the SNR of the image?

1.13. For the case of X-rays passing through tissue with a constant linear attenuation coefficient ($\mu_{\text{tissue}} > \mu_{\text{water}}$), does the CT number increase or decrease as a function of distance through the tissue due to beam hardening?

1.14. Draw the CT projection obtained from the setup shown in Figure 1.44. Assume that the spherical sample has a uniform attenuation coefficient throughout its volume.

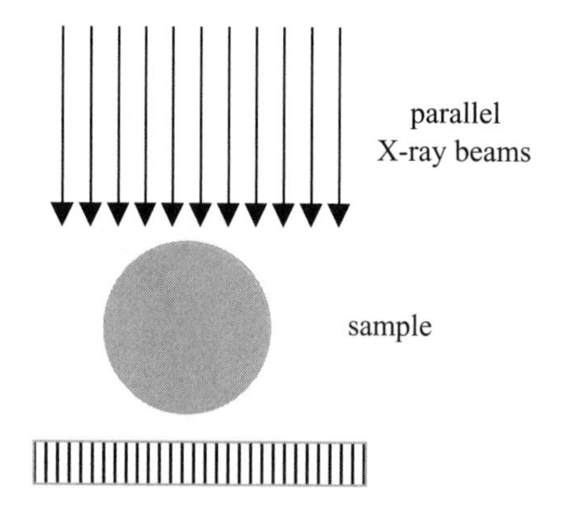

FIGURE 1.44. *Illustration for Exercise 1.14.*

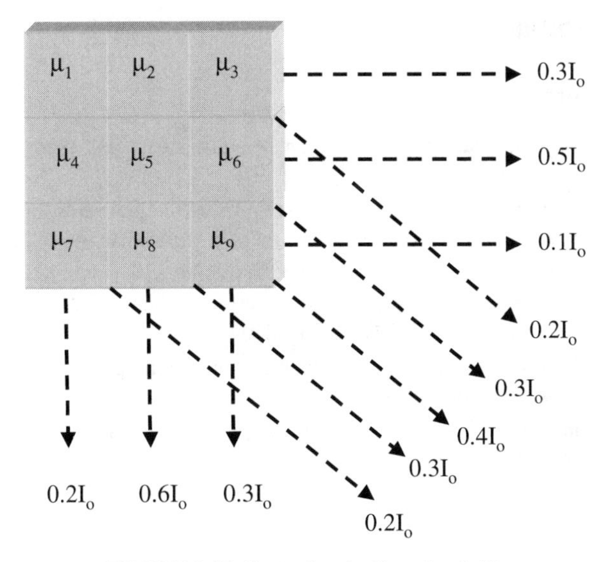

FIGURE 1.45. *Illustration for Exercise 1.16.*

1.15. Considering the effects of beam hardening, draw the actual CT projection that would be obtained from the sample in Exercise 1.14. Sketch the final image that would be formed from filtered backprojection of all of the projections acquired in a full scan of the sample in Exercise 1.14.

1.16. For the set of projections shown in Figure 1.45, perform one series of a ray-by-ray iteration on the horizontal, the diagonal, and the vertical projections. Calculate the minimum squared error after each iteration.

1.17. For the object shown in Figure B1 (Appendix B), draw the projections that would be acquired at angles $\phi = 0, 45, 90, 135$, and $180°$.

1.18. For the object shown in Figure 1.46, sketch the sinogram for values of ϕ from 0 to 360°.

FIGURE 1.46. *Illustration for Exercise 1.18.*

FURTHER READING

Original Papers

W. R¨ontgen, Uber eine neue Art von Strahlen,*Sitz. Ber. Phys. Med. Würzburg* **9,** 132–141 (1895).

J. Radon, Uber die Bestimmung von Funktionen durch ihre Integralwerte l¨angs gewisser Mannigfaltigkeiten, *Ber. Verh. Sächs. Akad. Wiss. Leipzig Math. Phys. Kl.* **69,** 262–277 (1917).

G. N. Ramachandran and V. Lakshminarayanan, Three-dimensional reconstruction from radiographs and electron micrographs: Applications of convolutions instead of Fourier transforms, *Proc. Natl. Acad. Sci. USA* **68,** 2236–2240 (1971).

G. N. Hounsfield, Computerised transverse axial scanning (tomography). Part 1: Description of system, *Br. J. Radiol.* **46,** 1016–1022 (1973).

J. Ambrose, Computerised transverse axial scanning (tomography). Part 2: Clinical application, *Br. J. Radiol.* **46,** 1023–1047 (1973).

L. A. Feldkamp, L. C. Davis, and J. W. Kress, Practical cone-beam algorithm, *J. Opt. Soc. Am. A* **1,** 612–619 (1984).

Books

Computed Tomography

W. A. Kalender, *Computed Tomography: Fundamentals, System Technology, Image Quality, Applications,* MCD, Munich, Germany (2001).

E. Seeram, *Computed Tomography: Physical Principles, Clinical Applications, and Quality Control,* Saunders, Philadelphia (2001).

Spiral and Multislice Computed Tomography

E. K. Fishman and R. B. Jeffrey, eds., *Spiral CT: Principles, Techniques and Applications,* Lippincott-Raven, Philadelphia (1998).

B. Marincek, P. R. Rose, M. Reiser, and M. E. Baker, eds., *Multislice CT: A Practical Guide,* Springer, New York (2001).

Review Articles

C. H. McCollough, Performance evaluation of a multi-slice CT system, *Med. Phys.* **26,** 2223–2230 (1999).

T. Fuchs, M. Kachelriess, and W. A. Kalender, Technical advances in multi-slice spiral CT, *Eur. J. Radiol.* **36,** 69–73 (2000).

J. Rydberg, K. A. Buckwalter, K. S. Caldemeyer, M. D. Phillips, D. J. Conces, Jr., A. M. Aisen, S. A. Persohn, and K. K. Kopecky, Multisection CT: Scanning techniques and clinical applications, *Radiographics* **20,** 1787–1806 (2000).

W. A. Kalender and M. Prokop, 3D CT angiography, *Crit. Rev. Diagn. Imaging* **42,** 1–28 (2001).

Specialized Journals

Journal of Computer Assisted Tomography

2

Nuclear Medicine

2.1. GENERAL PRINCIPLES OF NUCLEAR MEDICINE

In contrast to X-ray, ultrasound, and magnetic resonance, nuclear medicine imaging techniques do not produce an anatomical map of the body, but instead image the spatial distribution of radiopharmaceuticals introduced into the body. The complementary role of nuclear medicine diagnoses arises from the fact that most pathological conditions are initiated by a change in the basic chemistry and biochemistry of tissue. In time, these chemical changes lead to deficiencies in organ function and changes in the physical properties of the tissue. Examples include cell swelling and the formation of edema, tumor enlargement and metastasis, and changes in tissue morphology. Imaging techniques that are sensitive to these early biochemical changes form an important part of clinical diagnosis. Nuclear medicine detects these early indicators of disease by imaging the uptake and biodistribution of radioactive compounds introduced into the body in very small amounts (typically nanograms) via inhalation into the lungs, direct injection into the bloodstream, subcutaneous administration or oral administration. These "radiopharmaceuticals," also termed radiotracers, are compounds consisting of a chemical substrate linked to a radioactive element. The chemical structure of the particular radiopharmaceutical determines the biodistribution of the complex within the body, and a large number of radiopharmaceuticals are used clinically in order to target specific organs. Abnormal tissue distribution or an increase or decrease in the rate at which the radiopharmaceutical accumulates in a particular tissue is a strong indicator of disease. Radiation, usually in the form of γ-rays, from the radioactive decay of the radiopharmaceutical is detected using an imaging device called a gamma camera.

Figure 2.1 shows the basic principles and instrumentation involved in image formation. The radiopharmaceutical is shown in Figure 2.1 to be localized in a specific

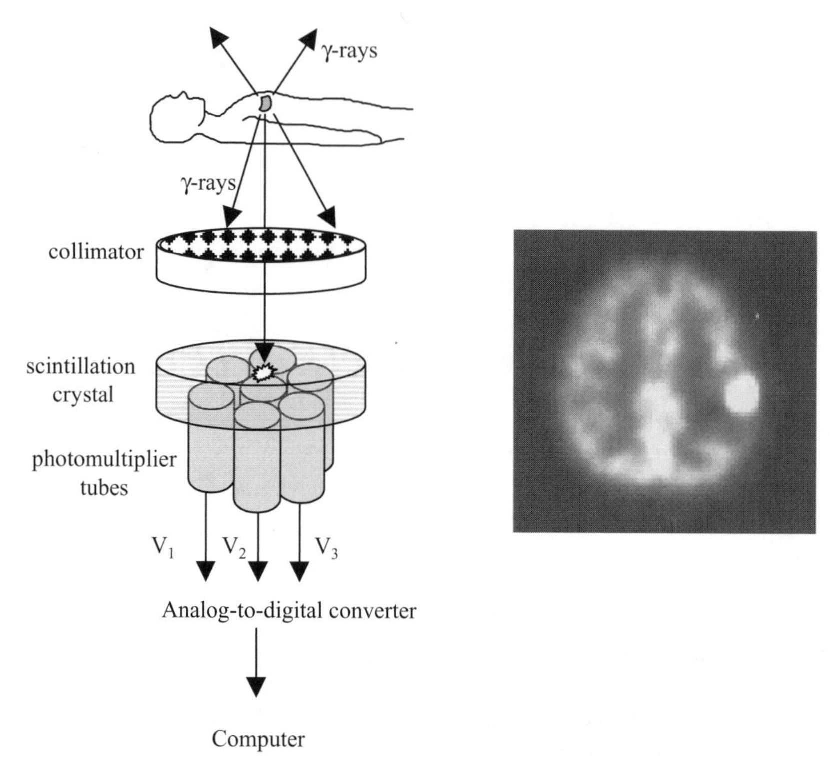

FIGURE 2.1. *(Left) A general schematic of the instrumentation required for the formation of nuclear medicine images using a gamma camera. (Right) A brain tumor shows up as an area of high signal intensity in one slice from a SPECT multislice dataset.*

organ in the body. Decay of the radioactive element produces γ-rays, which emanate in all directions. Attenuation of γ-rays in tissue occurs via exactly the same mechanisms as for X-rays, namely coherent scattering, Compton scattering, and photoelectric interactions. In order to determine the position of the source of the γ-rays, a collimator is placed between the patient and the detector so that only those components of radiation that have a trajectory at an angle close to 90° to the detector plane are recorded. Rather than using film, as in planar X-ray imaging, to record the image, a scintillation crystal is used to convert the energy of the γ-rays that pass through the collimator into light. These light photons are in turn converted into an electrical signal by photomultiplier tubes (PMTs). The image is formed by analyzing the spatial distribution and the magnitude of the electrical signals from each PMT. Planar nuclear medicine images are characterized, in general, as having a poor SNR and low spatial resolution (~5 mm), but extremely high sensitivity, being able to detect very small amounts of radioactive material, and very high specificity because there is no background radiation in the body.

Three-dimensional nuclear medicine images can be produced using the principle of tomography. A rotating gamma camera is used in a technique called single photon emission computed tomography (SPECT). As in X-ray CT, the increase in image dimensionality increases the diagnostic power of the technique significantly. This is particularly true in cases where the radiopharmaceutical is distributed in more than one overlying organ. The image on the right of Figure 2.1 shows a scan of a brain tumor using SPECT, with the tumor showing an increased uptake of the particular radiopharmaceutical compared to the surrounding healthy tissue. The most recently developed technique in nuclear medicine is positron emission tomography (PET), which is based on positron-emitting radiopharmaceuticals. Due to the nature of the processes involved in positron annihilation and subsequent emission of two γ-rays, covered in detail in Section 2.11, PET has a sensitivity advantage over SPECT of between two and three orders of magnitude.

2.2. RADIOACTIVITY

Radioactivity is an intrinsic property of particular isotopes that have unstable nuclei. Isotopes of a particular element have the same number of protons, but vary in the number of neutrons in the nucleus. The phenomenon of radioactivity refers to the process whereby various forms of radiation are emitted as a result of a spontaneous change in the composition of the nucleus. Whether or not an isotope is radioactive depends upon the stability of its nucleus, which in turn is dictated by the relationship between the atomic number (Z, the number of protons) and atomic mass (A, the sum of the number of protons and neutrons). Strong neutron–neutron, neutron–proton, and proton–proton forces are attractive over very short distances, whereas electromagnetic forces between protons are repulsive in nature, and so the stability of a particular nucleus is determined by the balance of these attractive and repulsive forces. For values of A less than 50 a stable configuration corresponds to a nucleus with equal numbers of neutrons and protons. For heavier nuclei, $A > 50$, the ratio of the number of neutrons to protons required for stability increases, as shown in Figure 2.2.

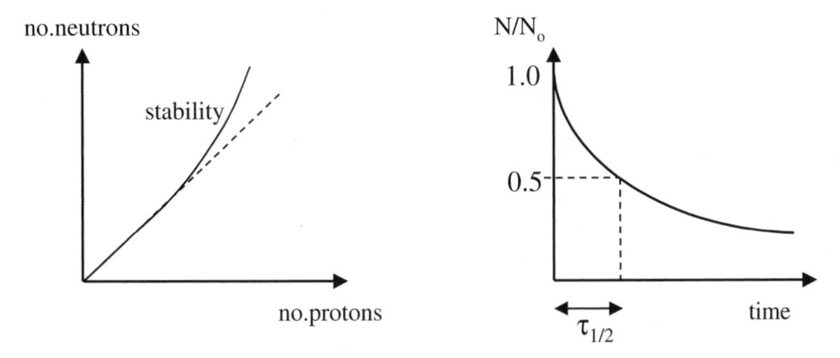

FIGURE 2.2. (Left) The solid line represents the number of protons and neutrons required for nuclear stability. The dashed line represents equal numbers of protons and neutrons. (Right) A graph showing the exponential radioactive decay of a radionuclide as a function of time. N is the number of nuclei at any given time, N_0 is the number at time $t = 0$, and $\tau_{1/2}$ is the half-life of the radionuclide.

The radioactivity, or activity, Q of a radionuclide is defined as the number of nuclear disintegrations per unit time. For N nuclei of a particular element

$$Q = -\frac{dN}{dt} = \lambda N \tag{2.1}$$

where λ is the decay constant. Radioactivity is measured in units of curies (Ci), or more conveniently, in millicuries, where 1 Ci equals 3.7×10^{10} disintegrations/second. Some older texts report measurements in becquerels (Bq), where 1 Bq is one disintegration/second. Equation (2.1) can be solved to give

$$N = N_0 \exp(-\lambda t) \tag{2.2}$$

where N_0 is the number of nuclei at time $t = 0$. The half-life $\tau_{1/2}$ of a particular element corresponds to the time required for the radioactivity to drop to one-half of its current value, as shown in Figure 2.2. The value of $\tau_{1/2}$ is independent of the value of N:

$$\tau_{1/2} = \frac{\ln 2}{\lambda} \tag{2.3}$$

When calculating the time dependence of radioactivity within the body for a nuclear medicine scan, the biological half-life of the radionuclide must also be considered. In many cases, excretion of the radionuclide from biological tissue is also an exponential process, which can be characterized by a decay constant λ_{bio} and corresponding half-life τ_{bio}. The effective half-life τ_{eff} of radioactivity within the body is given by

$$\frac{1}{\tau_{\text{eff}}} = \frac{1}{\tau_{1/2}} + \frac{1}{\tau_{\text{bio}}} \tag{2.4}$$

The value of τ_{eff} is always less than the shorter of the two half-lives $\tau_{1/2}$ and τ_{bio}.

2.3. THE PRODUCTION OF RADIONUCLIDES

There are four basic methods for producing radionuclides: neutron capture, nuclear fission, charged-particle bombardment, and the use of radionuclide generators. The first two methods use a small nuclear reactor specifically designed for radionuclide production. Many elements that were formerly produced using neutron capture are now created using nuclear fission, which uses fast neutrons with energies up to 100 MeV. In terms of clinical nuclear medicine, the most important nuclear fission reaction is the creation of ^{99}Mo, the chemical precursor used in the technetium generator described in Section 2.5:

$${}^{1}_{0}\text{n} + {}^{235}_{92}\text{Ur} \rightarrow {}^{236}_{92}\text{Ur} \rightarrow {}^{99}_{42}\text{Mo} + {}^{133}_{50}\text{Sn} + 4\,{}^{1}_{0}\text{n}$$

The ^{133}Sn subsequently decays to form ^{133}Xe, which is used in nuclear medicine studies of the lung. Another commonly used radionuclide, ^{131}I, is also formed by nuclear fission of ^{235}Ur.

The third method, charged-particle bombardment, uses a cyclotron. Cyclotrons work by ionizing hydrogen or deuterium gas using a radiofrequency field in the center of the cyclotron. These negatively charged ions are then accelerated in a spiral trajectory toward the outside of the circularly shaped cyclotron. Two superconducting magnets situated at the top and bottom of the cyclotron are used to contain the ion beam. At the outer edge of their trajectory, the ions exit the cyclotron and are magnetically steered through a thin copper "stripping foil." This foil removes electrons from the ions, leaving protons or deuterium nuclei to collide with the target, which is stationed within a thick boronated-polyethylene block. This block absorbs the scattered neutrons produced during bombardment. The proton or deuteron nuclei collide with a particular target to produce the desired radioactive isotopes. Commonly used radionuclides produced using a cyclotron include ^{201}Tl, ^{67}Ga, ^{111}In, and ^{123}I. A small on-site cyclotron is also used for production of radionuclides for positron emission tomography, covered in Section 2.11.

Finally, the most convenient method of radionuclide production is via an on-site generator. This unit can be delivered and removed from a medical facility, usually on a weekly basis. The radionuclide is produced continuously from the generator and is usually "milked" daily. A detailed description of the most commonly used system, the technetium generator, is given in Section 2.5.

2.4. TYPES OF RADIOACTIVE DECAY

Radioactive elements can decay via a number of mechanisms, of which the most common and important in nuclear medicine are α-particle decay, β-particle emission, γ-ray emission, and electron capture, described in detail below. Additional mechanisms involving positron emission are outlined later in this chapter. The most useful radionuclides for diagnostic imaging are those that emit γ-rays or X-rays because these forms of radiation can pass through tissue and reach a detector situated outside the body. A useful parameter in quantifying the attenuation of radiation as it travels through tissue is the half-value layer (HVL), which corresponds to the thickness of tissue that absorbs one-half of the radioactivity produced. A value of HVL less than several centimeters means that not only does very little radiation escape from the body, but patient radiation dose is also very high.

An α-particle consists of a helium nucleus—two protons and two neutrons—with a net positive charge. Typical particle energies are between 4 and 8 MeV. The α-particle has a tissue HVL of only a few millimeters, and is therefore not directly detected in nuclear medicine. This form of radioactive decay occurs mainly for radionuclides with an atomic number greater than 150.

A β-particle is an electron, and is emitted with a continuous range of energies. Radioactive decay occurs via the conversion of a neutron into a proton, with emission of a high-energy β-particle and an antineutrino. Kinetic energy is shared in a random manner between the β-particle and antineutrino, and hence the electron has a continuous range of energies. A 1-MeV β-particle has an HVL of 0.4 mm in tissue, a value rising to 4 mm for a 5-MeV β-particle.

Although radionuclides that produce predominantly α- or β-particles cannot be used for diagnosis using nuclear medicine scans, they can be used as radiotherapeutic agents if they can be targeted to, for example, tumors. Within the tumor the radioactivity destroys the diseased tissue and stops the cancer from proliferating. In addition, due to the low HVL values, very little radiation will reach the healthy tissue which lies outside the tumor.

No radionuclide can decay solely by γ-ray emission, but certain decay schemes result in the formation of an intermediate species that exists in a metastable state, with a reasonably long half-life. The radionuclide ^{99m}Tc, which is the most widely used radionuclide, used in over 90% of studies, exists in such a metastable state. It is formed from ^{99}Mo according to the scheme shown below. Roughly 90% of the metastable ^{99m}Tc nuclei follow this decay path:

$$^{99}_{42}\mathrm{Mo} \xrightarrow{\tau_{1/2}\ 66\ \mathrm{h}} \beta + {}^{99m}_{43}\mathrm{Tc} \xrightarrow{\tau_{1/2}\ 6\ \mathrm{h}} {}^{99g}_{43}\mathrm{Tc} + \gamma$$

The energy of the emitted γ-ray is 140 keV. Below an energy of 100 keV most γ-rays are absorbed in the body via photoelectric interactions, in direct analogy to X-ray attenuation in tissue, and so radionuclides used in nuclear medicine should emit γ-rays with energies greater than this value. Above an energy of 200 keV, γ-rays penetrate the thin collimator septa used in gamma cameras to reject unwanted, scattered γ-rays. Therefore, the ideal energy of a γ-ray for imaging lies somewhere between 100 and 200 keV.

The final mechanism of radioactive decay is electron capture (with subsequent γ-ray or X-ray emission), in which an orbital electron from the K or L shell is captured by the nucleus, producing a corresponding gap in the orbital shell. Electrons from outer shells fill the gap in a cascade process, which produces characteristic X-rays. The capture of the orbital electron also results in internal bremsstrahlung radiation being produced. Several clinically useful radionuclides decay via this mechanism: examples include iodine, thallium, and indium:

$$^{123}_{53}\mathrm{I} + {}^{0}_{-1}e \xrightarrow{13\ \mathrm{h}} {}^{123}_{52}\mathrm{Te} + \gamma \quad (159\ \mathrm{keV})$$

$$^{201}_{81}\mathrm{Tl} + {}^{0}_{-1}e \xrightarrow{73\ \mathrm{h}} {}^{201}_{80}\mathrm{Hg} + \gamma \quad (167\ \mathrm{keV}) + \text{X-rays} \quad (68\text{–}82\ \mathrm{keV})$$

$$^{111}_{49}\mathrm{In} + {}^{0}_{-1}e \xrightarrow{67\ \mathrm{h}} {}^{111}_{48}\mathrm{Cd} + \gamma \quad (171\ \mathrm{keV})$$

For clinical imaging, an ideal radionuclide should have a half-life that is short enough to limit the radiation dose to the patient, yet long enough such that the radioactivity is not exhausted by the time the nuclide has distributed within the body. Radioactive decay should be via monochromatic γ-ray emission to a stable nuclear state, and there should be no emission of α- or β-particles, which would result in large patient

TABLE 2.1. Properties of Common Radionuclides Used in Nuclear Medicine

Radionuclide	Half-life	γ-ray Energy (keV)
^{99m}Tc	6.02 h	140
^{67}Ga	3.2 d	93, 185, 300, 394
^{201}Tl	3.0 d	68–82 (X-rays)
^{133}Xe	5.3 d	81
^{111}In	2.8 d	171, 245
^{131}I	8 d	364
^{123}I	13 h	159

radiation doses. Table 2.1 lists the properties of the most commonly used radionuclides in nuclear medicine.

2.5. THE TECHNETIUM GENERATOR

A number of radionuclides fulfill many of the criteria outlined in the previous section for an ideal radiopharmaceutical for nuclear medicine. Most of these radionuclides, however, have to be produced from an off-site cyclotron or nuclear reactor. One exception is ^{99m}Tc, which can be produced from an on-site generator. The radionuclide ^{99m}Tc has a half-life of 6.02 h, is generated from a long-lived parent, ^{99}Mo, emits a monochromatic 140-keV γ-ray with very minor β-particle emission, and has an HVL of 4.6 cm. In combination with the advantages afforded by on-site production, these properties result in ^{99m}Tc being used in more than 90% of nuclear medicine studies.

The on-site technetium generator consists of an alumina ceramic column with radioactive ^{99}Mo absorbed on its surface in the form of ammonium molybdenate. The column is housed within a lead shield for safety considerations. The ^{99m}Tc is obtained by flowing an eluting solution of saline through the generator. The solution washes out the ^{99m}Tc, which binds very weakly to the alumina, leaving the ^{99}Mo behind. Suitable radioassays are then carried out to determine the concentration and the purity of the eluted ^{99m}Tc. Typically, the technetium is eluted every 24 h and the generator is replaced once a week. A simple mathematical model, presented below, describes the dynamic operation of the technetium generator.

The number of ^{99}Mo atoms, denoted by N_1, decreases with time from an initial maximum value N_0 at time $t = 0$. This radioactive decay produces N_2 atoms of ^{99m}Tc, which decay to form N_3 atoms of ^{99}Tc, the final stable product:

$$\begin{array}{ccccc} ^{99}\text{Mo} & \xrightarrow{\lambda_1} & ^{99m}\text{Tc} & \xrightarrow{\lambda_2} & ^{99}\text{Tc} \\ (N_1) & & (N_2) & & (N_3) \end{array}$$

The values of λ_1 and λ_2 are 2.92×10^{-6} and 3.21×10^{-5} s^{-1}, respectively. In the following analysis, for simplicity, the time dependence of N_1, N_2, and N_3 is assumed, rather than explicitly stated as $N_1(t)$, etc. The decay process can be represented by three simple differential equations:

$$\frac{dN_1}{dt} = -\lambda_1 N_1, \qquad \frac{dN_2}{dt} = \lambda_1 N_1 - \lambda_2 N_2, \qquad \frac{dN_3}{dt} = +\lambda_2 N_2 \tag{2.5}$$

From the first equation, the value of N_1 can be calculated as

$$N_1 = N_0 e^{-\lambda_1 t} \tag{2.6}$$

The equation for dN_2/dt can be rearranged to give

$$\frac{dN_2}{dt} + \lambda_2 N_2 = \lambda_1 N_1 \tag{2.7}$$

First, the homogeneous equation is solved by setting the right-hand side of equation (2.7) equal to zero, which results in

$$\text{(homogeneous)} \qquad N_2 = Ce^{-\lambda_2 t} \tag{2.8}$$

For the particular solution, N_2 can be expressed as

$$\text{(particular)} \qquad N_2 = De^{-\lambda_1 t} \tag{2.9}$$

Solving for D gives

$$D = \frac{\lambda_1 N_0}{\lambda_2 - \lambda_1} \tag{2.10}$$

Combining the homogeneous and particular components gives

$$N_2 = Ce^{-\lambda_2 t} + \frac{\lambda_1 N_0}{\lambda_2 - \lambda_1} e^{-\lambda_1 t} \tag{2.11}$$

Applying the boundary condition that $N_2 = 0$ at $t = 0$, we obtain

$$C = -\frac{\lambda_1 N_0}{\lambda_2 - \lambda_1} \tag{2.12}$$

The final solution for N_2 is therefore

$$N_2 = \frac{\lambda_1 N_0}{\lambda_2 - \lambda_1}(e^{-\lambda_1 t} - e^{-\lambda_2 t}) \tag{2.13}$$

The radioactivity of ^{99m}Tc, Q_2, is thus given by

$$Q_2 = \frac{\lambda_1 \lambda_2 N_0}{\lambda_2 - \lambda_1}(e^{-\lambda_1 t} - e^{-\lambda_2 t}) \tag{2.14}$$

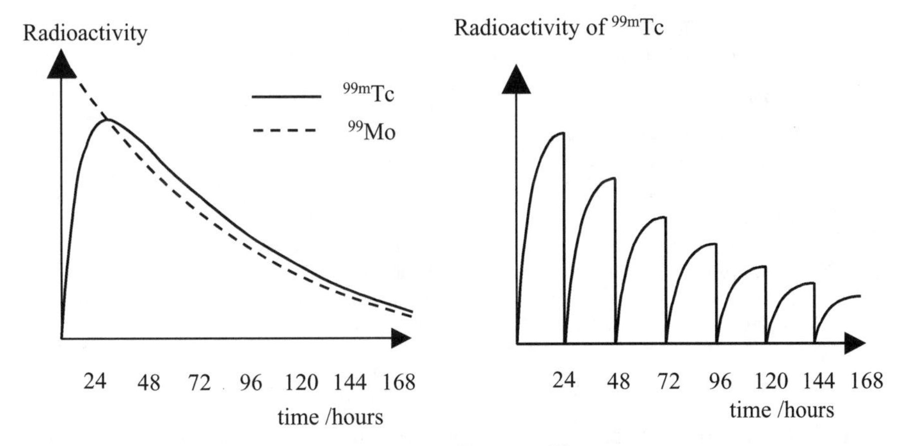

FIGURE 2.3. (Left) A plot of the radioactivity of ^{99}Mo and ^{99m}Tc as a function of time. (Right) A graph of the radioactivity of ^{99m}Tc in the technetium generator in the case where the ^{99m}Tc is removed every 24 h.

The time dependence of both Q_1 and Q_2 is plotted in the left part of Figure 2.3. The fact that the half-life (66 h) of the "parent" element, ^{99}Mo, is an order of magnitude longer than that (6 h) of the "daughter" isotope, ^{99m}Tc, results in an equilibrium state being established in which the ratio of the amounts of the two species is constant, that is, the decay rate of the daughter nucleus is governed by the half-life of the parent, rather than by its own. In practice, as already mentioned, the generator is "milked" every 24 h to remove the ^{99m}Tc. Figure 2.3 also shows the corresponding dynamic change in Q_2 for a 7-day period.

2.6. THE BIODISTRIBUTION OF TECHNETIUM-BASED AGENTS WITHIN THE BODY

The ^{99m}Tc eluted from the generator is in the form of sodium pertechnetate, $NaTcO_4$. If this compound is injected into the body, it concentrates in the thyroid, salivary glands, and stomach, and can be used for scanning these organs. The majority of radiopharmaceuticals, however, are prepared by reducing the pertechnetate to ionic technetium (Tc^{4+}) and then complexing it with a chemical ligand that binds to the metal ion. The properties of this ligand are chosen to have high selectivity for the organ of interest with minimal distribution in other tissues. The ligand must bind the metal ion tightly so that the radiopharmaceutical does not fragment in the body. General factors which effect the biodistribution of a particular agent include the strength of the binding to blood proteins such as human serum albumin (HSA), the lipophilicity and ionization of the chemical ligand (because transport across membranes is fastest for lipophilic and nonionized species), and the means of excretion from the body, for example, via the liver or kidney. Some commonly used

TABLE 2.2. ^{99m}Tc Radiopharmaceuticals and Corresponding Clinical Applications

Radiopharmaceutical	Clinical Application
^{99m}Tc-macroaggregated albumin	Pulmonary perfusion
^{99m}Tc-diphosphonate	Skeletal
^{99m}Tc-glucoheptonate	Brain tumors
^{99m}Tc-sulfur colloid	Liver and spleen, sentinel node location
^{99m}Tc-DTPA	Renal, pulmonary ventilation
^{99m}Tc-HMPAO	Brain perfusion
^{99m}Tc-Sestamibi	Myocardial perfusion
^{99m}Tc-MAG$_3$	Renal

^{99m}Tc-based radiopharmaceuticals are listed in Table 2.2; further examples are described in Section 2.10.

2.7. INSTRUMENTATION: THE GAMMA CAMERA

The gamma camera, shown in Figure 2.4, is the instrumental basis for all nuclear medicine imaging studies. The roles of each of the separate components are covered in the following sections.

2.7.1. Collimators

Many types of collimator are used in nuclear medicine, but the most common geometry is a parallel-hole collimator, which is designed such that only γ-rays traveling at angles close to 90° to the collimator surface are detected. The collimator thus reduces the contribution from γ-rays that have been Compton-scattered in tissue; these contain no useful spatial information, and reduce the image CNR. The collimator is usually constructed from thin strips of lead, through which transmission of γ-rays is negligible. The normal pattern of the lead strips is a hexagonally based "honeycomb" geometry, as shown in Figure 2.5.

The dimensions and the arrangement of the lead strips determine the contribution made by the collimator to the overall spatial resolution of the gamma camera. In Figure 2.5, if two point sources are placed a distance less than R apart, then they cannot be resolved. The value of R is given by

$$R = \frac{d\,(L+z)}{L} \tag{2.15}$$

where L is the length of the septa, d is the distance between septa, and z is the distance between the γ-ray source and the front of the collimator. Therefore, the spatial resolution can be improved by increasing the length of the septa in the collimator, or minimizing the value of z, that is, positioning the gamma camera as close to the patient as possible.

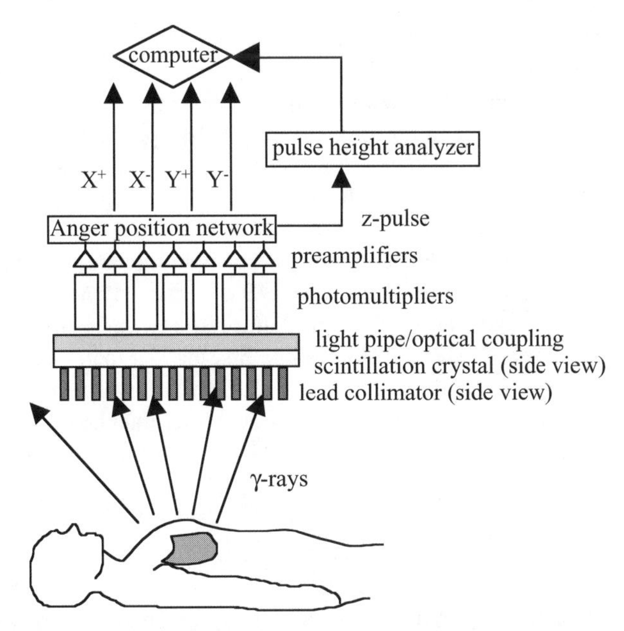

FIGURE 2.4. *Schematic diagram of a gamma camera positioned above the patient. The distribution of the radiopharmaceutical is indicated by the shaded region within the body.*

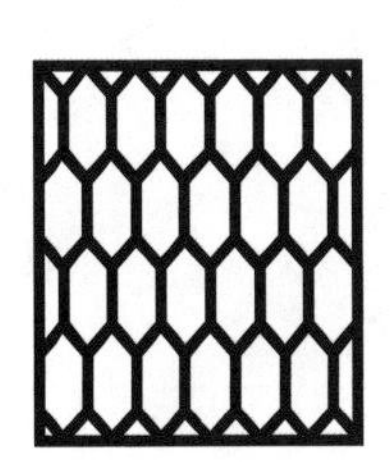

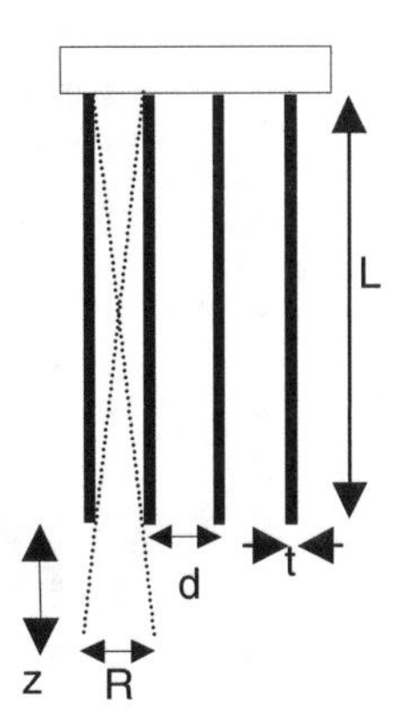

FIGURE 2.5. *(Left) A top view of a hexagonal geometry lead collimator placed directly on the surface of the scintillation crystal. (Right) A side view of the collimator and crystal: the values of L, t, d, and z determine the closest separation R at which two sources of radioactivity can be resolved.*

An important fact to note from equation (2.15) is that the spatial resolution depends upon the depth within the body of the organ in which the radiopharmaceutical source accumulates. Regions of radioactivity closer to the surface are represented on the image at a higher spatial resolution than those deeper in the body. This depth dependence results in images that can show geometric distortion, and great care must be taken in image interpretation in such cases.

There are two general classes of collimators, referred to as high resolution (HR) and high sensitivity (HS). In HR collimators the septa thickness is approximately 0.4 mm and the septa length is 24 mm. An HS collimator typically has the same septa length, 24 mm, as an HR collimator, but a reduced septa thickness between 0.15 and 0.2 mm. For both HR and HS collimators, the fact that the septal length is much greater than the septal thickness means that the vast majority of γ-rays from the radiopharmaceutical are absorbed by the septa rather than being detected by the scintillation crystal. The geometric efficiency, G, of the collimator is given by

$$G = k\left(\frac{d^2}{L(d+t)}\right)^2 \tag{2.16}$$

where k is a constant related to the collimator geometry. There are a number of other types of collimators, shown in Figure 2.6, that can be used to magnify, or alternatively reduce the size of, the image. A converging collimator, for example, can be used for imaging small organs close to the surface of the body. An extreme form of the converging collimator is a "pinhole collimator," which is used for imaging very small

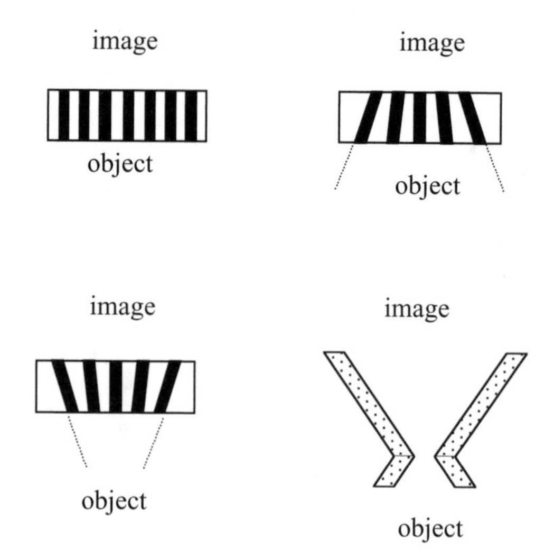

FIGURE 2.6. *Representations of four different forms of collimator used in nuclear medicine. (Top left) A parallel-hole collimator: the object and the image are the same size. (Top right) A diverging collimator, using which the image is smaller than the object. (Bottom left) A converging collimator produces a magnified image. (Bottom right) A pinhole collimator results in a greatly magnified image.*

organs. A pinhole collimator increases significantly the magnification and the spatial resolution of the image, but also results in some geometric distortion, particularly at the edges of the image. It is used primarily for thyroid and parathyroid imaging. In contrast, a diverging collimator reduces the size of the image compared to the physical dimensions of the object and is used to image a structure larger than the size of the detector.

2.7.2. The Scintillation Crystal and Coupled Photomultiplier Tubes

The most common γ-ray detector is based on a single crystal of thallium-activated sodium iodide, NaI(Tl). The thallium creates imperfections in the crystal structure of the NaI such that atoms within the crystal can be excited to elevated energy levels. When a γ-ray strikes the crystal, it loses energy through photoelectric and Compton interactions with the crystal. The electrons ejected by these interactions lose energy in a short distance by ionizing and exciting the scintillation molecules. Deexcitation of these excited states within the scintillation crystal occurs via emission of photons with a wavelength of 415 nm (visible blue light), corresponding to a photon energy of $\sim$4 eV. The intensity of the light is proportional to the energy of the incident γ-ray. The light emission decay constant, which is the time for the excited states to return to equilibrium, is 230 ns for NaI(Tl). This means that count rates of 10^4–10^5 γ-rays per second can be recorded accurately. The linear attenuation coefficient of NaI(Tl) at 140 keV has a high value, 2.22 cm^{-1}, and so 90% of the γ-rays that strike the scintillation crystal are absorbed in a 1 cm thickness. Overall, approximately 13% of the energy deposited in the crystal via γ-ray absorption is emitted as visible light. One disadvantage of the NaI(Tl) crystal is that it is hygroscopic, and so must be hermetically sealed.

The choice of crystal thickness in nuclear medicine involves the same tradeoff between spatial resolution and sensitivity as was described in Section 1.5.3 for intensifying screens in X-ray imaging. When a γ-ray strikes the NaI(Tl) crystal, light is produced from a very small volume determined by the range, typically 1 mm, of the photoelectrons or Compton-scattered electrons. The thicker the crystal, the broader is the light spread function and the poorer is the spatial resolution. For obtaining ^{99m}Tc or ^{201}Tl nuclear medicine images, the optimal crystal thickness is approximately 0.6 cm. However, this value is too small for detecting, with high sensitivity, the higher energy γ-rays associated with radiopharmaceuticals containing gallium, iodine, and indium and so a compromise crystal thickness of 1 cm is generally used in these cases.

The second step in forming the nuclear medicine image involves detection of the light photons emitted by the crystal by hexagonal PMTs, which are closely coupled to the scintillation crystal. This geometry gives efficient packing, and also has the property that the distance from the center of one PMT to that of each neighboring PMT is the same: this property is important for determination of the spatial location of the scintillation event using an Anger position network, as covered in Section 2.7.3. Arrays of 61, 75, or 91 PMTs, each with a diameter of between 25 and 30 mm, are typically used. The basic design of a PMT is shown in Figure 2.7. Light photons pass through the transparent window of the PMT and strike the photocathode, which is made of a bialkali material with a spectral sensitivity matched to the light-emission

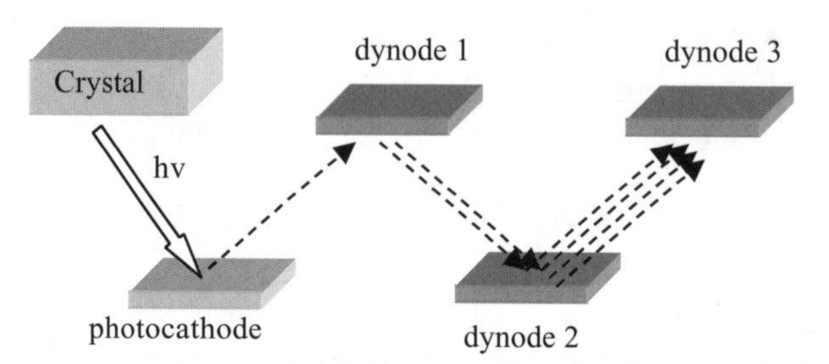

FIGURE 2.7. *A schematic of a photomultiplier tube. Light emitted by the scintillation crystal is converted into a current at the output of the photomultiplier tube. Only 3 dynodes are shown; typically up to 10 are present. For every electron striking a dynode, a significantly greater number of electrons is emitted.*

characteristics of the scintillation crystal. Provided that the photon energy is greater than the photoelectric work function of the photocathode, free electrons are generated in the photocathode via photoelectric interactions. These electrons have energies between 0.1 and 1 eV. A bias voltage of between 300 and 5000 V applied between the first anode (also called a dynode) and the photocathode attracts these electrons toward the anode. If the kinetic energy of this incident electron is above a certain value, typically 100–200 eV, when it strikes the anode a large number of electrons are emitted from the anode for every incident electron: the result is effectively noise-free amplification. A series of 10 successive accelerating dynodes produces between 10^5 and 10^6 electrons for each photoelectron, creating an amplified current at the output of the PMTs. This current then passes through a series of low-noise preamplifiers and is digitized using an A/D converter.

Each PMT should ideally have an identical energy response, that is, the output current as a function of the energy of the γ-ray. If this is not the case, then artifacts are produced in the image. For planar nuclear medicine scans, a variation in uniformity of up to 10% can be tolerated; however, for SPECT imaging, covered later in this chapter, this value should be less than 1%. In practice, calibration of the PMTs is performed using samples of uniform and known radioactivity, and automatic data correction algorithms are applied to the data. More recently, continuous monitoring of individual PMTs during the nuclear medicine scan has become possible using a light-emitting diode (LED) calibration source for each PMT.

New types of gamma cameras, based on multiple-crystal detectors, are currently being developed, and may become standard in the near future. In one such design, a two-dimensional array of long, thin crystals is situated in front of a single position-sensitive PMT (PSPMT). The signal from the PSPMT is digitized using a high-speed A/D converter, with this signal carrying information on the energy of the detected γ-ray, as well as the x and y coordinates of the scintillation event. In this setup, each crystal in the two-dimensional array represents one pixel in the reconstructed nuclear medicine scan. In a further development of the crystal-array concept, the NaI(Tl) crystals can be replaced by a semiconductor, cadmium zinc telluride (CZT), which has a much greater energy resolution and can measure much higher count rates.

2.7.3. The Anger Position Network and the Pulse Height Analyzer

The PMTs situated closest to a given γ-ray-induced scintillation in the crystal produce the largest output current. By comparing the magnitudes of the currents from all of the PMTs, the location of individual scintillations within the crystal can be estimated. This calculation is most easily carried out using an Anger logic circuit, named after one of the pioneers in development of the gamma camera, Hal Anger. This network produces four output signals, X^+, X^-, Y^+, and Y^-, the relative magnitudes and signs of which define the location of the scintillation event in the crystal. Figure 2.8 shows two of the four channels of such a network.

In addition to recording the individual components X^+, X^-, Y^+, and Y^-, the summed signal $(X^+ + X^- + Y^+ + Y^-)$, termed the "z-signal," is sent to a pulse-height analyzer (PHA). The PHA compares the z-signal to a threshold value, which for a ^{99m}Tc scan corresponds to that produced by a γ-ray with energy 140 keV. If the z-signal is below this threshold, it is rejected as having originated from a γ-ray that has been Compton-scattered in the body and therefore has no useful spatial information. In practice, rather than a single threshold value being used, a range of values of the z-signal is accepted. The reason is that even monochromatic 140-keV γ-rays that do not undergo significant scattering in the patient give a statistical distribution in the size of the z-signal. Causes of this distribution include some γ-rays being scattered only by very small angles in the patient, Compton scattering of the γ-rays within the scintillation crystal itself, and spatial nonuniformities in the crystal. The energy resolution of the system is defined as the full-width half-maximum (FWHM) of the photopeak, shown in Figure 2.9, and typically is about 14 keV (or 10%) for most gamma cameras. The narrower the FWHM of the system, the better it is at discriminating between unscattered and scattered γ-rays. The threshold level for accepting the "photopeak" is set to a slightly larger value, typically 15%. For example, a 15% window around a 140-keV photopeak means that values of 129.5–150.5 keV are accepted as corresponding to unscattered γ-rays.

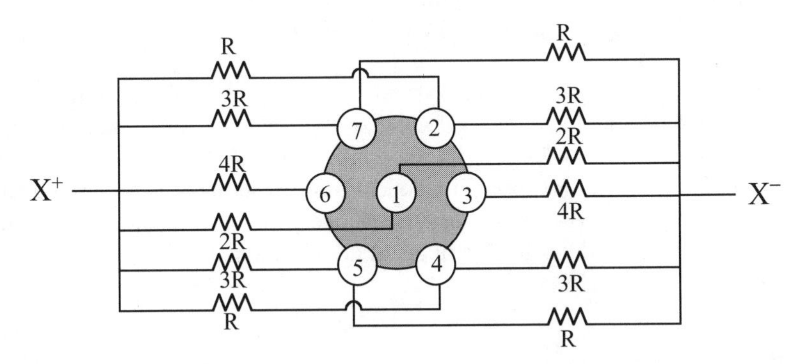

FIGURE 2.8. A version of an electronic network used for estimating the location at which a particular γ-ray strikes the scintillation crystal. For simplicity, only the X^+ and X^- channels are shown in their entirety and only seven PMTs (1–7) are drawn. The magnitude and polarity of the outputs X^+ and X^- determine the position estimate in the x direction.

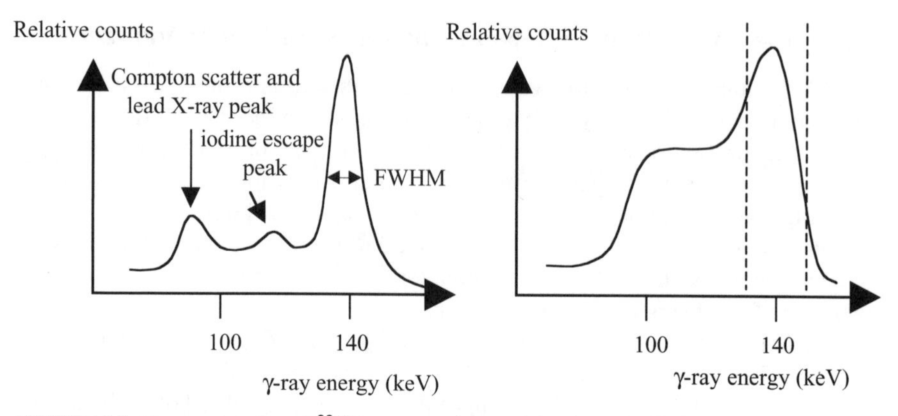

FIGURE 2.9. Energy spectra of ^{99m}Tc γ-rays detected by the scintillation crystal. (Left) The situation when only the gamma camera is used, with no patient. (Right) A broadened spectrum is obtained with the patient in place. The dashed vertical lines represent the range of values accepted by the pulse height analyzer.

Figure 2.9 compares the energy spectrum for ^{99m}Tc for a gamma camera in the absence and in the presence of a patient. In the former case, a number of distinct peaks are visible in addition to the expected 140-keV primary γ-ray peak. The iodine escape peak arises from γ-ray photoelectric interactions in the crystal, resulting in the release of iodine characteristic X-rays, which have an energy of 28.5 keV. The γ-rays reaching the scintillation crystal, therefore, have a residual energy of 111.5 (140 – 28.5) keV. The lead X-ray peak arises from the 140-keV γ-rays interacting with the K-shell electrons of lead in the collimator, giving rise to characteristic X-rays at 75 and 88 keV. Compton scattering of the γ-rays in the scintillation crystal results in a peak at 90 keV. In the presence of the patient, the energy spectrum of the detected γ-rays broadens considerably, due almost entirely to Compton scattering in the patient.

If the z-signal lies within the accepted range, then the values of the X^+, X^-, Y^+, and Y^- signals are used by the computer to estimate the position of the scintillation event, and this is recorded in a two-dimensional data matrix for subsequent image filtering and display.

If the geometric efficiency of the system is high and the injected dose of radiopharmaceutical is large, then the total number of γ-rays that strike the scintillation crystal can exceed the recording capabilities of the system. This is because of the finite recovery times required for various components of the gamma camera. If scintillation events occur at time intervals less than these recovery times, then they cannot be fully recorded. The overall "dead time" τ of the system is defined by

$$\tau = \frac{N - n}{nN} \tag{2.17}$$

where N is the true count rate (number of scintillations per second) and n is the observed count rate. Specifications for standard gamma cameras typically have a 20% loss in the number of counts recorded.

2.8. IMAGE CHARACTERISTICS

As outlined in the introduction to this chapter, the characteristics of nuclear medicine scans are a low SNR and poor spatial resolution, but an extremely high CNR, compared to other imaging modalities. Various forms of data postprocessing are used to increase the image SNR, although this degrades further the spatial resolution.

2.8.1. Signal-to-Noise Ratio

Radioactive decay is a statistical process in that there is no way to predict exactly which atom will decay at a particular time. The number of disintegrations per unit time fluctuates around an average value described by a Poisson statistical distribution, which is covered in Section 5.3.1. The SNR is proportional to the square root of the total number of counts and therefore the greater the number of γ-rays detected, the higher is the SNR. Factors which affect the SNR include the following:

1. The radioactive dose administered: The number of γ-rays detected is proportional to the dose of radiopharmaceutical, but there are clearly patient safety limits to the dose that can be used. There is also an upper limit in the number of counts that can be recorded per unit time, beyond which the dead time of the system means that further increases in the counts does not improve the SNR. Compared to imaging with X-rays, typically 10,000 times fewer counts are detected.
2. The effectiveness of the radiopharmaceutical at targeting a specific organ: The higher the organ specificity of the radiopharmaceutical, the higher is the accumulated dose in that particular organ and the greater is the SNR.
3. The total time over which the image is acquired: The greater the time, the larger is the number of γ-rays detected. The time is limited by patient comfort and the radioactive and biological half-lives of the radiopharmaceutical.
4. Tissue attenuation: The closer the organ being imaged is to the surface of the patient, the less is the degree of γ-ray attenuation. For different radionuclides, the higher the energy of the γ-ray emitted, the lower is the attenuation in tissue and the higher is the image SNR.
5. The intrinsic sensitivity of the gamma camera: For a given system, increasing the scintillation crystal thickness increases the SNR because more γ-rays are detected (however, this decreases the spatial resolution). Similarly, decreasing the length or thickness of the lead septa increases the SNR. The geometry of the collimator, that is, pinhole, converging, diverging, etc., also affects the image SNR.
6. Postacquisition image filtering: Due to the relatively low SNR of nuclear medicine images, processing of the final image to aid diagnosis is standard clinical practice. Normally this processing consists of applying a low-pass filter to the image, as covered in Section 5.5. This filter reduces the contribution of high spatial frequencies, that is, reduces the noise level, but also blurs the image. The degree to which the image is low-pass-filtered depends on the SNR of the acquired image. Because the intrinsic image spatial resolution is relatively poor, quite strong filtering can be applied without introducing significant blurring.

2.8.2. Spatial Resolution

There are four major contributions to the spatial resolution of a nuclear medicine scan:

1. The intrinsic spatial resolution of the gamma camera (excluding the collimator) R_{gamma}: This reflects the uncertainty in the exact location at which light is produced in the scintillation crystal. The degree of uncertainty is dictated by the thickness of the crystal and also by the intrinsic resolution of the Anger position encoder. The thicker the crystal, the broader is the light spread function (Section 1.5.3) and the poorer is the spatial resolution. A typical value of R_{gamma} lies in the range 3–5 mm.
2. The geometry of the collimator: From equation (2.15), the spatial resolution resulting from the use of a parallel-hole collimator is determined by the length and the spacing between, the lead septa. In addition, the extent to which the spatial resolution depends upon the depth within the body at which the radiopharmaceutical accumulates is also determined by these parameters. Finally, the spatial resolution depends on the choice of parallel, converging, diverging, or pinhole collimator.
3. The degree of Compton scattering of γ-rays within the patient: The deeper the targeted organ lies within the body, the greater is the number of γ-rays that will be Compton-scattered, the lower is the CNR, and the poorer is the spatial resolution. The number of these scattered γ-rays that is detected depends upon the geometry of the collimator, with a tradeoff between the SNR and spatial resolution.
4. Postacquisition image filtering: As covered in the previous section.

Considering the first three terms, the overall spatial resolution is given by

$$R_{\text{system}} = \sqrt{R^2_{\text{gamma}} + R^2_{\text{coll}} + R^2_{\text{Compton}}} \tag{2.18}$$

where R_{coll} and R_{Compton} are the spatial resolutions corresponding to factors 2 and 3 above, respectively. Typical values for the overall system spatial resolution are approximately 1–2 cm at large depths within the body and 5–8 mm close to the collimator surface. In practice, the actual form of the PSF has two main contributions. The contributions from the collimator and gamma camera affect the FWHM of the PSF, as shown in Figure 2.10, but the PSF also has long "tails," with these tails attributable mainly to Compton scattering in the patient.

2.8.3. Contrast-to-Noise Ratio

The intrinsic image contrast is extremely high in nuclear medicine because there is no background signal from tissues in which the radiopharmaceutical has not distributed. In this case, the image CNR is essentially equal to the image SNR. However, the presence of Compton-scattered γ-rays does contribute to some degradation of the image SNR. If the spatial resolution is poor, then the CNR is reduced because image

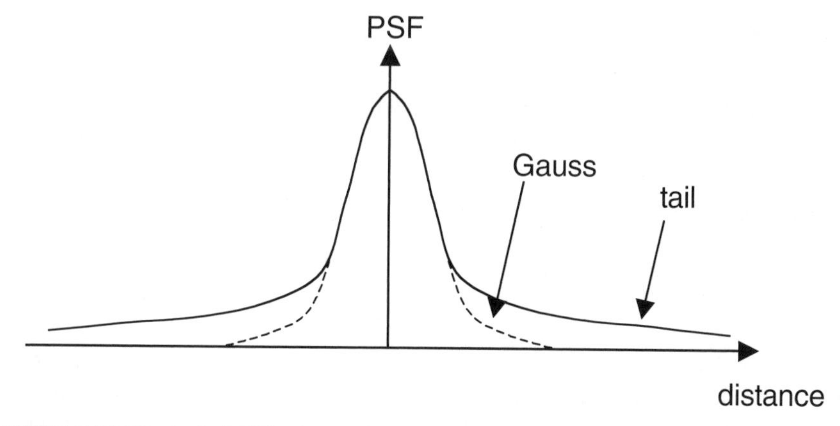

FIGURE 2.10. *The typical PSF of a nuclear medicine scan. The contribution from Compton scattering within the patient gives the PSF a long tail. A Gaussian function, which would result if only the contributions from the gamma camera and collimator were considered, is also shown for comparison.*

blurring causes signal "bleed" from areas of high signal intensity to those where no signal should be present. This phenomenon is referred to as the partial volume effect, and is particularly pronounced for small structures. Postacquisition processing using low-pass filters to increase the SNR also affects the CNR: these filters can either increase the CNR if the SNR increase outweighs the loss in spatial resolution, or can decrease the CNR if the loss in spatial resolution is dominant.

2.9. SINGLE PHOTON EMISSION COMPUTED TOMOGRAPHY

The technique of SPECT applies tomographic principles in order to produce a series of two-dimensional nuclear medicine scans from adjacent slices of tissue. The relationship between planar nuclear medicine, also called "planar scintigraphy," and SPECT is therefore identical to that between planar X-ray imaging and CT. SPECT has an improved CNR over planar scintigraphy by up to a factor of five or six because sources of radioactivity are not superimposed. The spatial resolution of SPECT is not intrinsically increased compared to planar scintigraphy, and in many cases is actually slightly degraded, a FWHM of 1 cm being typical. In general, about five times as many counts are needed in SPECT as in planar scintigraphy in order to obtain an equivalent image SNR. SPECT uses much of the same instrumentation and many of the same radiopharmaceuticals as planar scintigraphy, and most SPECT machines can, in fact, also be used for planar and dynamic nuclear medicine scans. SPECT is the standard acquisition modality for imaging brain and myocardial perfusion and for oncological investigations, and can also be used to increase the image quality of static bone and renal scans. Improved quantitation of absolute concentrations of radiopharmaceuticals is also possible because corrections for attenuation and scatter can be readily implemented.

2.9.1. Instrumentation for SPECT

SPECT can be performed using either multidetector or rotating gamma camera systems. In the former, a large number of scintillation crystals and associated electronics are placed around the patient. The primary advantage of the multidetector system is its high sensitivity, resulting in high spatial resolution and rapid imaging. However, system complexity and associated cost have meant that these types of systems are not widely used in the clinic. The latter approach, using a rotating gamma camera, is preferred for routine clinical imaging because it also can be used for planar scintigraphy. Data are collected from multiple views obtained as the detector rotates about the patient's head.

The simplest setup involves a single gamma camera which rotates in a plane around the patient, collecting a series of signal projections, which, after correction for scatter and attenuation, can be filtered and backprojected to form the image, as described in Appendix B. Because the array of PMTs is two-dimensional in nature, the data can be reconstructed as a series of adjacent slices, as shown in Figure 2.11. An obvious improvement to this setup is to increase the number of cameras in the system because the sensitivity per slice is approximately proportional to the number of

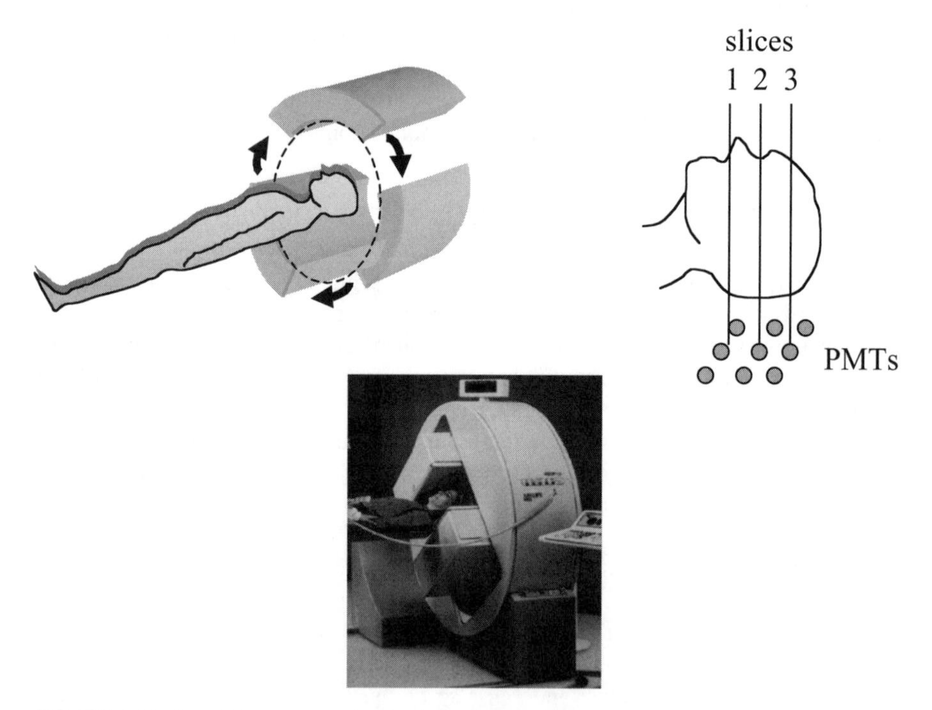

FIGURE 2.11. (Top left) A schematic of a three-head rotating gamma camera for SPECT. (Top right) Multiple adjacent slices can be reconstructed from the data recorded by different PMTs. (Bottom) A photograph of a two-head SPECT system.

cameras. Two- and three-camera systems, depicted in Figure 2.11, are now commonly used. There is also an improvement in spatial resolution with multihead systems, typical numbers being 6–10 mm FWHM for three-head systems, compared to 14–17 mm FWHM for single-head. The rotational orbit of the camera can either be circular or elliptical, with elliptical orbits maintaining the shortest distance between the patient and detector for body scans thus achieving the highest possible spatial resolution. A 360° rotation is generally needed in SPECT because the effects of γ-ray scatter and tissue attenuation and the dependence of the spatial resolution on the source-to-detector distance all mean that projections acquired at 180° to one another are not identical. A focused, rather than parallel-hole, collimator is often used in SPECT. This geometry increases the sensitivity of the scan without significantly decreasing the spatial resolution of the system. Typical geometries of the collimator are either a cone beam, where the collimator holes converge to a point, or a fan beam, in which the holes converge to a line parallel to the axis of camera rotation. The disadvantages involved in using such collimator geometries include the increased complexity of data reconstruction. The position network used in an SPECT scanner is digital, rather than analog as in planar scintigraphy, with the output from each PMT being digitized directly, and estimation of the location of the γ-ray scintillation event is performed by computer.

In a SPECT brain scan, each image of a multislice dataset is formed from typically 500,000 counts, with a spatial resolution of $\sim$7 mm. Myocardial SPECT has a lower number of counts, typically 100,000 per image, and a spatial resolution about one-half that of the brain scan. The data matrix acquired is usually either 64×64 or 128×128. Increasing the resolution from 64×64 to 128×128 improves the spatial resolution of the image, but decreases the SNR because there are four times fewer counts contributing to each pixel in the reconstructed image. Projections can either be acquired in a "stop-and-go" mode or acquired during continuous rotation of the gamma camera. The latter method is much more time efficient, but the speed of rotation must be chosen carefully so that minimal image blurring occurs.

The intrinsic three-dimensional nature of the SPECT images means that the final data can be displayed in any desired orientation. Visualization algorithms such as volume rendering can also be used to analyze the data: this particular approach is used, for example, to make volumetric cardiac measurements.

2.9.2. Scatter and Attenuation Correction

Although similar methods of data acquisition are used in SPECT and CT, and backprojection algorithms form the basis of image reconstruction in both techniques, there is an important difference in that scatter and attenuation correction are required for SPECT data. Because the geometry of the X-ray beam geometry in CT is well-defined by tight source collimation, unlike the situation in SPECT, where obviously no source collimation is possible, the contribution of scattered radiation to the image is potentially much greater in SPECT. It is also worth reemphasizing the different roles of tissue attenuation in CT and SPECT. In CT, the reconstructed image is effectively an estimate of the spatial distribution of the X-ray attenuation coefficients. In SPECT, the reconstructed image is an estimate of the spatial distribution of injected radiopharmaceutical. Spatially dependent γ-ray attenuation coefficients give rise to artifacts in the reconstructed image, and so should be corrected.

In the absence of tissue attenuation, a measured SPECT projection can be represented as

$$p(r, \phi) = c_e \int f(x, y)\, ds \tag{2.19}$$

where c_e is a constant which relates the magnitude of the detected signal to the actual amount of radioactivity in the body. If tissue attenuation is included, then equation (2.19) becomes

$$p(r, \phi) = c_e \int f(x, y) \exp\left[-\int \mu(u, v)\, ds'\right] ds \tag{2.20}$$

where the exponent refers to the attenuation factor for detected photons originating from position (x, y) and traveling along a line perpendicular to the scintillation crystal. Equation (2.22) is extremely difficult to solve analytically, involving an attenuated inverse Radon transform, and so attenuation correction is an important part of SPECT data processing.

The first step in data processing is scatter correction. The number of scattered γ-rays varies from pixel to pixel, and so a position-dependent scatter correction needs to be performed. One such method uses a dual-energy window detection method. One window is centered at the photopeak, with a "subwindow" set to a lower energy. The main window contains contributions from both scattered and unscattered γ-rays, but the subwindow should have contributions only from scattered γ-rays. The main window typically has a fractional width W_m of 20%, that is, between 126 and 154 keV for ^{99m}Tc. The subwindow has a fractional width W_s of ~7% centered at 121 keV. The true number of primary γ-rays C_{prim} can be calculated from the total count C_{total} in the main window and the count C_{sub} in the subwindow:

$$C_{prim} = C_{total} - \frac{C_{sub} W_m}{2 W_s} \tag{2.21}$$

Figure 2.12 shows the effect of a pixel-by-pixel scatter correction.

The second step in processing the data is attenuation correction, which can be performed using either of two methods. In the first realization, the assumption is made that the γ-ray attenuation coefficient in tissue is uniform throughout the entire body. The only requirement for correction is an accurate estimate of the physical dimensions and the boundaries of the area being imaged, information which can be measured by CT or magnetic resonance imaging (MRI). The assumption of a spatially invariant attenuation coefficient works well when, for example, imaging the brain, but introduces image artifacts in applications such as cardiac imaging in which tissue attenuation is highly spatially dependent.

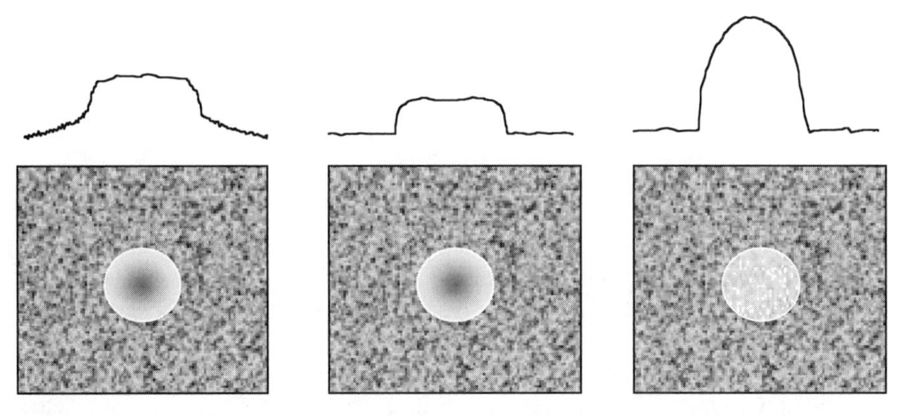

FIGURE 2.12. *Implementation of image corrections for SPECT. (Left) An uncorrected image of a cylinder containing a uniform distribution of radiopharmaceutical. Attenuation artifacts cause the signal intensity in the center of the image to be much less than that around the edges. A one-dimensional projection of the data is shown at the top of the image. The projection also shows that the noise level due to scattered γ-rays is higher closer to the object than further away, as would be expected. (Center) The image and the projection after scatter correction. (Right) The image and the projection after attenuation correction, showing the expected hemispherical profile.*

The second technique applies a spatially variant correction based on a measured estimate of tissue attenuation properties. This measurement uses a transmission scan with tubes of known concentration of radioactive gadolinium (^{153}Gd) placed at the focal line of each fan-beam collimator. The isotope ^{153}Gd is long-lived and emits γ-rays with energies of $\sim$100 keV. The patient is placed in the SPECT scanner and a "transmission scan" is performed, which detects the spatial variation in the ^{153}Gd radiation transmitted through the patient. This scan is then used to estimate the spatial distribution of the tissue attenuation coefficient. After acquisition of the transmission scan, the patient is injected with a radiopharmaceutical and a normal diagnostic scan is performed. If required by time constraints, the transmission calibration scan and the diagnostic images can be acquired simultaneously using a single ^{153}Gd source placed at the focal line of only one of the collimators, with one detector acquiring transmission data and the other two measuring the distribution of the radiopharmaceutical. The effect of attenuation correction on an SPECT image is shown on the right of Figure 2.12.

2.9.3. Image Reconstruction

Filtered backprojection of the SPECT data is the most common reconstruction method. A low-pass filter, typically a Butterworth filter, is used in the filtered backprojection algorithm. The general expression for a Butterworth filter is given by

$$|H(j\omega)|^2 = \frac{1}{1+(j\omega)^{2n}} \tag{2.22}$$

where n is the order of the filter. The higher the value of n, the sharper is the filter. From the Nyquist sampling theorem the maximum spatial frequency in the image ν_{max} is given by

$$\nu_{max} = \frac{1}{2\Delta x} \tag{2.23}$$

where Δx is the pixel size. The filter used in the backprojection is defined with the cutoff frequency as a function of this Nyquist frequency, for example, a 10-pole Butterworth filter with bandwidth 0.4 Nyquist. For multislice SPECT data, spatial filtering is also applied along the slice direction.

In addition to filtered backprojection, iterative reconstruction methods are also available on commercial machines. These iterative methods can often give better results than filtered backprojection because accurate attenuation corrections based on transmission source data can be built into the iteration process, as can the overall MTF of the collimator and gamma camera. The method of backprojection is not particularly well-suited to the incorporation of attenuation and scatter corrections.

2.10. CLINICAL APPLICATIONS OF NUCLEAR MEDICINE

The major clinical applications of nuclear medicine are the measurement of blood perfusion in the brain, the diagnosis of tumors in various organs, and the assessment of cardiac function. The following descriptions are not exhaustive, but outline the development of a wide variety of different radiopharmaceuticals for the detection of many different types of disease.

2.10.1. Brain Imaging

Planar scintigraphy is used in brain scanning to detect tumors using either injected ^{99m}Tc-diethylenetriaminetetraacetic acid (DTPA) or ^{99m}Tc-glucoheptonate. As described earlier, in Section 1.15.1, in healthy brain tissue the blood brain barrier (BBB) selectively filters the blood supply to the brain, allowing only a limited number of naturally occurring substrates, such as glucose, to enter brain tissue. If the brain is damaged, the BBB is disrupted such that injected radiopharmaceuticals can now enter the brain tissue. Because blood flow is often higher in tumors than in healthy tissue, injected radiopharmaceuticals tend to show higher uptake in tumors than surrounding tissue, as seen in Figure 2.13. Planar scintigraphy is also used to confirm brain death. If the brain is functionally dead, then the carotid arteries are visualized on nuclear medicine scans, but are cut off at the base of the skull. The sagittal and venous sinuses are not visualized.

SPECT studies are performed to measure blood perfusion in the brain, most commonly using ^{99m}Tc-HMPAO (Ceretec), the chemical structure of which is shown in Figure 2.14. Ceretec is a neutral complex, which passes through the BBB due to its low molecular weight, relative lipophilicity, and electrical neutrality. Within cells,

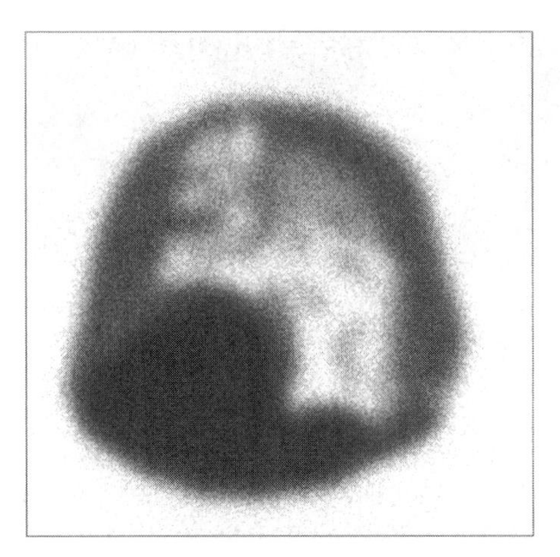

FIGURE 2.13. *A glioblastoma shows increased uptake on an anterior scan using injected ^{99m}Tc-glucoheptonate.*

the agent is metabolized into a more hydrophilic species, which cannot easily diffuse back out of the cell. The spatial distribution of the radiopharmaceutical is proportional to the regional cerebral blood flow (rCBF), and so the agent accumulates in types of tumors that have enhanced blood flow. Peak activity occurs 1–2 min after injection, with typically 4–7% of the dose accumulating in the brain, most of which remains in the brain for time periods up to 24 h. Brain perfusion studies are also carried out using Neurolite, the chemical structure of which is shown in Figure 2.14. Neurolite is a neutral, lipophilic ^{99m}Tc(V) complex and is also able to penetrate the BBB. This agent undergoes ester hydrolysis in tissue, resulting in the formation of one free acid group: having formed a charged complex, the agent is unable to diffuse back across the BBB.

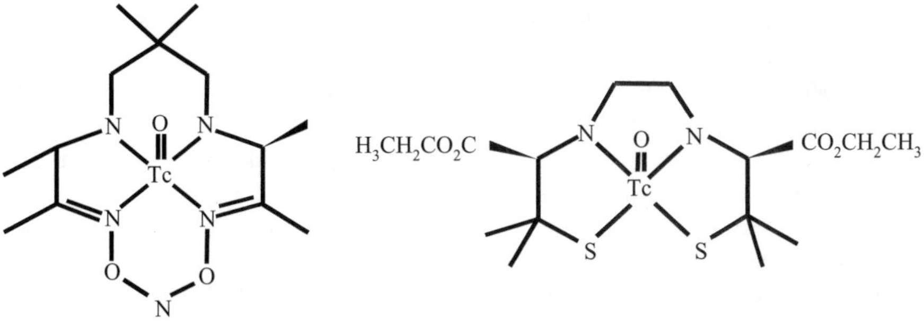

$H_3CH_2CO_2C$ $CO_2CH_2CH_3$

Ceretec Neurolite

FIGURE 2.14. *The chemical structures of two agents used for brain scanning: (Left) Ceretec, ^{99m}Tc-D,L-HMPAO (hexamethyl propylene amine oxime: 3,6,6,9-tetramethyl-4,8-diazaundecane-2,10-dione dioxime). (Right) Neurolite, ^{99m}Tc-L,L-ECD, where ECD= ethyl-cysteine dimer.*

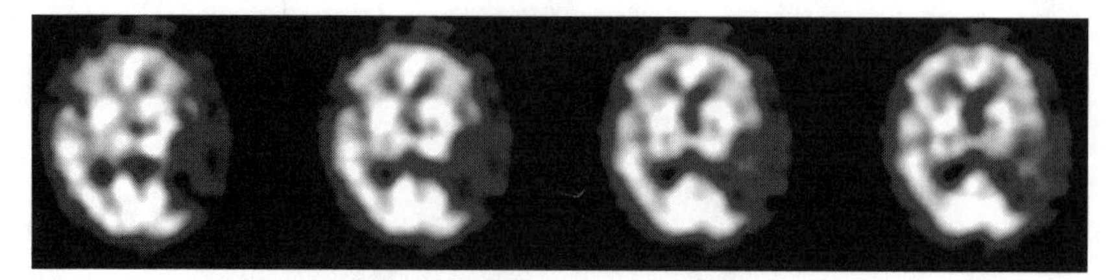

FIGURE 2.15. *Multislice SPECT brain perfusion images of a patient who has extensive brain damage from a stroke. A striking perfusion deficit can be seen in the lower right side of the brain.*

Ceretec is used to diagnose a large range of diseases that cause altered perfusion in the brain. The normal brain has symmetric blood perfusion patterns in the two hemispheres, with higher blood flow in cortical gray matter than white matter. Diseases that cause altered perfusion patterns include epilepsy, cerebral infarction, schizophrenia, and dementia. One commonly studied form of dementia is Alzheimer's disease, which is characterized by bilateral decreased flow in the temporal and parietal lobes with normal flow in the primary sensorimotor and visual cortices. Brain tumors can also be visualized using SPECT via increased blood flow to the lesion resulting in higher signal from the tumor. In contrast to this situation, stroke patients often show a complete lack of blood flow in the affected area of the brain, as seen in Figure 2.15.

Brain tumors can also be identified using SPECT imaging of labeled amino acids such as ^{123}I-α-methyl-L-tyrosine (IMT), which is taken up in tumors by a specific amino acid transport system. This agent accumulates in tumors to a much higher degree than in surrounding cortical gray matter due to this active transport mechanism.

2.10.2. Bone Scanning and Tumor Detection

Whole-body scanning using ^{99m}Tc phosphonates such as methylenediphosphonate (MDP) or hydroxymethylenediphosphonate (HMDP, Osteoscan) can be used to detect bone tumors and also soft-tissue tumors that cause deformation and remodeling of bone structure. The mode of concentration of these agents in bone is thought to involve the affinity of diphosphonate for the metabolically active bone mineral hydroxyapatite, which exhibits increased metabolic turnover during bone growth. The usual response of bone to a tumor is to form new bone at the site or in the periphery of the tumor. For example, spinal tumors, which consist of metastatic lesions growing in the spinal marrow space, cause the bone structure of the spine to remodel. This results in local uptake of the radiopharmaceutical. Scanning starts 2–3 h after injection of the radiopharmaceutical, to allow accumulation within the skeletal structure, and 10 or more scans are used to cover the whole body (Figure 2.16). If any suspected tumor sites show up, then more-localized scans can be acquired. Bone infarctions or aggressive bone metastases often show up as signal voids in the nuclear medicine scan because bone necrosis has occurred and there is no blood flow to deliver the radiopharmaceutical to that region.

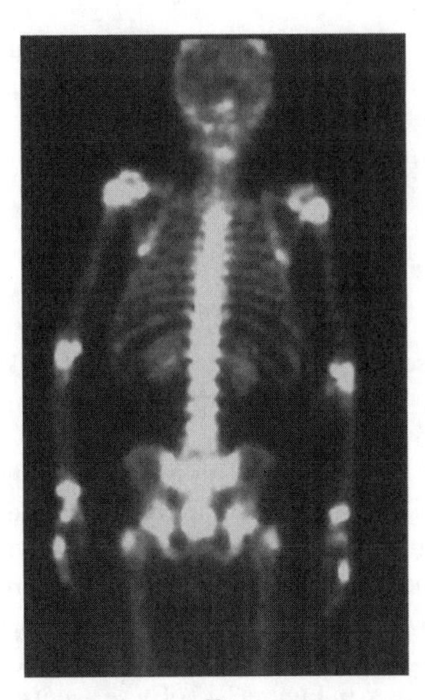

FIGURE 2.16. *A whole-body bone scan using ^{99m}Tc-MDP. A background from scattered radiation can be seen throughout the body.*

Gallium (^{67}Ga) citrate is another agent used for tumor detection because it concentrates in certain viable primary and metastatic tumors as well as focal sites of infection, although the exact mechanism of biodistribution is not well understood. Typical applications of ^{67}Ga scanning include diagnosis of Hodgkin's disease, lung cancer, non-Hodgkin's lymphoma, malignant melanoma, and leukemia. Also used in tumor detection is ^{201}Tl, accumulating mainly in viable tumor tissue. It is used in the form of thallious chloride, and can be used to detect thyroid cancer, primary bone tumors (unlike ^{99m}Tc-MDP, ^{201}Tl does not show activity secondary to bone healing), and in differentiating benign from malignant breast lesions. Combined ^{201}Tl and ^{67}Ga scans can be used for the specific diagnosis of Karposi's sarcoma, which is often associated with AIDS, because this sarcoma is usually ^{201}Tl-positive and ^{67}Ga-negative.

Radiopharmaceuticals can also be designed to target specific sites present during the cell cycle of the cancerous tissue. For example, it is well established that somatostatin receptors are overexpressed in a number of human tumors. A radiopharmaceutical, ^{111}In-DTPA-octreotide (where octreotide is a metabolically stable analog of somatostatin containing eight amino acids), has been designed to target these tumors, which include endocrine pancreatic tumors, carcinoids and paragangliomas, lymphomas, and breast cancer. The long half-life, 67 h, of ^{111}In means that imaging is typically performed 24 h after injection to allow the fraction of the radiopharmaceutical dose that distributes nonselectively within tissue to be excreted. Two γ-rays with energies 172 and 247 keV are emitted by this radionuclide, and both are detected in order to increase SNR of the image.

Monoclonal antibodies and fragments have also been used to target tumors. One example is Oncoscint, which is an ^{111}In(III)-labeled IgG murine monoclonal antibody. This agent targets the cell surface mucin-like glycoprotein antigen TAG-72, which is found in colorectal and ovarian carcinomas.

2.10.3. Cardiac Imaging

Cardiac SPECT scans are performed to measure blood flow patterns in the heart and to detect coronary artery disease and myocardial infarcts. Unlike most other applications, the cardiac SPECT system usually contains only two rotating gamma cameras, with the detectors situated at 90° to one another. Typically, only a 180° rotation is used to form the image because the heart is positioned close to the front of the thorax and well to the left of the body, and therefore views in which the detector is far away from the heart would essentially contribute only scattered γ-rays.

The most common type of scan measures myocardial perfusion and is referred to as a cardiac stress test. This procedure is usually carried out using radiopharmaceuticals such as ^{99m}Tc-sestamibi (Cardiolite) or ^{99m}Tc-tetrafosmin (Myoview), the chemical structures of which are shown in Figure 2.17. These agents are uni-positively charged complexes, a feature which results in their concentrating in heart muscle. The degree of lipophilicity of the agents is also an important aspect in their uptake into the heart. If the lipophilicity is too low, this impedes uptake, but if the lipophilicity is too high, then the agent is bound strongly to blood proteins and the uptake is also low.

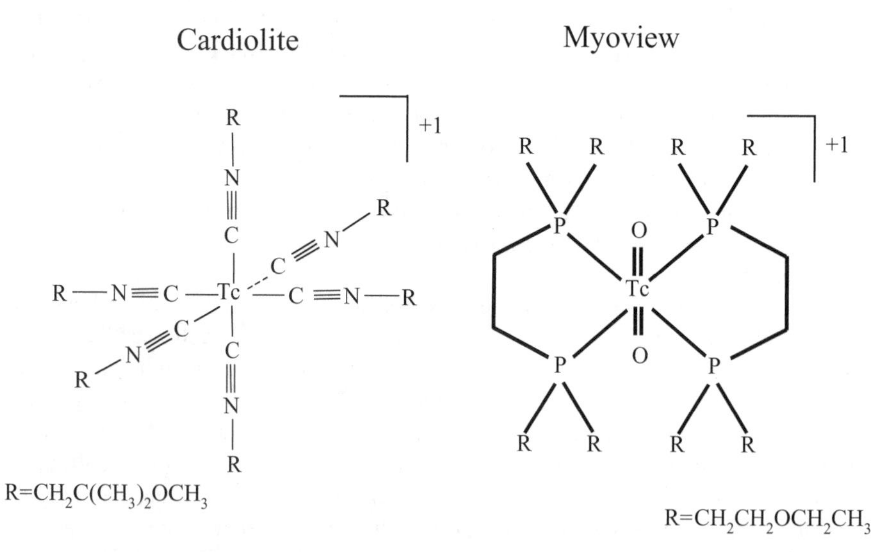

FIGURE 2.17. *The chemical structures of two radiopharmaceuticals used for myocardial perfusion SPECT. (Left) Cardiolite, ^{99m}Tc-hexakis(2-methoxy-1,2-methylpropyl) isonitrile. (Right) Myoview, ^{99m}Tc-trans-dioxotechnetium(V) (1,2-bis(ethoxyethyl)phosphino)ethane.*

The first stage of the stress test involves injecting a relatively low dose, ~8 mCi, of radiopharmaceutical while the patient is exercising. Exercise continues for about 1 min after injection to ensure clearance of the tracer from the blood. Regional uptake of the radiopharmaceutical is proportional to local blood flow, with about 5% of the dose going to the heart. Exercise increases the oxygen demand of the heart causing normal coronary arteries to dilate, with blood flow increasing to a value typically three to five times that at rest. If the coronary arteries are narrowed or blocked (stenosis), however, they cannot dilate and so the blood flow cannot increase sufficiently to satisfy the oxygen demand of the heart. This results in mild myocardial ischemia, which shows up as an area of low signal intensity on the SPECT scan.

If the stress test gives abnormal results, then a SPECT scan is taken at rest a few hours later, with a larger dose, typically 20–25 mCi. Healthy patients exhibit uniform uptake of the radiopharmaceutical throughout the left ventricular myocardium, but myocardial infarcts appear as "cold spots," that is, as areas of low image intensity. Figure 2.18 shows a series of short-axis slices from a myocardical SPECT scan along with a schematic of the heart to show the orientation of the images. The multislice data can also be reconstructed and displayed as oblique-, long-, or short-axis views of the heart, greatly aiding diagnosis.

^{201}Tl-based agents such as thallious chloride are also used in SPECT imaging in order to measure myocardial perfusion. The hydrogenated Tl^{+} ion is roughly the

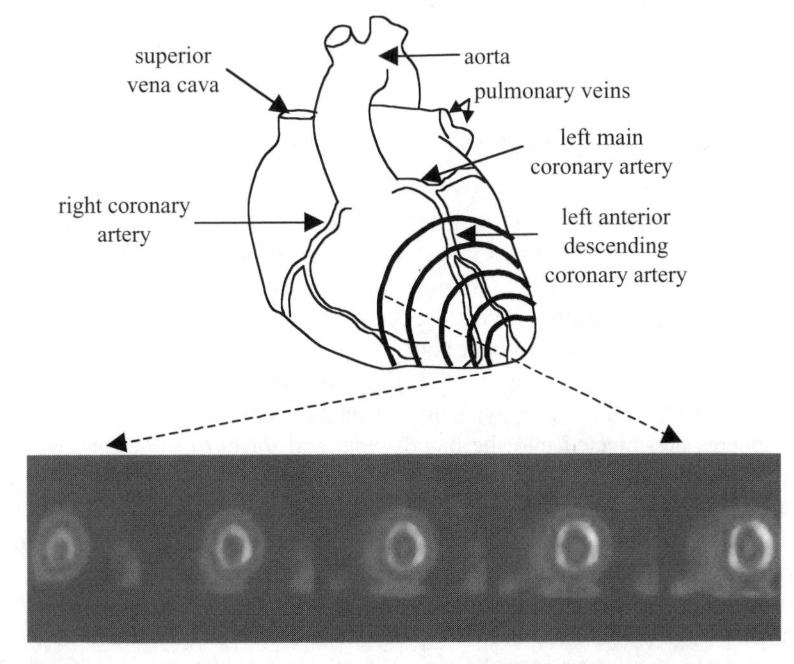

FIGURE 2.18. *(Top) A schematic of the heart showing the major veins and arteries. The dark rings correspond to the positions of the short-axis SPECT images shown below. (Bottom) Multislice images acquired 1 h after injection of Cardiolite during exercise.*

same size as the potassium ion (K^+) and therefore behaves similarly in the body, entering cells via the sodium/potassium pump. A typical imaging protocol involves injection during exercise, a rest period of 3–4 h, reinjection, and a delay of 4–8 h before imaging. About 5% of the injected dose goes to the myocardium, and again regional uptake of the radiopharmaceutical is proportional to the local blood flow. A dual energy window is used, with a 10% window centered at 80 keV and a 20% window centered at 167 keV. The disadvantage of imaging ^{201}Tl compared to ^{99m}Tc is the lower SNR (typically 3–10 times fewer counts per unit time are recorded) and the need for an off-site cyclotron to produce the radionuclide.

A further class of agents used to assess cardiac disease comprises radiopharmaceuticals that are formed from fatty acids. Fatty acids are a major source of energy in normal myocardium, but fatty acid oxidation is suppressed in ischemic and postischemic myocardium. Therefore, the biodistribution of a radiolabeled fatty acid is indicative of the metabolic state of the myocardium. Radioactive iodinated analogs of fatty acids such as 15-(*p*-iodophenyl)-3-(*R*, *S*)-methylpentadecanoic acid (BMIPP) are used most commonly. Regional uptake of BMIPP can be compared to myocardial perfusion studies, such as described previously, to detect the presence of perfusion/metabolism mismatches. These mismatches correspond to diseases such as reversible myocardial ischemia, in which cardiac function is still present, but blood flow to a particular region has been reduced. Because the tissue is still functioning metabolically, myocardial revascularization, in which blood flow to the region is surgically increased, can potentially restore full cardiac function.

2.10.4. The Respiratory System

The roles of the lungs are to add oxygen to, and remove carbon dioxide from, the blood supply to the rest of the body. These processes occur at the blood–air interface in the alveoli of the lungs. Blood flows to the lungs through the pulmonary arteries and veins and via the bronchial arteries. Air enters the lungs via the pharynx into the trachea. Different respiratory diseases can either cause disruptions to blood flow (perfusion), air flow (ventilation), or both.

Perfusion studies of the lung use ^{99m}Tc-labeled microspheres of macroaggregated albumin (MAA), with particles typically between 30 and 40 μm in diameter. These microspheres are injected into the bloodstream and travel to the right side of the heart and pulmonary artery. Within a few seconds of injection, 90–95% of the dose becomes trapped in the pulmonary capillaries and precapillary arterioles. The particles are distributed uniformly within the lung if there is no occlusion in the pulmonary arterial system. If the pulmonary artery or one of its branches is occluded, then radioactivity is absent from this region.

In ventilation studies, radioactive ^{133}Xe gas is dissolved in saline and injected intraveneously into the patient, who must hold his/her breath for approximately 30 s during the scan. When the gas reaches the pulmonary artery it is expired into the lung

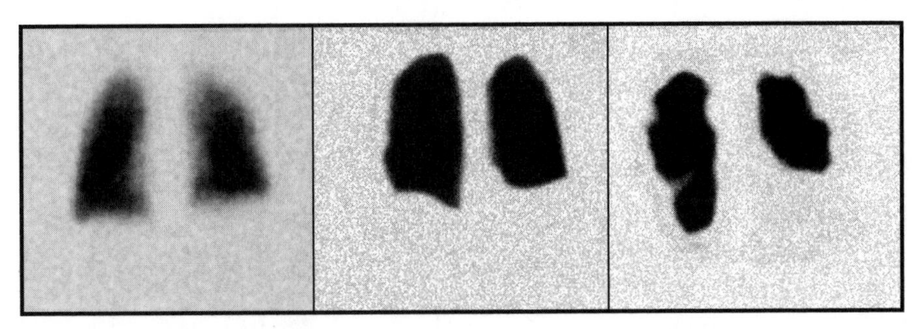

FIGURE 2.19. *(Left) A perfusion scan from a healthy patient using ^{99m}Tc-labeled MAA, which shows homogeneous perfusion throughout the lung. (Center) A ventilation scan from a patient using ^{133}Xe, showing normal ventilation. (Right) A perfusion scan using MAA, which shows an inhomogeneous distribution of radioactivity, indicative of a pulmonary embolism.*

because ^{133}Xe is relatively insoluble in blood. Only those areas of the lungs in which pulmonary artery circulation is intact give a signal on the nuclear medicine scan: any airway blockage results in a signal void. Recently, aerosolized Tc-labeled DTPA has found increasing use in ventilation studies.

Perfusion (Q) and ventilation (V) scans are often carried out in the same examination. A so-called "V/Q mismatch," in which ventilation is normal, but perfusion is abnormal, is indicative of the presence of an obstruction such as a pulmonary embolism. The embolus blocks blood flow to the lungs, but ventilation is normal because there is no corresponding blockage in the airway. An example of planar scintigraphy images corresponding to such a case is shown in Figure 2.19. The opposite situation, in which perfusion is normal, but ventilation is abnormal, suggests an obstructive airway disease. If both perfusion and ventilation are abnormal, referred to as a V/Q-matched abnormality, this is indicative of diseases such as bronchitis, asthma, or pulmonary edema.

2.10.5. The Liver and Reticuloendothelial System

The functions of the liver include detoxification of the blood supply, formation of bile, and the metabolism and synthesis of a variety of proteins. The most common diseases of the reticuloendothelial system (RES) are cirrhosis and fatty infiltrations of the liver, the presence of tumors (hepatomas) and abscesses, obstructions to hepatobiliary clearance, and hemangiomas.

The radiopharmaceutical used most often to image the liver is a ^{99m}Tc-labeled sulfur colloid. This colloid consists of small particles with diameters ($\sim$100 nm) less than the size of the capillary junctions in the liver. The particles in the colloid are phagocytized by the RES, and the radiopharmaceutical concentrates in the Kupffer cells in the liver as well as in the spleen and bone marrow. In normal patients, between 80% and 90% of the Kupffer cells are located in the liver, between 5% and 10% in the spleen, and the remainder in the bone marrow. When a disease such as cirrhosis

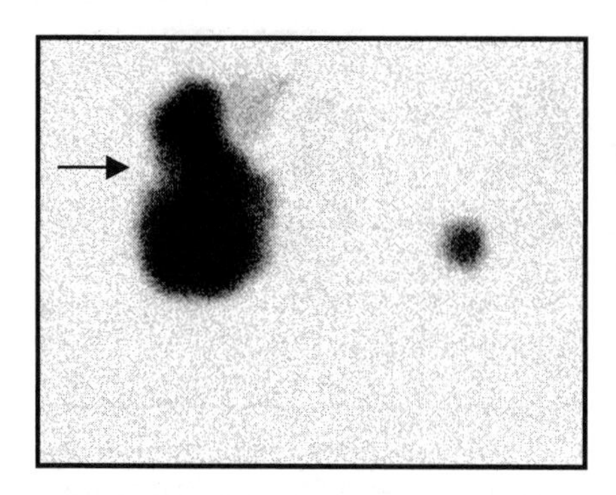

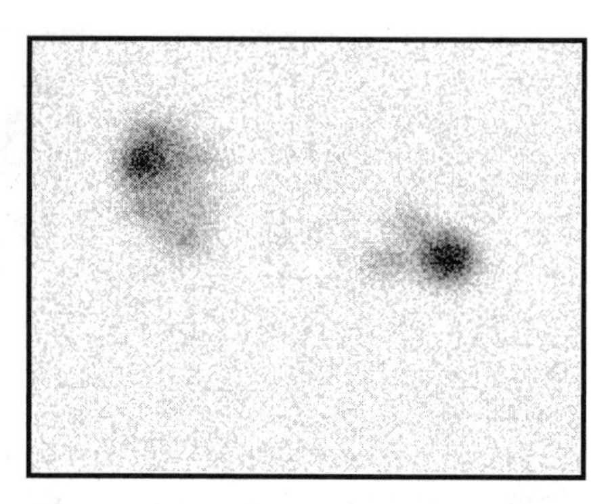

FIGURE 2.20. *Transverse SPECT images of the liver showing a cavernous hemangioma. (Left) In the ^{99m}Tc-labeled sulfur-colloid scan there is an area, shown by the arrow, which has a sharply reduced uptake of the agent. (Right) In the ^{99m}Tc-labeled RBC scan an increased vascularity, compared to the surrounding liver, in the hemangioma is indicated by a higher signal intensity.*

of the liver is present, then the liver is unable to phagocytize the particles fully, and an increased level of radioactivity is seen in the spleen and the bone marrow. The colloids are preferentially localized in normal tissue, with almost no radioactivity found in abnormal lesions (focal nodular hyperplasia is an exception), and so diseases such as metastatic tumors, cysts, abscesses, and hematomas can be visualized by the lack of radioactivity in these areas, so-called "cold spots" in the image

A second radiopharmaceutical, ^{99m}Tc-labeled red blood cells (RBCs), is often used to determine whether a lesion detected using the ^{99m}Tc-labeled sulfur colloid is vascular (blood flow present) or avascular (blood flow absent) in nature. The radio-labeled RBCs mimic the body's own RBCs and circulate in the bloodstream for a long period of time. Therefore, areas of the nuclear medicine scan that show activity are indicative of the presence of blood flow. An example of a nuclear medicine study using both of these ^{99m}Tc-labeled agents is shown in Figure 2.20.

2.10.6. Renal Imaging

Radiopharmaceuticals used in brain scanning, such as ^{99m}Tc-DTPA and ^{99m}Tc-glucoheptonate, can also be used to image renal function because these agents are excreted through the kidneys. The agent ^{99m}Tc-glucoheptonate shows greater retention in the cortex of the kidney than in the medulla, as does another agent used for renal scanning, ^{99m}Tc-O(dmsa)$_2$ (^{99m}Tc-dimercaptosuccinic acid). In contrast, the radiopharmaceutical ^{99m}TcO-MAG$_3$ (^{99m}TcO-mercaptoacetyltriglycine) preferentially accumulates in the medulla, and is used as a renal tubular imaging agent. Whichever agent is used, the normal diagnostic procedure is to acquire a time series of images in order to build up a profile of the increase and subsequent decay of the radiopharmeutical concentration. Abnormal kinetics during one or both of the stages is indicative of specific physiological defects in the kidneys. For example, a prolonged retention of the agent in one or both of the kidneys is associated with renal artery stenosis. Renal infarction, on the other hand, is associated with a very slow buildup of the agent.

2.11. POSITRON EMISSION TOMOGRAPHY

Positron emission tomography (PET) is one of the fastest growing imaging modalities in modern clinical diagnosis. Similar to SPECT, PET is a tomographic technique that is used to measure physiology and function, rather than gross anatomy. The fundamental difference between the two imaging techniques is that the injected or inhaled radiopharmaceuticals used in PET emit positrons, which, after annihilation with an electron in tissue, result in the formation of two γ-rays. The fact that two γ-rays are detected, rather than one as in SPECT, allows the instrumentation used in PET to be designed to produce images with much higher SNR and spatial resolution than in SPECT.

PET is used clinically mainly in oncology, cardiology, and neurology. The spatial distribution, extent of uptake, rate of uptake, and rate of washout of a particular radiopharmaceutical are all quantities which can be used to distinguish diseased from healthy tissue. The major disadvantages of PET revolve around its high cost, typically $1.5–2.5 million for a system, and the need to have a cyclotron on-site to produce positron-emitting nuclides, because the half-lives of these nuclides are so short. As a result, there are currently fewer than 200 PET scanners in the United States.

2.11.1. General Principles

As outlined above, PET is a diagnostic imaging technique used to map the biodistribution of positron-emitting radiopharmaceuticals within the body. These radiopharmaceuticals must be synthesized using a cyclotron, and are structural analogs of a biologically active molecule, such as glucose, in which one or more of the atoms has been replaced by a radioactive atom. Examples of such radiopharmaceuticals include fluorodeoxyglucose (FDG), which contains ^{18}F, and [^{11}C]palmitate. Isotopes such as ^{11}C, ^{15}O, ^{18}F, and ^{13}N undergo radioactive decay by emitting a positron, that is a positively charged electron (e^+), and a neutrino (ν):

$$^{A}_{Z}X \rightarrow {}_{Z-1}^{A}X + e^{+} + \nu$$

The positron travels a short distance ($\sim$1 mm) in tissue in a random direction before annihilating with an electron. This annihilation results in the formation of two γ-rays, each with an energy of 511 keV, which travel in opposite directions at an angle of 180° to one another:

$$e^{+} + e^{-} \rightarrow \gamma + \gamma$$

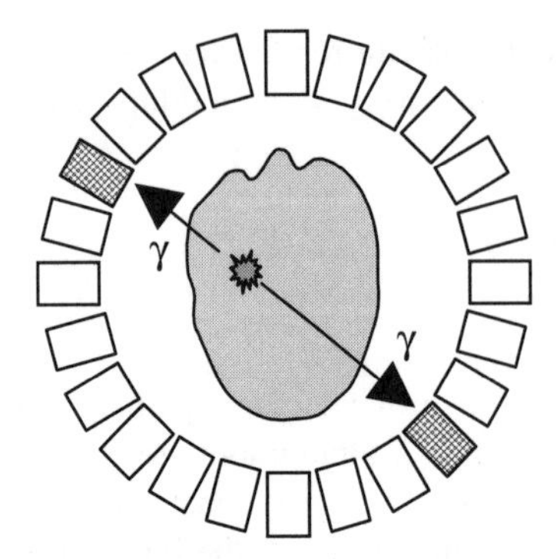

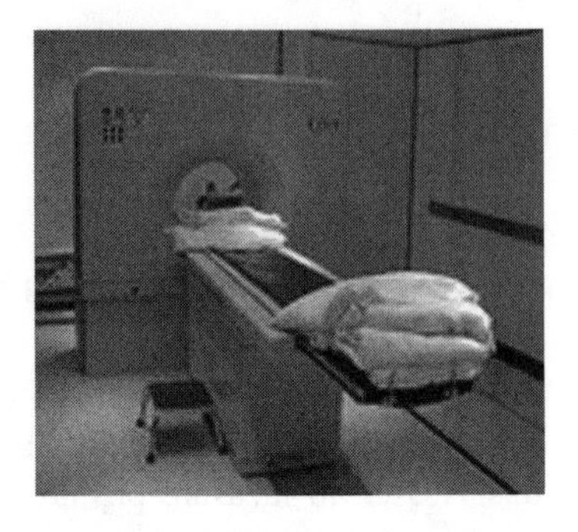

FIGURE 2.21. *(Left) A schematic of a PET head scanner, showing an annihilation coincidence between two detectors. (Right) A commercial PET scanner with patient bed for positioning. © 2002 Philips Medical Systems.*

Because two "antiparallel" γ-rays are produced and both must be detected, a PET system consists of a complete ring of scintillation crystals surrounding the patient, as shown in Figure 2.21. Because the two γ-rays are created simultaneously, both are detected within a certain time window, the value of which is determined by the diameter of the detector ring and the location of the radiopharmaceutical within the body. The location of the two crystals that actually detect the two antiparallel γ-rays defines a line along which the annihilation must have occurred. This process of line definition is referred to as annihilation coincidence detection (ACD) and forms the basis of signal localization in PET. This process should be contrasted with that in SPECT, which requires collimation of single γ-rays. The difference in these localization methods is the major reason for the much higher detection efficiency (typically $\sim$1000-fold) in PET than in SPECT. Image reconstruction in PET is via filtered backprojection, as described previously. Because the γ-ray energy of 511 keV in PET is much higher than the 140 keV of γ-rays in conventional nuclear medicine, different materials such as bismuth germanate are used for the scintillation crystals. The higher γ-ray energy means that less attenuation of the γ-rays occurs in tissue, a second factor which results in the high sensitivity of PET. The spatial resolution in PET depends upon a number of factors including the number and size of the individual crystal detectors: typical values of the overall system spatial resolution are $\sim$3–5 mm.

2.11.2. Radionuclides Used for PET

All the radionuclides used in PET are produced by a cyclotron. The most commonly used radionuclides are ^{18}F, ^{11}C, ^{15}O, and ^{13}N, which are incorporated into biologically active molecules before being injected into or inhaled by the patient. These radionuclides can all be produced from relatively small cyclotrons using protons with an energy of ~10 MeV or deuterons with an energy ~5 MeV. Typical reactions are as follows:

$$^{12}C \xrightarrow{\text{proton}} {}^{11}C + \text{proton} + \text{neutron}$$
$$^{14}N \xrightarrow{\text{proton}} {}^{11}C + {}^{4}_{2}He$$
$$^{16}O \xrightarrow{\text{proton}} {}^{11}N + {}^{4}_{2}He$$
$$^{13}C \xrightarrow{\text{proton}} {}^{13}N + \text{neutron}$$
$$^{15}N \xrightarrow{\text{proton}} {}^{15}O + \text{neutron}$$
$$^{14}N \xrightarrow{\text{deuterium}} {}^{15}O + \text{neutron}$$
$$^{18}O \xrightarrow{\text{deuterium}} {}^{18}F + \text{neutron}$$
$$^{20}Ne \xrightarrow{\text{deuterium}} {}^{18}F + {}^{4}_{2}He$$

The radioactive properties of these four radionuclides are summarized in Table 2.3.

After production of the particular radionuclide it must be incorporated, via rapid chemical synthesis, into the corresponding radiopharmaceutical. For speed and safety considerations the synthesis should ideally be carried out robotically. Such robotic units are available commercially for synthesizing ^{18}FDG, $^{15}O_2$, $C^{15}O_2$, $C^{15}O$, and $H_2{}^{15}O$.

Other, less commonly used nuclei are produced by larger, higher current cyclotrons, including (half-lives are listed in parentheses) ^{52}Fe (8.3 h), ^{55}Co (17.5 h), ^{61}Cu (3.3 h), ^{62}Cu (9.7 min), ^{64}Cu (12.7 h), ^{62}Zn (9.2 h), ^{63}Zn (38.5 min), ^{70}As (52.6 min), ^{71}As (65.3 min), ^{76}Br (16.2 h), ^{82}Rb(1.27 min), ^{86}Y (14.7 h), ^{89}Zr (78.4 h), ^{110}In (4.9 h), ^{120}I (81 min), ^{124}I (4.2 days), and ^{122}Xe (20.1 h).

2.11.3. Instrumentation for PET

The major differences in PET instrumentation compared to that in SPECT are the scintillation crystals needed to detect 511-keV γ-rays efficiently and the additional circuitry needed for coincidence detection.

2.11.3.1. Scintillation Crystals. Detection of the antiparallel γ-rays uses a large number of scintillation crystals, which are usually formed from bismuth germanate (BGO). The crystals are placed in a circular arrangement surrounding the patient, and the crystals are coupled to a smaller number of PMTs. Coupling each crystal to a single

TABLE 2.3. Properties of the Most Common Radionuclides Used for PET

Radionuclide	Half-life (min)
^{11}C	20.4
^{15}O	2.07
^{13}N	9.96
^{18}F	109.7

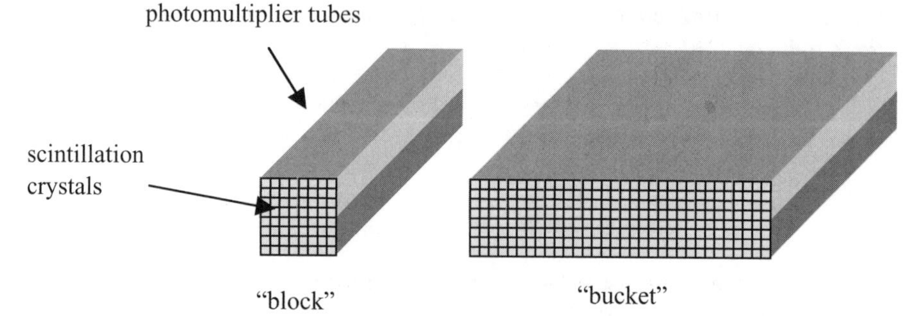

FIGURE 2.22. *(Left) A "block" of 8 × 8 crystals is coupled to four PMTs (differential shading of the PMTs is for illustrative purposes only and does not imply any differences in their physical characteristics). (Right) A "bucket" of detectors consists of four blocks and contains 256 crystals.*

PMT would give the highest possible spatial resolution, but would also increase the cost prohibitively. Typically, each "block" of scintillation crystals consists of an 8 × 8 array cut from a single BGO crystal, with the cuts filled with light-reflecting material. The dimensions of each block are roughly 6.5 mm in width and height and 30 mm in depth. Each block of 64 individual crystals is coupled to four PMTs, as shown in Figure 2.22. Localization of the detected γ-ray to a particular crystal is performed in the same way, outlined in Section 2.7.3, as in conventional nuclear medicine. Four of these blocks of crystals are arranged to form a "bucket," with a 0.6-mm gap between the blocks. The full detector ring may have up to 32 such buckets, that is, 8192 crystals in total.

The properties of various materials that are or have been used as scintillation crystal detectors in PET are shown in Table 2.4. In terms of the parameters in Table 2.4, the ideal detector crystal would:

1. Have a high density, which results in a large effective cross-section for Compton scattering, and a correspondingly high γ-ray detection efficiency
2. Have a large effective atomic number, which also results in a high γ-ray detection efficiency due to γ-ray absorption via photoelectric interactions
3. Have a short decay time to allow a short coincidence time to be used, with a reduction in accidental coincidences (Section 2.11.4.2) and an increased SNR in the reconstructed PET image
4. Have a high light output (emission intensity) to allow more crystals to be coupled to a single PMT, reducing the complexity and cost of the PET scanner
5. Have an emission wavelength near 400 nm; this wavelength represents the point of maximum sensitivity for standard PMTs
6. Have an index of refraction near 1.5 to ensure efficient transmission of light between the crystal and the PMT; optical transparency at the emission wavelength is also important
7. Be nonhygroscopic to simplify the design and construction of the many thousands of crystals needed in the complete system

TABLE 2.4. Properties of Various Detectors Employed in PET[a]

Material	Decay Time (ns)	Emission Intensity	Density (g/cm^3)	$\lambda_{emitted}$ (nm)	η	A_{eff}	Hygroscopic
BGO	300	0.15	7.13	480	2.15	75	No
GSO(Ce)	60_{prim}, 600_{sec}	0.3	6.71	430	1.85	59	No
BaF_2	0.8_{prim}, 600_{sec}	0.12	4.88	220, 310	1.49	53	No
CsF	4	0.05	4.64	390	1.48	53	Yes
CaF_2(Eu)	900	0.4	3.18	435	1.44	17	No
LSO(Ce)	40	0.75	7.40	420	1.82	65	Yes
NaI(Tl)	230_{prim}, 1000_{sec}	1	3.67	410	1.85	51	Yes

[a] A_{eff} is the effective atomic number, η is the refractive index, and decay times are expressed as primary and secondary decays. The emission intensity is reported relative to a value of 1.0 for NaI(Tl). GSO(Ce) is cerium-doped gadolinium orthosilicate (Gd_2SiO_5), and LSO(Ce) is cerium-doped lutetium orthosilicate (Lu_2SiO_5).

The combination of the high density and large effective atomic number of BGO results in its high linear attenuation coefficient, 0.96 cm^{-1}, compared to lower values for LSO(Ce), 0.87 cm^{-1}, and NaI(Tl), 0.35 cm^{-1}. This means, for example, that a NaI(Tl) crystal would have to be 2.7 times as thick as one constructed from BGO to give same detection efficiency. The major disadvantage of BGO is its low emission intensity at 480 nm. This means that a maximum of 16 crystal elements can be coupled to each PMT, whereas the number for LSO(Ce) can be up to 144. Indeed, in the future, LSO(Ce) may well become the material most used for PET scintillation crystals. Its major disadvantage is lutetium's natural radioactivity, which must be corrected for in image reconstruction.

The size of the crystal is also an important design criterion. In general, the narrower the width of the crystal, the higher is the intrinsic spatial resolution of the system. However, there is a lower limit on the size, below which the spatial resolution can actually worsen. This is because there is little or no physical collimation of the γ-rays in PET, and so a γ-ray that strikes a very thin crystal at a relatively large incident angle can be scattered and penetrate several adjacent crystals. This process can degrade the system spatial resolution significantly. One way to minimize this effect is to make the diameter of the detector ring larger, so that the incident angles become smaller. However, this leads to a decrease in the system sensitivity. In practice, a typical value of the crystal width for BGO is ~1 cm.

2.11.3.2. Annihilation Coincidence Detection Circuitry. In a PET scan a large number of annihilation coincidences are detected. Some of these are true coincidences, but there are many mechanisms by which "false" coincidences can be recorded. Several of these mechanisms are outlined in Section 2.11.4.2. The ACD circuitry is designed to maximize the ratio of true-to-false recorded coincidences. In Figure 2.23 an injected radiopharmaceutical is located in the forward right part of the brain. A positron is emitted and annihilates with an electron, and two antiparallel γ-rays are produced. The first γ-ray reaches crystal number 2 and produces a number of photons. These photons are converted into an amplified electrical signal, at the output of the PMT, which is fed into a PHA. If the voltage is within a predetermined

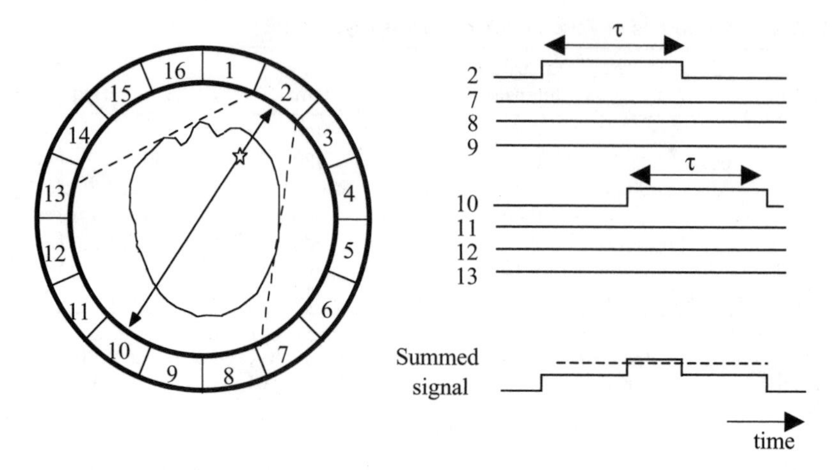

FIGURE 2.23. The principle of annihilation coincidence detection. (Left) The two γ-rays reach detectors 2 and 10, triggering respective logic pulses of length τ seconds. (Right) If both logic pulses are sent to the coincidence detector within the system coincidence resolving time 2τ, then the summed signal lies above the threshold value (dashed line) and a coincidence is recorded.

range, then the PHA generates a "logic pulse," which is sent to the coincidence detector. Typically, this logic pulse is 6–10 ns long. Variations in the exact location of the γ-ray within the crystal, and also the decay time of the excited states created in the BGO crystal, create a random "time jitter" in the delay between the γ-ray striking the crystal and the leading edge of the logic pulse being sent to the coincidence detection circuitry. In Figure 2.23, the first γ-ray having been detected by crystal 2, only those crystals numbered between 7 and 13 can detect the second γ-ray from the annihilation. When the second γ-ray is detected and produces a voltage that is accepted by the associated PHA, a second logic pulse is sent to the coincidence detector. The coincidence detector adds the two logic pulses together and passes the summed signal through a separate PHA, which has a threshold set to a value just less than twice the amplitude of each individual logic pulse. If the logic pulses overlap in time, then the system accepts the two γ-rays as having evolved from one annihilation and records a line integral between the two crystals. The PET system can be characterized by its "coincidence resolving time," which is defined as twice the length of the logic pulse, and usually has a value between 12 and 20 ns.

2.11.4. Image Reconstruction

Basic image reconstruction in PET is essentially identical to that in SPECT, with both iterative algorithms and those based on filtered backprojection being used to form the image from individual line projections. However, prior to reconstruction, the data must be corrected for attenuation effects and, more importantly, for accidental and multiple coincidences.

2.11.4.1. Attenuation Correction. The HVL for γ-rays with energies of 511 keV is about 7 cm in soft tissue, which means that there is considerable attenuation of γ-rays originating from deep within the body or brain. In order to obtain accurate quantitative images of the distribution of the radiopharmaceutical, this effect must be corrected. There are two basic methods, which are very similar to those described for SPECT imaging in Section 2.9.2. The first technique is based on assuming a spatially uniform attenuation coefficient throughout the body, and the second on empirical attenuation measurements. In organs such as brain, there is relatively little variation in the attenuation coefficient of different tissue components, and an average value can be used. Significant errors may occur, however, if air-filled areas such as the sinuses are located in the image FOV. In cases where the assumption of uniform attenuation coefficient is not valid, for example, in cardiac PET studies, an external ring source of positron emitters, usually containing germanium-68, is used for a transmission-based calibration. The difference between the number of disintegrations detected in the presence and the absence of the patient allows the spatially variant tissue attenuation factor to be estimated.

2.11.4.2. Corrections for Accidental, Multiple and Scattered Coincidences. The main sources of noise in PET are accidental and scattered coincidences. If two detectors i and j are considered, then

$$C_{ij}^{\mathrm{O}} = C_{ij}^{\mathrm{T}} + C_{ij}^{\mathrm{S}} + C_{ij}^{\mathrm{A}} \tag{2.24}$$

where C_{ij}^{O} is the observed coincidences between detectors i and j, C_{ij}^{T} is the true number of coincidences, C_{ij}^{S} is the number of scattered coincidences, and C_{ij}^{A} is the number of accidental coincidences. A very detailed account of these phenomena can be found in the book by Cho, pp. 212–221, cited in Further Reading at the end of this chapter. The term due to accidental coincidences is usually much higher than that due to scattered coincidences.

Accidental coincidences refer to events in which the line integral formed by the detection of the two γ-rays is assigned incorrectly. One way in which this can occur is shown in Figure 2.24.

A second mechanism for accidental coincidences, similar to that shown in Figure 2.24, occurs if the first γ-ray is not recorded because it is attenuated within tissue via a photoelectric interaction. The second and the third steps leading to the recording of this accidental coincidence are identical to those shown in Figure 2.24. Other ways in which accidental coincidences can arise include contributions from γ-rays from a radiopharmaceutical distributed in an area that is out of the plane of the detector ring, and the presence of background radiation. The rate at which these accidental coincidences (C_{ij}^{A}) are recorded for a given detector pair (i, j) is given by

$$C_{ij}^{\mathrm{A}} = 2\tau R_i R_j \tag{2.25}$$

where R_i and R_j are the single count rates in the individual detectors i and j, respectively, and τ is the length of the logic pulse. Typically, the ratio of coincidences to

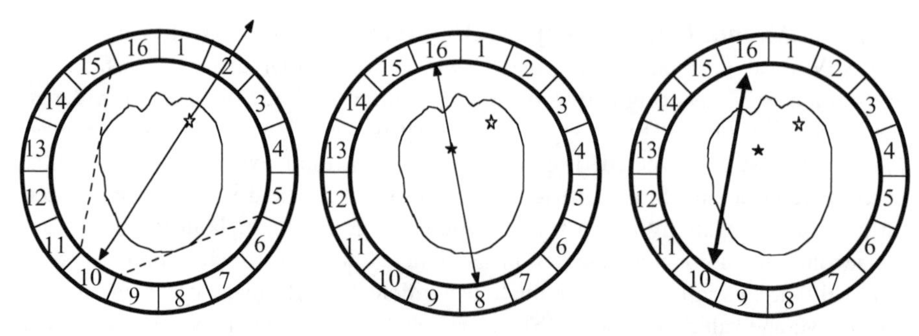

FIGURE 2.24. *An illustration of one mechanism, due the finite quantum yield of a scintillation crystal, by which an accidental coincidence can be recorded. (Left) A positron annihilation (open star) occurs and two γ-rays are emitted. The first γ-ray to reach the detector passes straight through crystal 2 without being detected. The second γ-ray is recorded by crystal 10. (Center) A short time after the first annihilation, a second positron annihilation (closed star) occurs and the first γ-ray from the latter event is detected by crystal 16. This event occurs within the coincidence resolving time of the system, triggered by crystal 10. (Right) The accidental coincidence is recorded as a true coincidence, and causes an incorrect line integral joining detectors 10 and 16 to be assigned.*

single counts is only 1:100. Equation (2.25) shows that the value of τ should be made as small as possible, to reduce the contribution of accidental coincidences, but not so short as to reject true coincidences.

There are two practical methods used to correct for accidental coincidences. The first method uses equation (2.25) and the measured values of R_i and R_j for each detector pair i and j to estimate the corresponding values of C_{ij}^{A}. These values are then subtracted from the acquired data before image reconstruction. The second method uses additional parallel timing circuitry, which splits the logic pulse from one of the detectors into two components. The first component is used in the standard mode to measure the total number of coincidences. The second component is delayed well beyond the coincidence resolving time so that only accidental coincidences are recorded. The accidental coincidences are then removed from the acquired data before the reconstruction process.

A multiple coincidence represents the combination of a true coincidence with one or more unrelated events. For example, in a triple coincidence, shown in Figure 2.25, two events are recorded during the coincidence resolving time, which is triggered by detection of the first γ-ray. Because it is not clear which of these later two events should be accepted, the data are discarded. Such triple coincidences represent a significant loss of counts, and result in an effective deadtime for the PET system. The deadtime loss (DTL), in units of counts per second, is estimated by measuring the number of triple coincidences over the scanning time T. In order to determine the true radioactivity level in the image, a correction for this deadtime must be made. The correction factor is given by

$$\text{correction factor} = \frac{\text{true coincidences} + (\text{DTL})\,T}{\text{true coincidences}} \tag{2.26}$$

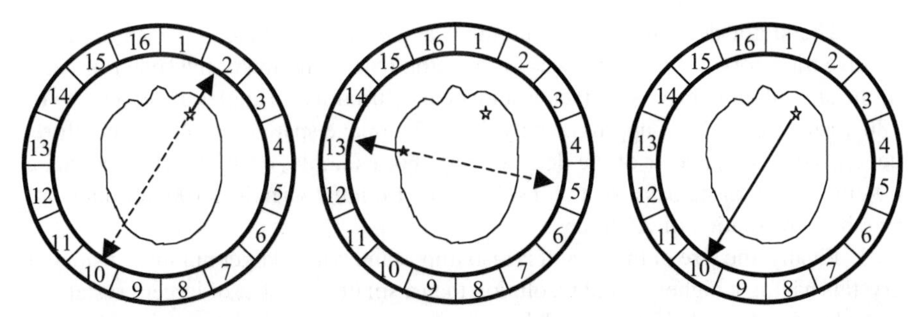

FIGURE 2.25. *A schematic showing the occurrence of a triple coincidence. (Left) The first γ-ray from the first annihilation (open star) is recorded by detector 2. (Center) Almost immediately after the first annihilation, a second one (closed star) takes place. Before the second γ-ray from the first annihilation reaches detector 10, the first γ-ray from the second annihilation reaches detector 13. (Right) Within the coincidence resolving time of the first annihilation, the second γ-ray from the first annihilation reaches detector 10, and a triple coincidence is recorded.*

Scattered coincidences occur if one, or both, of the γ-rays from the positron annihilation undergoes Compton scattering in the body. The net result is that a slightly erroneous line integral is recorded. Because the γ-rays lose only small amounts of energy in these Compton interactions, scatter rejection on the basis of the energy of the detected γ-rays is impractical. The most common method of correcting for scatter is very similar to that used in SPECT, covered in Section 2.9.2. The amount of scatter in the image is measured in areas outside the patient, and these values are extrapolated mathematically to estimate the amount of scatter inside the patient. This function is then subtracted from the raw data to give the corrected image.

2.11.5. Image Characteristics

Many of the factors which affect the SNR and CNR in PET are identical to those in SPECT. The roles of radiopharmaceutical dose, targeting efficiency, image acquisition time, γ-ray attenuation in the patient, system sensitivity, and image postprocessing are exactly the same as outlined in Section 2.8.1 and 2.8.3. However, in contrast to SPECT, the PSF in PET is essentially constant throughout the patient. This is because the inherent "double detection" of two γ-rays traveling at an angle of 180° to one another eliminates the depth dependence of the PSF. Other factors which influence the spatial resolution of the PET image include the following:

1. The finite distance which the positron travels before annihilation with an electron effectively defines a "sphere of uncertainty" with regard to the original position of the disintegration of the radiopharmaceutical. The distance increases with the energy of the positron. Typical values of the maximum positron energy and corresponding FWHM distances traveled are: ^{18}F (640 keV, 1 mm), ^{11}C (960 keV, 1.1 mm), ^{13}N (1.2 MeV, 1.4 mm), ^{15}O (1.7 MeV, 1.5 mm), and ^{82}Rb (3.15 MeV, 1.7 mm).

2. The slight deviation from a nominal angle of 180° which characterizes the relative trajectories of the two γ-rays is a factor. Due to motion of the center of mass of the annihilation there is, in fact, a statistical distribution in angles about a mean of 180°, with a FHWM of approximately 0.3°. The image spatial resolution, therefore, depends on the diameter of the detector ring. For example, from this effect alone, a 60-cm-diameter ring has a spatial resolution of 1.6 mm, whereas a 100-cm-diameter ring has a resolution of 2.6 mm.

3. Finally, the size of the crystal is also important, with a larger number of smaller crystals having a higher spatial resolution than a smaller number of larger crystals. A contribution of one-half the crystal diameter to the overall spatial resolution is a good approximation.

The overall spatial resolution is the combination of all three components, analogous to equation (2.18), and is typically 3–4 mm for a small ring system and 4–6 mm for a larger, whole-body imager. The relatively poor spatial resolution, but high specificity in PET has led to a growing increase in "fusing" PET images with those obtained from CT, which have a high spatial resolution. A wide variety of software algorithms for three-dimensional image registration and fusion are becoming available commercially.

2.11.6. Multislice and Three-Dimensional PET Imaging

Multislice capability can be introduced into PET imaging, as for CT, by having a number of detector rings stacked alongside one another, as shown in Figure 2.26. Each ring typically consists of 16 buckets of 8 × 8 blocks of scintillation crystals. The number of rings in a high-end multislice PET scanner can be up to 48. Retractable septa (lead or tungsten) are positioned between each ring: these are kept in position for multislice operation and retracted for imaging in three-dimensional mode.

Image planes can be formed between two crystals in the same ring (direct planes), and also from crystals in adjacent rings (cross planes). For a system with n rings, there

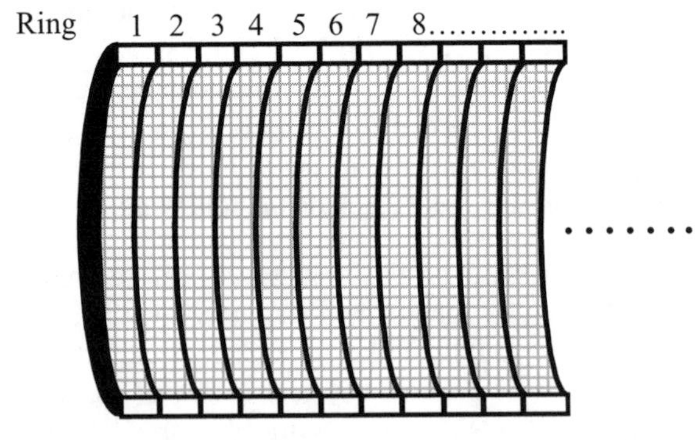

FIGURE 2.26. *A cutaway view of a multislice PET system. The retractable septa between adjacent rings are shown as thick black lines.*

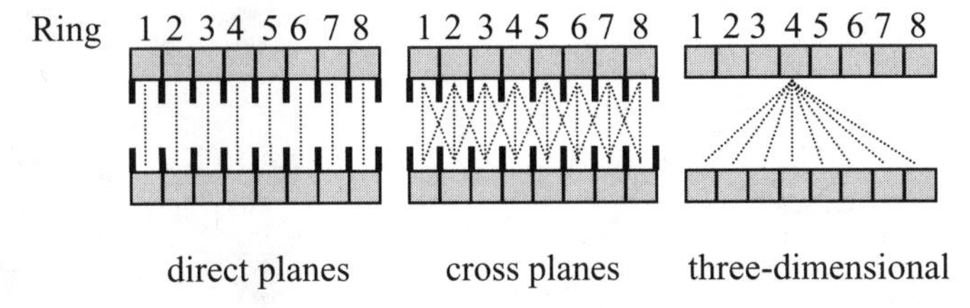

FIGURE 2.27. *Various data acquisition modes in multislice (direct planes and cross planes) and three-dimensional PET.*

are n direct planes and $n - 1$ cross planes, making a total of $2n - 1$ image planes, as shown in Figure 2.27. If the septa are removed, then an $n \times n$ three-dimensional dataset can be acquired. The sensitivity of a three-dimensional scan is approximately 10 times higher than that of the corresponding multislice dataset due to the absence of the septa. However, the amount of scatter is also increased, though to a much lesser extent.

2.11.7. Clinical Applications of PET

Major additions in the clinical uses of PET have been seen recently, almost entirely due to their new status as approved procedures by Medicare, for example, in the United States. PET is used mainly for the diagnosis, staging, and evaluation of treatment efficacy for tumors in the breast, lung, head, and neck, and also colorectal cancer. PET is used to provide quantitative information on metabolic and physiological changes in three major areas: brain imaging, cardiac studies, and tumor imaging.

2.11.7.1. Brain Imaging. Brain scans using PET can measure both regional cerebral blood flow (rCBF) and tissue metabolism. The former quantity is usually measured with ^{15}O-labeled water and the latter with FDG. Diseases in which brain perfusion in localized areas is either increased or reduced compared to normal patients can be diagnosed by mapping the distribution of ^{15}O, the concentration of which is proportional to brain perfusion.

In the body, the radiopharmaceutical FDG is metabolized in exactly the same way as naturally occuring 2-deoxyglucose. Once injected, FDG is actively transported across the BBB into the cells in brain tissue. Inside the cell, FDG is phosphorylated by glucose hexokinase to give FDG-6-phosphate. This chemical is trapped inside the cell because it cannot react with G-6-phosphate dehydrogenase, which is the next step in the glycolytic cycle. The amount of intracellular FDG is therefore proportional to both the rate of initial glucose transport and subsequent intracellular phosphorylation. A high glucose metabolic rate, which is found for many types of malignant gliomas and astrocytomas, for example, results in a high signal intensity on the image, as shown in Figure 2.28. In other applications, areas of the brain with reduced glucose metabolism can often be identified as focal centers for epilepsy.

Another agent, 3,4-dihydroxy-6-fluoro-DL-phenylananine, [^{18}F]DOPA, measures L-DOPA uptake and the rate of dopamine synthesis in the brain. Alzheimer's disease

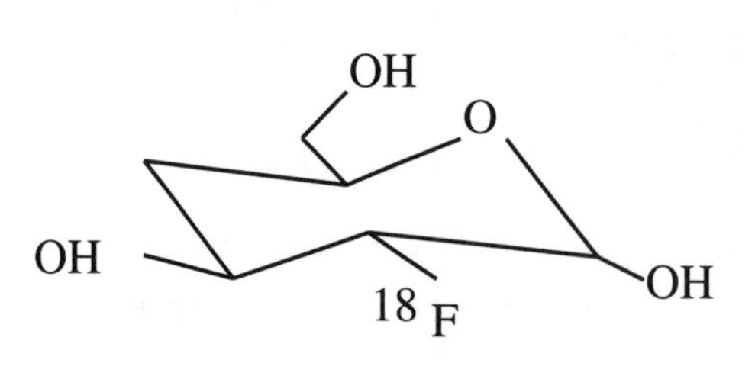

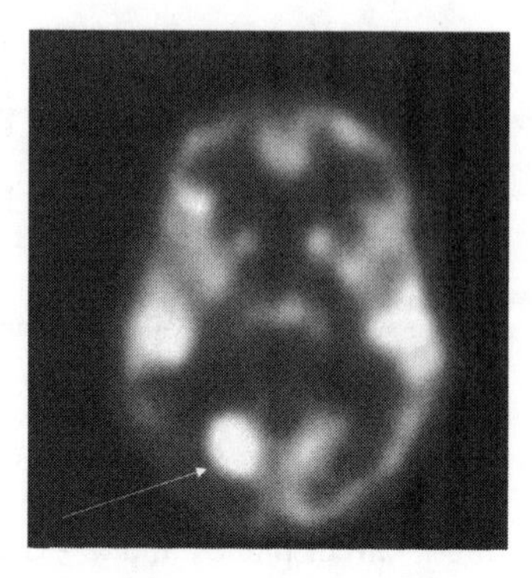

FIGURE 2.28. (Left) The chemical structure of 2-deoxy-2-[^{18}F]fluoroglucose (FDG). (Right) A PET brain scan using FDG of a patient with an astrocytoma, which shows up as an area of significantly increased signal intensity.

and Parkinson's disease can be diagnosed at an early stage by a reduction in dopamine synthesis. It is also possible to perform neuroscience investigations to determine particular areas of the brain that are involved in specific cognitive tasks because increases in regional cerebral blood flow are associated with neural activity. Measurements of these changes in blood flow are made mainly with $H_2{}^{15}O$, but can also be performed with FDG.

2.11.7.2. Cardiac Studies. In cardiac studies, both blood flow and metabolism can be measured using PET. Blood flow can be assessed using $^{13}NH_3$, with metabolism being studied by [^{11}C]palmitate or FDG. In healthy myocardium, long-chain fatty acids are the principal energy source, whereas in ischemic tissue, glucose plays a major role in residual oxidative metabolism and the oxidation of long-chain fatty acids is reduced substantially. [^{11}C]Palmitate is a labeled long-chain fatty acid, and is used for assessing myocardial fatty acid metabolism. Myocardial infarction, for example, causes a decrease in the regional uptake of [^{11}C]palmitate.

One example of the clinical application of cardiac PET is the assessment of whether a heart transplant or bypass surgery should be carried out on a particular patient. A measured absence of both blood flow and metabolism in parts of the heart shows that the tissue has died, and so a heart transplant may be necessary. If blood flow is absent in an area, but the tissue maintains even a reduced metabolic state, then the tissue is still alive and bypass surgery would be more appropriate. Illustrative images of both situations are shown in Figure 2.29. Many other agents, such as [^{11}C]acetate, ^{11}CO, and ^{82}Rb-based radiopharmeuticals, are also used in cardiac studies.

2.11.7.3. Tumor Imaging. Malignant cells, in general, have higher rates of aerobic glucose metabolism than healthy cells. Therefore, in PET scans using FDG the tumors show up as areas of increased signal intensity. For a cancer, and particularly

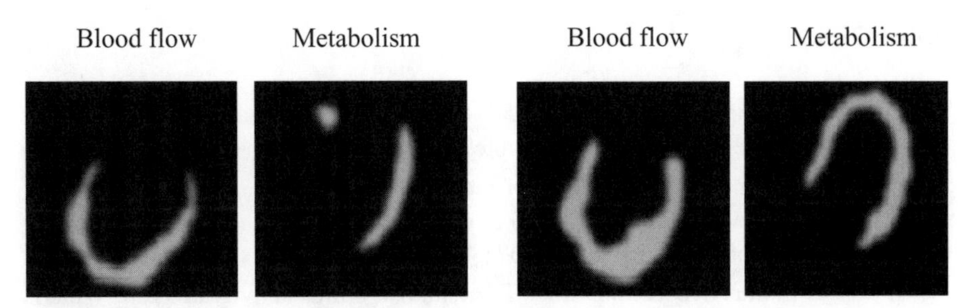

FIGURE 2.29. *Myocardial PET imaging. (Left) A scan using $^{13}NH_3$ indicates that blood flow is absent in the area of the myocardium shown at the top of the image, and the scan using [^{11}C]palmitate shows that metabolism is also absent in this tissue. This patient would require a heart transplant. (Right) The corresponding scans for a patient who could undergo bypass surgery. Although the $^{13}NH_3$ scan again shows an area of no blood flow, the corresponding region in the [^{11}C]palmitate metabolic scan shows activity.*

metastatic cancer, in which the lesions may have spread from their primary focus to secondary areas, a whole-body PET scan is performed. The patient is injected intravenously with ~10 mCi of FDG and placed in the scanner approximately 30 min after injection. Data are acquired for between 30 min and 2 h. Due to the limited physical size of the scanner, the complete image is a usually a composite of three or more separate scans. A typical scan of a patient with metastatic cancer is shown in Figure 2.30.

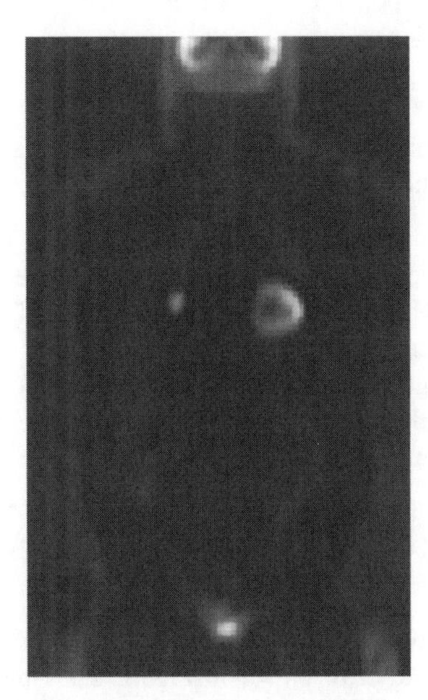

FIGURE 2.30. *A composite whole-body FDG PET scan, showing accumulation of the agent in a small lung tumor. High levels of FDG can be seen in brain, heart, and bladder.*

EXERCISES

2.1. **(a)** In a sample of 1000 atoms, if 50 atoms decay in 5 s, what is the radioactivity, measured in mCi, of the sample?

(b) In order to produce a level of radioactivity of 1 mCi, how many nuclei of ^{99m}Tc ($\lambda = 3.22 \times 10^{-5}\text{s}^{-1}$) must be present? What mass of the radionuclide does this correspond to? (Avogadro's number is 6.02×10^{23}.)

(c) A radioactive sample of ^{99m}Tc contains 10 mCi activity at 9 am. What is the radioactivity of the sample at 3 p.m. on the same day?

2.2. In a nuclear medicine scan using ^{99m}Tc, the image SNR for a 30-min scan was 50:1 for an injected radioactive dose of 1 mCi (3.7×10^7 disintegrations per second). Imaging began immediately after injection.

(a) If the injected dose were doubled to 2 mCi, what would be the image SNR for a 30-min scan?

(b) If the scan time were doubled to 60 min with an initial dose of 1 mCi, what would be the image SNR?

2.3. In the technetium generator, show mathematically that if $\lambda_2 >> \lambda_1$, then the radioactivities of the parent and daughter nuclei become equal in value at long times.

2.4. Using the equations derived in the analysis of the technetium generator, plot graphs of the activity of parent and daughter nuclei for the following cases:

(a) $\tau_{1/2}(\text{parent}) = 600\,\text{h}$, $\tau_{1/2}(\text{daughter}) = 6\,\text{h}$.

(b) $\tau_{1/2}(\text{parent}) = 6\,\text{h}$, $\tau_{1/2}(\text{daughter}) = 6\,\text{h}$.

(c) $\tau_{1/2}(\text{parent}) = 0.6\,\text{h}$, $\tau_{1/2}(\text{daughter}) = 6\,\text{h}$.

2.5. Calculate the spatial resolution of the pinhole collimator in Figure 2.31 in terms of the variables shown in the figure.

2.6. Three parameters which affect the image SNR in nuclear medicine are the thickness of the detector crystal, the length of the lead septa in the antiscatter grid, and the FWHM of the energy window centered around 140 keV. For each parameter, does an increase in the value of the particular parameter increase or decrease the image SNR? In each case, name one other image characteristic (e.g., CNR, spatial resolution) that is affected, and explain whether this image characteristic is improved or degraded.

2.7. Compton scattering in the patient results in a broad range of γ-ray energies between 90 and 140 keV, as shown in Figure 2.9. Explain the reason for the 90-keV value.

2.8. The energy spectrum of detected γ-rays contains components at energies greater than 140 keV, as shown in Figure 2.9. Suggest possible origins of this phenomenon.

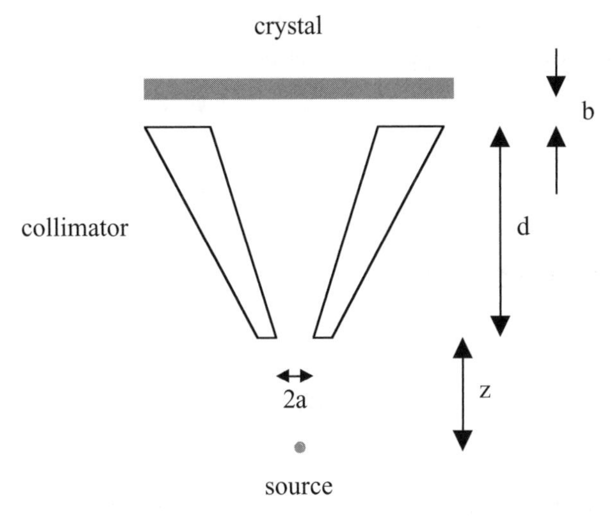

FIGURE 2.31. *Illustration for Exercise 2.5.*

2.9. Isosensitive imaging is a technique that acquires nuclear medicine scans from opposite sides of the patient and then combines the signals to remove the depth dependence of the signal intensity. By considering the attenuation of γ-rays in the patient, show how this technique works, and what mathematical processing of the two scans is necessary.

2.10. For a 128×128 data matrix, how many total counts are necessary for a 1% pixel-by-pixel uniformity level in a SPECT image?

2.11. Two ways of reducing the statistical noise in the image are to double the total imaging time and double the mass of tracer injected. Considered separately, by what factor would each of these reduce the noise in the image?

2.12. Take the following image intensities as a template:

$$\begin{matrix} 1 & 1 & 1 & 1 & 1 \\ 1 & 2 & 2 & 2 & 1 \\ 1 & 2 & 3 & 2 & 1 \\ 1 & 2 & 2 & 2 & 1 \\ 1 & 1 & 1 & 1 & 1 \end{matrix}$$

Calculate the image intensities after applying each of the two convolution kernels shown below. To which class of filter does each convolution kernel belong?

$$\begin{matrix} +1 & +1 & +1 \\ +1 & +4 & +1 \\ +1 & +1 & +1 \end{matrix} \qquad \begin{matrix} -1 & -1 & -1 \\ -1 & +9 & -1 \\ -1 & -1 & -1 \end{matrix}$$

2.13. Using the rest mass of the electron, show that the energies of the two γ-rays produced by the annihilation of an electron with a positron are 511 keV.

2.14. PET scans often show an artificially high level of radioactivity in the lungs. Suggest one mechanism by which this might occur.

FURTHER READING

Original Papers

Nuclear Medicine Instrument Design

B. Cassen, L. Curtis, C. Reed, and R. Libby, Instrumentation for ^{131}I used in medical studies, *Nucleonics* **9,** 46–50 (1951).

H. O. Anger, Scintillation camera, *Rev. Sci. Instrum.* **29,** 27–33 (1958).

D. E. Kuhl and R. Q. Edwards, Image separation radioisotope scanning, *Radiology* **80,** 653–661 (1963).

H. O. Anger, Scintillation camera with multichannel collimators, *J. Nucl. Med.* **5,** 515–531 (1964).

SPECT and PET Instrument Development

J. S. Robertson, R. B. Marr, M. Rosenblum, V. Radeka, and Y. L. Yamamoto, Thirty-two-crystal positron transverse section detector, in *Tomographic Imaging in Nuclear Medicine* (G. S. Freedmen, ed.), pp. 142–153, Society of Nuclear Medicine, New York (1973).

D. E. Kuhl, R. Q. Edwards, A. R. Ricci, R. J. Yacob, T. J. Mich, and A. Alavi, The Mark IV system for radionuclide computed tomography of the brain, *Radiology* **121,** 405–413 (1976).

R. J. Jaszczak, P. H. Murphy, D. Huard, and J. A. Burdine, Radionuclide emission computed tomography of the head with ^{99m}Tc and a scintillation camera, *J. Nucl. Med.* **18,** 373–380 (1977).

J. W. Keyes, N. Orlandea, W. J. Heetderks, P. F. Leonard, and W. L. Rogers, The Humongotron—a scintillation-camera transaxial tomograph, *J. Nucl. Med.* **18,** 381–387 (1977).

Z. H. Cho and M. R. Farukhi, Bismuth germanate as a potential scintillation detector in positron cameras, *J. Nucl. Med.* **18,** 840–844 (1977).

M. M. Ter-Pogossian, N. A. Mullani, J. Hood, C. S. Higgins, and M. Curie, A multi-slice positron emission computed tomograph (PETT IV) yielding transverse and longitudinal images, *Radiology* **128,** 477–484 (1978).

Radioisotopes

B. M. Gallagher, A. Ansari, H. Atkins, V. Casella, D. R. Christman, J. S. Fowler, T. Ido, R. R. MacGregor, P. Som, C. N. Wan, A. P. Wolf, D. E. Kuh, and M. Reivich, Radiopharmaceuticals XXVII. ^{18}F-Labeled 2-deoxy-2-fluoro-D-glucose as a radiopharmaceutical for measuring regional myocardial glucose metabolism *in vivo:* Tissue distribution and imaging studies in animals, *J. Nucl. Med.* **18,** 990–996 (1977).

Books

Physics and Instrumentation

R. A. Powsner and E. R. Powsner, *Essentials of Nuclear Medicine Physics,* Blackwell Science, London (1998).

R. Chandra, *Nuclear Medicine Physics: The Basics,* Lippincott, Williams and Wilkins, Philadelphia (1998).

F. A. Mettler, M. J. Guberteau, and B. Mettler, *Essentials of Nuclear Medicine Imaging,* Saunders, Philadelphia (1998).

J. H. Thrall and H. A. Ziessman, *Nuclear Medicine: The Requisites,* Mosby St. Louis (2001).

Z-H Cho, J. P. Jones, and M. Singh, "Foundations of medical imaging," J. Wiley, New York (1993).

Applications

R. L. Van Heertum and R. S. Tikofsky, eds., *Functional Cerebral SPECT and PET Imaging,* Lippincott, Williams and Wilkins, Philadelphia (2000).

Review Articles

C. M. T. Medley and G. C. Vivian, Radionuclide developments, *Br. J. Radiol.* **70,** S133–S144 (1997).

S. Liu and D. S. Edwards, ^{99m}Tc-Labeled small peptides as diagnostic radiopharmaceuticals, *Chem. Rev.* **99,** 2235–2268 (1999).

S. S. Jurisson and J. D. Lydon, Potential technetium small molecule radiopharmaceuticals, *Chem. Rev.* **99,** 2205–2218 (1999).

C. J. Anderson and M. J. Welch, Radiometal-labeled agents (non-technetium) for diagnostic imaging, *Chem. Rev.* **99,** 2219–2234 (1999).

M. C. Groch and W. D. Erwin, SPECT in the year 2000: Basic principles, *J. Nucl. Med. Technol.* **28,** 233–244 (2000).

C. L. Melcher, Scintillation crystals for PET, *J. Nucl. Med.* **41,** 1051–1055 (2000).

M. C. Groch and W. D. Erwin, Single-photon emission computed tomography in the year 2001: Instrumentation and quality control, *J. Nucl. Med. Technol.* **29,** 9–15 (2001).

L. Bouwens, R. Van de Walle, J. Nuyts, M. Koole, Y. D'Asseler, S. Vandenberghe, I. Lemahieu, and R. A. Dierckx, Image-correction techniques in SPECT, *Comput. Med. Imag. Graph.* **25,** 117–126 (2001).

F. J. Beekman, C. Kamphuis, M. A. King, P. P. van Rijk, and M. A. Viergever, Improvement of image resolution and quantitative accuracy in clinical single photon emission computed tomography, *Comput. Med. Imag. Graph.* **25,** 135–146 (2001).

C. L. Melcher, Scintillation crystals for PET, *J. Nucl. Med.* **41,** 1051–1055 (2000).

T. G. Turkington, Introduction to PET instrumentation, *J. Nucl. Med. Technol.* **29,** 1–8 (2001).

S. Thobois, S. Guillouet, and E. Broussolle, Contributions of PET and SPECT to the understanding of the pathophysiology of Parkinson's disease. *Neurophysiol Clin.* **31,** 321–340 (2001).

W. Becker and J. Meller, The role of nuclear medicine in infection and inflammation, *Lancet Infect. Dis.* **1,** 326–333 (2001).

T. Inoue, N. Oriuchi, K. Tomigyoshi, and K. Endo, A shifting landscape: What will be next FDG in PET oncology? *Ann. Nucl. Med.* **16,** 1–9 (2002).

Specialized Journals

Clinical Positron Imaging

European Journal of Nuclear Medicine and Molecular Imaging

Journal of Nuclear Medicine

Journal of Nuclear Medicine Technology

Journal of Radioanalytical and Nuclear Chemistry

Nuklearmedizin [in German]

3

Ultrasonic Imaging

3.1. GENERAL PRINCIPLES OF ULTRASONIC IMAGING

Ultrasonic imaging is a noninvasive, easily portable, and relatively inexpensive diagnostic modality which finds extensive use in the clinic. Operating typically at frequencies between 1 and 10 MHz, it produces images via the backscattering of mechanical energy from boundaries between tissues and from small structures within tissue. Lower frequencies of 1–3 MHz are used for studies of deep-lying structures, such as the liver, and higher frequencies of 5–10 MHz for imaging regions closer to the body surface. In addition to obtaining anatomical information from images, ultrasound is also used widely to measure blood flow in vessels via a Doppler shift in the backscattered frequency from blood. This technique can be used, for example, to detect abnormalities arising from compromised blood flow in stenotic arteries. Ultrasonic imaging is an extremely fast technique, with real-time imaging capabilities using frame rates in excess of 30 per second. It also has high intrinsic spatial resolution, particularly at high frequencies, and involves no ionizing radiation. The weaknesses of the technique include the relatively poor soft-tissue contrast and the fact that gas and bone impede the passage of ultrasound waves, meaning that certain organs cannot easily be imaged. This latter consideration is often referred to as ultrasonic imaging having a limited "acoustic window." The major clinical applications of ultrasound include many aspects of obstetrics and gynecology involving the assessment of fetal health, acquiring electrocardiographs and the general assessment of heart function, intra-abdominal imaging of the liver, kidneys, gallbladder and spleen, many musculoskeletal applications, the detection of compromised blood flow in veins and arteries, and the tracking of needle biopsies.

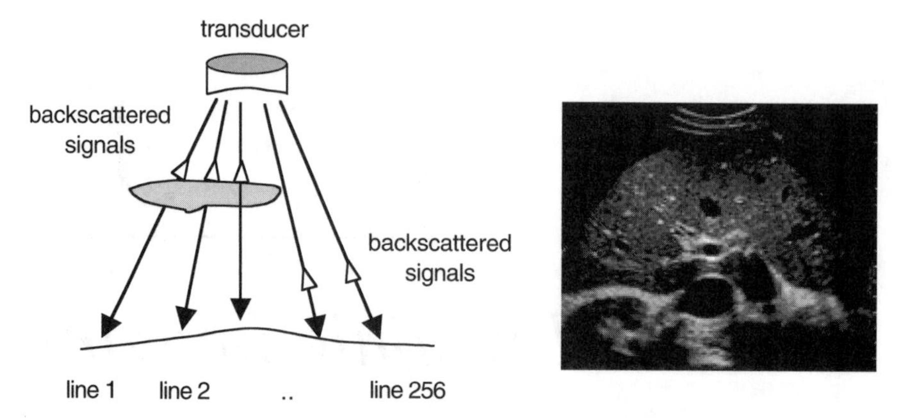

FIGURE 3.1. (Left) The basic principles of ultrasonic imaging. An ultrasound transducer transmits mechanical energy into the body. Part of the energy is backscattered from tissue boundaries and small structures and is detected by the transducer. By scanning through the body with a number of adjacent ultrasound beams, an image is formed. (Right) A two-dimensional image of the liver (©2000 ATL Ultrasound). The brightness of each pixel in the image is representive of the amount of energy backscattered at that point.

The basic principle of ultrasonic imaging is shown in Figure 3.1. A short pulse, typically 1–5 μs long, of energy is transmitted into the body using an ultrasound transducer. The transducer is focused to produce a narrow ultrasound beam, which propagates as a pressure wave through tissue at a speed of approximately 1540 m/s. The initial trajectory of this beam is represented by line 1 in Figure 3.1. When the ultrasound wave encounters tissue surfaces, boundaries between tissues, or structures within organs, a part of the energy of the pulse is scattered in all directions, with a certain fraction of the energy being backscattered along the original transmission path and returning to the transducer. As well as transmitting energy into tissue, the transducer also acts as the signal receiver, and converts the backscattered pressure waves into voltages, which, after amplification and filtering, are digitized. Using the measured time delay between pulse transmission and echo reception and the propagation velocity of 1540 m/s, one can estimate the depth of the feature. After all of the echoes have been received from the first beam trajectory, the direction of the beam is electronically steered to acquire a second line of data adjacent to the first. This process is repeated to acquire between 64 and 256 lines, typically, per image. The time required to acquire the echoes for each line is sufficiently short, on the order of 100–300 μs, depending on the required depth of view, that complete ultrasonic images can be acquired in tens of milliseconds, allowing dynamic imaging studies to be performed.

3.2. WAVE PROPAGATION AND CHARACTERISTIC ACOUSTIC IMPEDANCE

The contrast, the signal intensity, and the noise characteristics in an ultrasonic image are all determined by the propagation properties of ultrasound through tissue and the

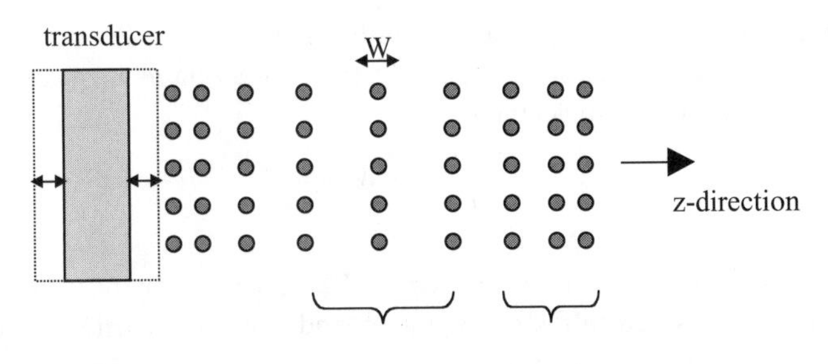

FIGURE 3.2. *Depiction of the processes involved in the transmission of an ultrasound wave through tissue.*

interactions that give rise to backscattered signals. Considerable insight into these processes can be gained by analyzing simple models of both tissue structure and the properties of the ultrasound wave, as outlined in this section.

A useful model of tissue is that of a lattice of small particles held together by elastic forces. Energy is coupled into the tissue using a transducer, which is assumed to expand and contract in thickness with a sinusoidal motion, as shown in Figure 3.2, at a frequency denoted by ω. As the ultrasound energy passes through the tissue, the particles move very short distances about a fixed mean position, whereas the ultrasonic energy propagates over much larger distances. The directions of particle vibration and wave propagation are the same in tissue, meaning that ultrasound can be classified as a longitudinal wave.

For the following analysis, it is assumed that the propagating wave has a planar wavefront, and that the tissue is perfectly homogeneous and does not attenuate the wave, that is, no energy is lost as the wave passes through tissue. The particle displacement W, shown in Figure 3.2, is related to the sound propagation velocity c by a second-order differential equation referred to as the one-dimensional, linearized, lossless wave equation for propagation of sound in fluids:

$$\frac{\partial^2 W}{\partial z^2} = \frac{1}{c^2}\frac{\partial^2 W}{\partial t^2} \tag{3.1}$$

The value of W is typically a few tenths of a nanometer. The value of c depends on the tissue density ρ and compressibility κ:

$$c = \frac{1}{\sqrt{\kappa\rho}} \tag{3.2}$$

The units of κ are $(\mathrm{Pa})^{-1}$, with the value of κ equal to the inverse of the bulk modulus of the tissue. The more rigid the tissue, the smaller is the value of κ, and therefore the greater is the velocity of the ultrasound wave within that tissue. This dependence of propagation velocity on tissue structural properties is potentially very useful for clinical diagnosis of, for example, a solid tumor mass surrounded by healthy, more compressible, tissue. The particle velocity in the z direction u_z is given by the time derivative of the particle displacement:

$$u_z = \frac{dW}{dt} \tag{3.3}$$

The value of u_z is typically 1–10 cm/sec, and is much lower than the value of c. The pressure p, measured in Pa, of the ultrasound wave at a particular point in the z direction is given by

$$p = \rho c u_z \tag{3.4}$$

Because the source undergoes sinusoidal motion, $p(t)$ and $u_z(t)$ can themselves be expressed as

$$\begin{aligned} p(t) &= p_0 e^{j\omega t} \\ u_z(t) &= u_0 e^{j\omega t} \end{aligned} \tag{3.5}$$

where p_0 and u_0 are the peak pressure and particle velocity, respectively. The propagating wave can be represented by a series of compression and rarefraction waves as shown in Figure 3.2. The intensity i of the ultrasound wave is defined as the amount of power carried by the wave per unit area, and can be expressed as the product of $p(t)$ and $u_z(t)$. The average intensity I, measured in watts/m^2, can be calculated by integrating $i(t)$ over the period T of one cycle of the ultrasound wave:

$$I = \frac{1}{T}\int_0^T p(t)u(t)\,dt = \frac{1}{2}p_0 u_0 \tag{3.6}$$

The value of the average intensity is an important measure because there are federal guidelines which limit the ultrasound intensity during a clinical scan. This subject is covered more fully in Section 3.12.

A particularly important parameter in ultrasonic imaging is the characteristic acoustic impedance Z of tissue, which is defined as the ratio of the pressure to the particle velocity:

$$Z = \frac{p}{u_z} \tag{3.7}$$

This equation can be considered as a direct analog to Ohm's law in electrical circuits, with the complementary physical constants being voltage/pressure, current/particle velocity, and resistance/characteristic impedance. The value of Z can also be expressed in terms of the physical properties of the tissue:

$$Z = \rho c = \rho \frac{1}{\sqrt{\rho\kappa}} = \sqrt{\frac{\rho}{\kappa}} \tag{3.8}$$

Table 3.1 lists values of Z for tissues relevant to clinical ultrasonic imaging.

TABLE 3.1. Acoustic Properties of Biological Tissues

	Characteristic Acoustic Impedance $\times 10^5$(g cm^{-2} s^{-1})	Speed of Sound (m s^{-1})
Air	0.0004	330
Blood	1.61	1550
Bone	7.8	3500
Fat	1.38	1450
Brain	1.58	1540
Muscle	1.7	1580
Vitreous humor (eye)	1.52	1520
Liver	1.65	1570
Kidney	1.62	1560

3.3. WAVE REFLECTION AND REFRACTION

Table 3.1 shows that soft tissues such as liver, kidney, and muscle have very similar values of Z, and that only air, that is, the lungs, and bone have acoustic properties that are significantly different. The relevance of the relative values of Z is outlined in Figure 3.3, which shows the interaction of an ultrasound wave with a boundary between two tissues with different acoustic impedances. The boundary is drawn as being flat, implying both that its dimensions are much greater than the ultrasound wavelength and also that any surface irregularities are much smaller than this wavelength. Under this condition, a certain fraction of the energy of the wave is reflected back toward the transducer, with the remaining fraction being transmitted through the boundary. It should be noted that the description of "reflection" is actually a special case of the general phenomenon of wave scattering, as described in more detail in Section 3.4.2.

In the simplest case, shown on the left of Figure 3.3, the angle between the incident wave and the boundary is 90°. The pressure reflection coefficient R_p, defined as the ratio of the pressures of the reflected (p_r) and incident (p_i) waves, is given by

$$R_p = \frac{p_r}{p_i} = \frac{Z_2 - Z_1}{Z_2 + Z_1} \tag{3.9}$$

The corresponding pressure transmission coefficient T_p, defined as the ratio of the pressures of the transmitted (p_t) and incident waves, can be calculated by applying two boundary conditions. First, the acoustic pressures on both sides of the boundary are equal, and second, the particle velocities normal to the boundary are equal. These conditions result in the relationship

$$T_p = R_p + 1 \tag{3.10}$$

and therefore

$$T_p = \frac{p_t}{p_i} = \frac{2Z_2}{Z_2 + Z_1} \tag{3.11}$$

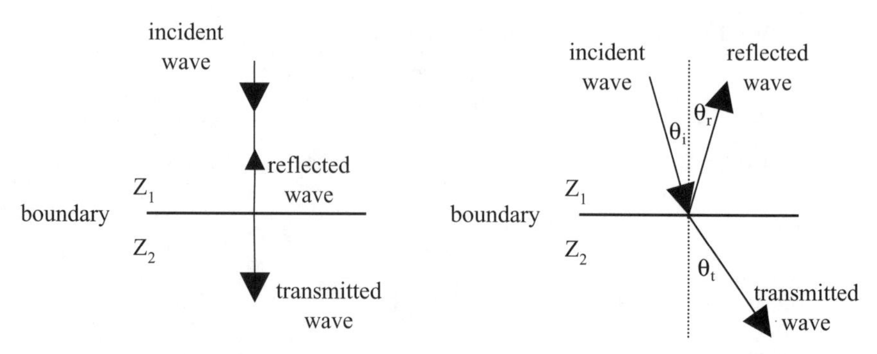

FIGURE 3.3. *The effect of a boundary between two tissues having acoustic impedances Z_1 and Z_2 on the propagation of an ultrasound wave. (Left) The incident wave is traveling at an angle of 90° with respect to the boundary and (right) the wave travels at an arbitrary angle $(90 - \theta_i)^\circ$ with respect to the boundary.*

If the ultrasound wave moves from a low to a high acoustic impedance, i.e., $Z_1 < Z_2$, then the reflected wave will undergo a 180° phase shift with respect to the incident wave.

The intensity reflection coefficient R_I and intensity transmission coefficient T_I are defined in terms of the intensity of the reflected (I_r), incident (I_i), and transmitted (I_t) waves:

$$R_I = \frac{I_r}{I_i} = R_p^2 = \frac{(Z_2 - Z_1)^2}{(Z_2 + Z_1)^2} \tag{3.12}$$

In this case, conservation of energy means that the two intensity coefficients are related by

$$T_I + R_I = 1 \tag{3.13}$$

and therefore

$$T_I = \frac{I_t}{I_i} = \frac{4Z_1Z_2}{(Z_1 + Z_2)^2} \tag{3.14}$$

Irrespective of whether the value of R_p or R_I is being considered, it is clear that the reflected signal detected by the transducer is maximized if the value of either Z_1 or Z_2 is zero. However, in this case, the ultrasound beam will not reach structures that lie deeper in the body. At an interface between bone and soft tissue, for example, a very large reflected signal, or "echo," results, making up approximately 40% of the incident intensity. This greatly attenuates the transmitted beam and makes imaging of structures behind bone extremely difficult. At a gas/soft tissue interface more than 99% of the intensity is reflected, making it impossible to scan through the lungs or gas in the bowel. At the other extreme, if Z_1 and Z_2 are equal in value, then no signal is detected from the boundary. Using values of Z in Table 3.1, it can be determined that, at boundaries between soft tissues, the intensity of the reflected wave is typically less than 0.1% of that of the incident wave.

In the case where the angle between the incident beam and boundary is not 90°, as shown on the right-hand side of Figure 3.3, the equations governing the angles of reflection and transmission are given by

$$\theta_\mathrm{i} = \theta_\mathrm{r} \tag{3.15}$$

$$\frac{\sin\theta_\mathrm{i}}{\sin\theta_\mathrm{t}} = \frac{c_1}{c_2} \tag{3.16}$$

where c_1 and c_2 are the speed of sound in tissues 1 and 2, respectively. If the values of c_1 and c_2 are not equal, then the transmitted signal is refracted. This angular deviation from the original direction of propagation can cause misregistration artifacts in the image (Section 3.7). The pressure and intensity reflection and transmission coefficients are given by

$$R_\mathrm{p} = \frac{p_\mathrm{r}}{p_\mathrm{i}} = \frac{Z_2\cos\theta_\mathrm{i} - Z_1\cos\theta_\mathrm{t}}{Z_2\cos\theta_\mathrm{i} + Z_1\cos\theta_\mathrm{t}} \tag{3.17}$$

$$T_\mathrm{p} = \frac{p_\mathrm{t}}{p_\mathrm{i}} = \frac{2Z_2\cos\theta_\mathrm{i}}{Z_2\cos\theta_\mathrm{i} + Z_1\cos\theta_\mathrm{t}} \tag{3.18}$$

$$R_\mathrm{I} = \frac{I_\mathrm{r}}{I_\mathrm{i}} = \frac{(Z_2\cos\theta_\mathrm{i} - Z_1\cos\theta_\mathrm{t})^2}{(Z_2\cos\theta_\mathrm{i} + Z_1\cos\theta_\mathrm{t})^2} \tag{3.19}$$

$$T_\mathrm{I} = \frac{I_\mathrm{t}}{I_\mathrm{i}} = \frac{4Z_2Z_1\cos^2\theta_\mathrm{i}}{(Z_2\cos\theta_\mathrm{i} + Z_1\cos\theta_\mathrm{t})^2} \tag{3.20}$$

3.4. ENERGY LOSS MECHANISMS IN TISSUE

In addition to reflection from tissue boundaries, there are a number of other mechanisms by which the ultrasound beam loses energy as it propagates through tissue. The two most important of these mechanisms are absorption of energy via tissue relaxation, and scattering of the ultrasound beam. The combination of these two mechanisms, together with reflection and refraction covered in the previous section, is referred to as ultrasonic attenuation.

3.4.1. Absorption

Absorption losses refer to the conversion of ultrasound mechanical energy into heat. There are two major mechanisms involved in this process: classical absorption and relaxation. The phenomenon of classical absorption occurs due to friction between particles as they are displaced by the passage of the ultrasound wave. This loss is characterized by an absorption coefficient, β_class. The value of β_class is proportional to the square of the frequency of the ultrasound wave:

$$\beta_{\text{class}} = Af^2 \tag{3.21}$$

where A is a constant containing a number of quantities including the coefficient of viscosity, the coefficient of shear viscosity, and the thermal conductivity.

The second absorption mechanism is termed "relaxation." Tissue can be characterized by a relaxation time τ, which is the time taken for a molecule to return to its original position after having been displaced by the ultrasound wave. For example, in Figure 3.2, compression of the particles corresponds to the passage of the positive half of the pressure wave, which forces the particles together. If the relaxation time of the molecule is of the same order as the period of the ultrasound wave, then at the time of the next positive pressure maximum the relaxation mechanism is acting to return the particles to their equilibrium separation. Thus, the actions of the pressure wave and relaxation mechanism are exactly opposite to one another. Intuitively, then, the maximum absorption of energy from the wave occurs when these two motions are exactly 180° out of phase. A useful analogy is that of pushing a swing: the minimum energy required occurs when the swing is stationary at its maximum height, and the maximum energy corresponds to pushing it in the opposite direction to its travel, which occurs when it is at its minimum height. The relaxation process is characterized by a relaxation absorption coefficient β_{r}. The frequency dependence of β_{r} is shown in Figure 3.4 and is given by

$$\beta_{\text{r}} = \frac{B_0 f^2}{1 + (f/f_{\text{R}})^2} \tag{3.22}$$

Tissue, being inhomogeneous in nature, consists of a broad range of values of τ and f_{R}. The total absorption coefficient β can be written as the sum of the classical and

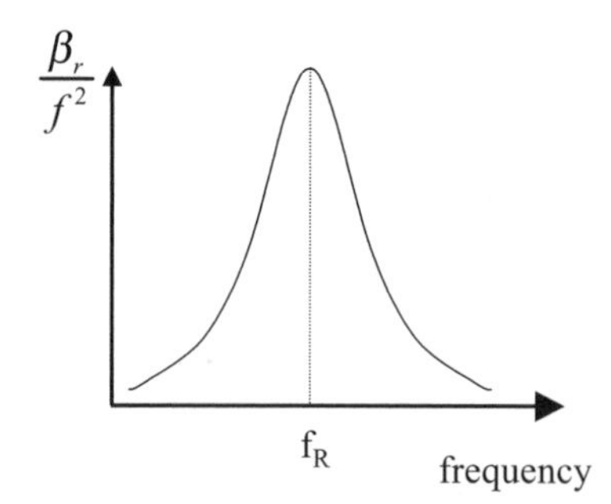

FIGURE 3.4. *The frequency dependence of the relaxation absorption coefficient β_{r}. The maximum occurs at a value $f_{\text{R}} = (2\pi\tau)^{-1}$.*

relaxation components:

$$\beta = \beta_{\text{class}} + \beta_{\text{r}} = Af^2 + \sum_n \frac{B_0 f^2}{1 + (f/f_{\text{R}})^2} \tag{3.23}$$

Measured values of absorption in many tissues have shown that there is an almost linear relationship between the total absorption coefficient and ultrasound operating frequency.

3.4.2. Scattering

As outlined in Section 3.3, reflection and refraction of the ultrasound beam occur at boundaries where the dimensions of the surfaces are large compared to the wavelength of the ultrasound beam. If the beam encounters tissue surface irregularities or particles within tissue that are the same size as or smaller than the ultrasound wavelength, then the wave is scattered in many directions. The angular dependence and the magnitude of the scattering are dependent upon the shape, the size, and the physical and acoustic properties (e.g., characteristic impedance, compressibility, density) of the scatterer. The scattering process is characterized in terms of a scattering cross section σ_{s}, which is defined as the power scattered per unit incident intensity. Scattering is extremely complicated, and there is no exact mathematical expression for the value of σ_{s} for an arbitrary scatterer geometry. However, for particles that are much smaller than the ultrasound wavelength, an approximate expression is given by

$$\sigma_{\text{s}} = \frac{64\pi^5}{9\lambda^4} r^6 \left[\left| \frac{\kappa_{\text{s}} - \kappa}{\kappa} \right|^2 + \frac{1}{3} \left| \frac{3(\rho_{\text{s}} - \rho)}{2\rho_{\text{s}} + \rho} \right|^2 \right] \tag{3.24}$$

where κ_{s} is the adiabatic compressibility of the scatterer and κ is that of the surrounding tissue, ρ_{s} is the density of the scatterer and ρ is that of the tissue, and r is the radius of the scatterer.

If the size of the scattering body is small compared to the wavelength, then scattering is relatively uniform in direction, with slightly more energy being scattered toward the transducer than away from it. This case is termed Rayleigh scattering, and is exemplified by the interaction of ultrasound with red blood cells, which have diameters on the order of 7 μm. This interaction forms the basis for ultrasonic Doppler blood velocity measurements, which are covered in Section 3.10. In this size regime, the value of σ_{s} increases as the fourth power of frequency. As the size of the particles increases to the same order of magnitude as the wavelength, as, for example, in liver, scattering becomes highly complex and is not well-defined.

3.4.3. Attenuation

Attenuation of the ultrasound beam as it propagates through tissue is the sum of the scattering and the absorption processes. Attenuation is characterized by an exponential decrease in both the pressure and the intensity of the ultrasound beam as a function of its propagation distance z:

$$\begin{aligned} I(z) &= I(z=0)\ \exp(-\mu z) \\ p(z) &= p(z=0)\ \exp(-\alpha z) \end{aligned} \tag{3.25}$$

where μ is the intensity attenuation coefficient and α the pressure attenuation coefficient, both measured in units of cm^{-1}, with μ being equal to 2α. The value of μ is often stated in units of decibels (dB) per cm, where the conversion factor between the two units is given by

$$\mu(\text{dB cm}^{-1}) = -\frac{1}{z} 10 \log \frac{I(z)}{I(z=0)} = 4.343\mu(\text{cm}^{-1}) \tag{3.26}$$

On the dB, logarithmic scale, the two coefficients μ and α become interchangeable:

$$\alpha(\text{dB cm}^{-1}) = -\frac{1}{z} 20 \log \frac{p(z)}{p(z=0)} = 8.686\alpha(\text{cm}^{-1}) = \mu(\text{dB cm}^{-1})$$

As seen previously, the processes of absorption and scattering are strongly dependent on frequency, and therefore one would expect the values of μ and α to be likewise. Somewhat surprisingly, given the complexity of the frequency dependence of the different mechanisms and the overall inhomogeneity of tissue, there is an approximately linear relationship between attenuation coefficient (in dB cm^{-1}) and frequency for most tissues. A typical attenuation coefficient for soft tissue is 1 dB cm^{-1} MHz^{-1}, that is, for an ultrasound beam at 3 MHz, the attenuation coefficient is 3 dB cm^{-1}. For fat there is a different frequency dependence, with the attenuation coefficient being given by approximately $0.7f^{1.5}$ dB cm^{-1}. The values of the attenuation coefficient for air and bone are much higher, 45 and 8.7 dB cm^{-1}, respectively, at a frequency of 1 MHz.

3.5. INSTRUMENTATION

The instrumentation for ultrasonic imaging consists of a transducer, either single-crystal or, much more commonly, an array of crystals, detection electronics, which includes modules for time-gain compensation and beam forming, and computers for data processing, image display, and data storage. In ultrasonic imaging the transducer acts both as a transmitter and a signal receiver. In transmission mode it converts an oscillating voltage applied from a power source into mechanical vibrations, which are transmitted as a series of pressure waves into the body. Signal reception is essentially exactly the reverse process of transmission, in which the backscattered pressure waves are converted into electrical signals. These are amplified, digitized, and processed to form the ultrasonic image.

3.5.1. Single-Crystal Transducers

A schematic diagram and a photograph of a transducer are shown in Figure 3.5. The critical component in the process of signal transduction from an applied electrical voltage into mechanical vibration, and vice versa, is a piezoelectric crystal. When an alternating voltage is applied across opposite surfaces of a crystal of piezoelectric material, the thickness of the crystal oscillates at the same frequency as the driving voltage, with the change in thickness being proportional to the magnitude and polarity of this voltage. The most common piezoelectric material used for ultrasound transducers is lead zirconate titanate (PZT). Many versions of this composite have been used in transducers. The two faces of the crystal are coated with a thin layer of silver and connected electrically. A plastic matching layer is added to the external face of the crystal to provide acoustic coupling between the crystal and the patient and also to protect the surface of the crystal.

The piezoelectric crystal is most commonly engineered into a disk, which either has a flat (plane-piston transducer) or concave (focused transducer) surface. The crystal has a natural resonant frequency f_0 given by

$$f_0 = \frac{c_{\text{crystal}}}{2d} \tag{3.27}$$

where c_{crystal} is the speed of sound in the crystal and d is its thickness. There are also resonant frequencies at the odd harmonics of f_0, that is, $3f_0$, $5f_0$, $7f_0$, etc. If the diameter of the crystal is much larger than its thickness, then longitudinal ultrasound waves are transmitted into the body. The speed of sound in a PZT crystal is

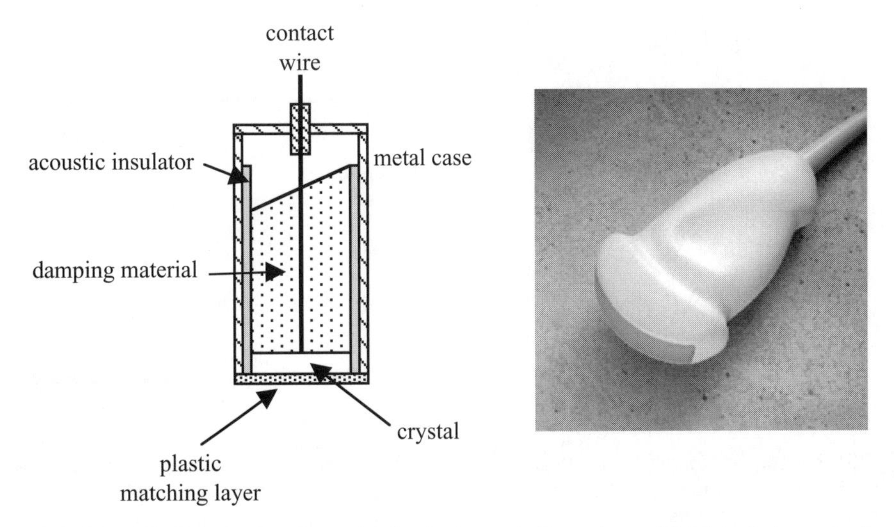

FIGURE 3.5. *(Left) A simple schematic of a single-crystal transducer. (Right) A photograph of a commercial transducer (©2000 ATL Ultrasound).*

roughly 4000 ms^{-1}, which translates into a thickness of 1.3 mm at a fundamental frequency of 1.5 MHz.

The other important component of the transducer is the damping material, typically an epoxy substrate impregnated with metal powder, which absorbs energy from the vibrating transducer. With the exception of continuous wave Doppler measurements (Section 3.10.2), ultrasonic imaging uses a series of pulses of ultrasound, which are produced by gating the voltage applied to the face of the crystal on and off. At the end of each voltage pulse, the crystal returns to a resting state, but in doing so, internal vibrational modes are set up. These modes result in a finite "ring-down time" before the crystal physically comes to rest. Since the mechanical vibrations of the crystal produce the ultrasound pressure wave, the pulse of ultrasound transmitted into the body is actually longer than the applied voltage pulse. If there is close coupling between an efficient damping material and the crystal, the length of the ultrasound pulse will be minimized. The scaling property of the Fourier transform, outlined in Appendix A, shows that efficient mechanical damping results in ultrasound waves being transmitted into the body with a broad range of frequencies, as shown in Figure 3.6. The bandwidth

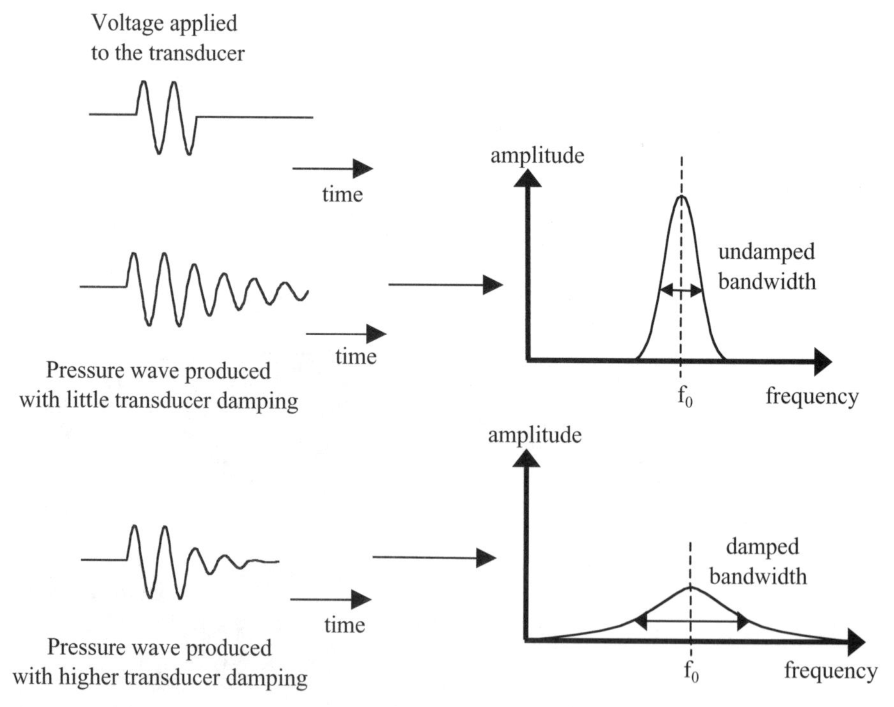

FIGURE 3.6. Time-domain and frequency-domain characteristics of damped transducers. A short pulse of alternating voltage is applied to the face of the crystal. With little mechanical damping, the crystal oscillates for a long time, producing a very sharp frequency spectrum with low bandwidth and high Q. With heavy damping, the crystal oscillations die out quickly, producing a much shorter pulse in the time domain and much broader bandwidth in the frequency domain.

(BW) of a transducer is usually stated at the 3-dB level, that is, the value of the BW is the difference between the frequencies at which the amplitude of the beam drops to 50% of its peak value. Alternatively, the quality factor Q of the transducer is often specified, where

$$Q = \frac{2\pi f_0}{\text{BW}} \tag{3.28}$$

Typical Q values for well-damped transducers are between 1 and 2. As will be covered in Section 3.5.1.3, the spatial resolution in the axial direction is proportional to the length of the ultrasound pulse, with a shorter pulse giving a better axial resolution. The number of "ring-down" cycles for a crystal is essentially independent of the resonant frequency of the crystal, and so higher ultrasound frequencies give shorter ring-down times and improved axial resolution. In addition to good axial spatial resolution, a large transducer bandwidth has advantages for harmonic and subharmonic imaging, which are covered in Section 3.11. The disadvantage of a low Q value is that, as shown in Figure 3.6, the ultrasound beam contains less energy at the fundamental frequency f_0.

The characteristic acoustic impedance of PZT is about 15 times that of skin or tissue, and so placing the piezoelectric crystal directly against the patient would result in a large amount of the energy being reflected back from the boundary. In order to maximize energy transfer into the body, it can be shown mathematically (Exercise 3.4) that a matching layer of material with an acoustic impedance Z_{ML} should be placed between the crystal (Z_c) and skin (Z_s), where Z_{ML} is given by

$$Z_{\text{ML}} = \sqrt{Z_c Z_s} \tag{3.29}$$

The thickness of this matching layer should be one-fourth of the ultrasound wavelength, again to maximize energy transmission through the layer in both directions (Exercise 3.7).

In order to overcome the problem of the characteristic acoustic impedance mismatch between PZT and the body, plastics such as polyvinyldifluoride (PVDF) are used in some transducers. These compounds have a value of Z much closer to that of water and can be made into thin, flexible sheets.

3.5.1.1. The Beam Geometry of a Single Transducer. The simplest transducer, termed a plane-piston, is one in which the piezoelectric crystal has a flat face. The properties of the transmitted ultrasound wave can be modeled by considering the transducer to be made up of a large number of point sources, each of which emits a spherical wave. The total pressure wave is a superposition of each of these individual components. If wave propagation is in the z direction, then the on-axis, or axial, intensity $I(z)$ of the wave is given by

$$I(z) \approx 2\rho c u_z^2 \sin^2\left[\frac{\pi}{2}\left(\frac{a^2/\lambda}{z}\right)\right] \tag{3.30}$$

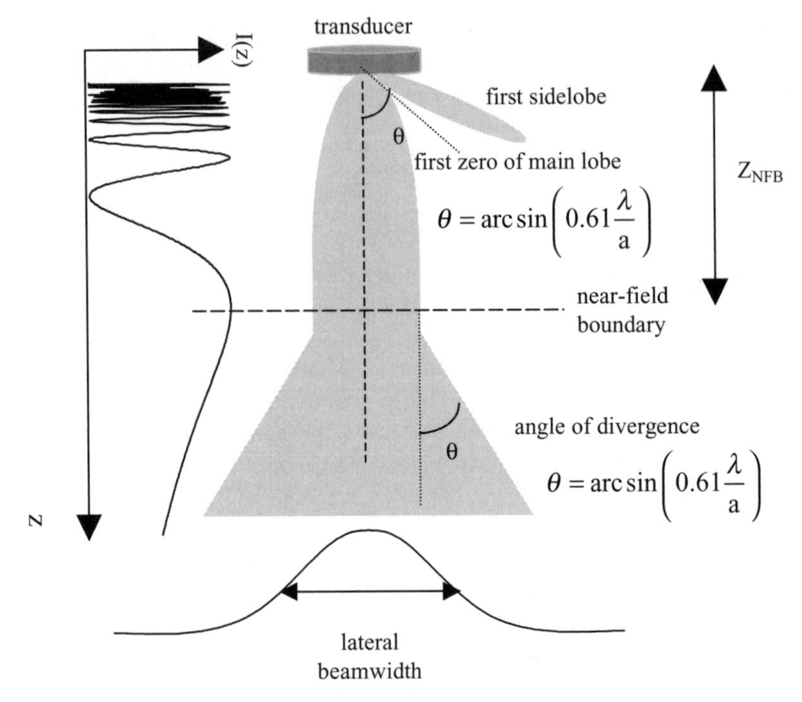

FIGURE 3.7. *A schematic diagram showing the axial and the lateral beam shapes from a single-crystal transducer. Also shown are the first side lobes of the main beam.*

where a is the radius of the crystal. A plot of $I(z)$ versus z is shown in Figure 3.7. The wavefront very close to the transducer face is extremely complicated. The last intensity (or pressure) maximum occurs at the so-called "near-field boundary" (NFB), also referred to as the "last axial maximum." Axial positions closer to the transducer than the NFB are referred to as being in the near-field, or Fresnel, zone, whereas those beyond the NFB comprise the far-field, or Fraunhofer, zone. The position of the NFB is given by

$$Z_{\text{NFB}} \approx \frac{a^2}{\lambda} \tag{3.31}$$

At the NFB, the field has a lateral beam width which is similar to the diameter of the transducer. Beyond the NFB, the beam diverges in the lateral direction and the axial intensity of the ultrasound beam decreases smoothly. In the far-field zone, the ultrasound wavefront can be well-approximated as planar.

In addition to the main beam, side lobes may also be present due to the transducer acting as a diffraction grating. These side lobes are undesirable because they remove energy from the main beam, and can also introduce artifacts into an image. The magnitude and the number of side lobes depend upon the ratio of the ultrasound wavelength to the transducer diameter. The greater this ratio, the fewer is the number of side lobes, but also the closer the NFB lies to the face of the transducer.

This simple model of the ultrasound beam strictly applies to continuous wave (CW) ultrasound, rather than pulsed ultrasound. However, the results are still useful because the general features of the beam geometry in pulsed ultrasound are very similar to those in CW ultrasound. The major difference is that the axial intensity profiles for pulsed ultrasound are not as sharp or as complex as for the CW case.

3.5.1.2. *Lateral Resolution and Depth of Focus.* A cross section of the ultrasound beam in the far-field region in Figure 3.7 shows that the lateral beamwidth can be well-approximated by a Gaussian function. The FWHM of this function is given by

$$\mathrm{FWHM} = 2\sqrt{2\ln 2}\sigma \cong 2.36\sigma \tag{3.32}$$

where σ is the standard deviation of the Gaussian function. The value of the FWHM of the beam determines the lateral resolution of the ultrasound image. As discussed in Section 5.2.2, two features in the object being imaged are just distinguishable when the separation between them in the lateral direction is equal to the FWHM of the beam. If two backscatterers are positioned closer than the FWHM of the beam, then they produce echoes in the received signal that are superimposed, as shown in Figure 3.8. The FWHM for a particular transducer at a certain depth can be measured experimentally by moving a small reflector across the ultrasound beam and measuring the intensity of the reflected signal as a function of the lateral position of the scatterer.

Because a single-crystal transducer typically has a diameter of between 1 and 5 cm, the intrinsic lateral resolution is very poor. Therefore, some form of beam focusing is normally used. Either a concave lens, usually constructed of plastic, can be placed in front of the crystal, or else the face of the crystal itself can be manufactured in a curved form.

The advantage of using a lens to focus is that lenses of different focusing powers can be used with a single transducer for many different applications. The lens is machined from a material in which the ultrasound propagation velocity is slower than that in tissue. The wavefront emanating from the lens does not conform exactly to the curvature of the lens, and its geometry can be calculated by considering the relative phase shifts that occur for each small element of the wavefront as it passes through the lens. The curvature of the lens is characterized by the aperture, or *f*-number, analogous to an optical lens used in photography. The *f*-number ($f\#$) is defined as

$$f\# = \frac{R}{2a} \tag{3.33}$$

where R is the radius of curvature and a is the radius of the lens. The focal distance F is defined as the distance, measured from the face of the transducer, at which the lateral beam width is narrowest. The plane perpendicular to the beam axis at this distance is called the focal plane, as shown in Figure 3.9. The value of F is related to

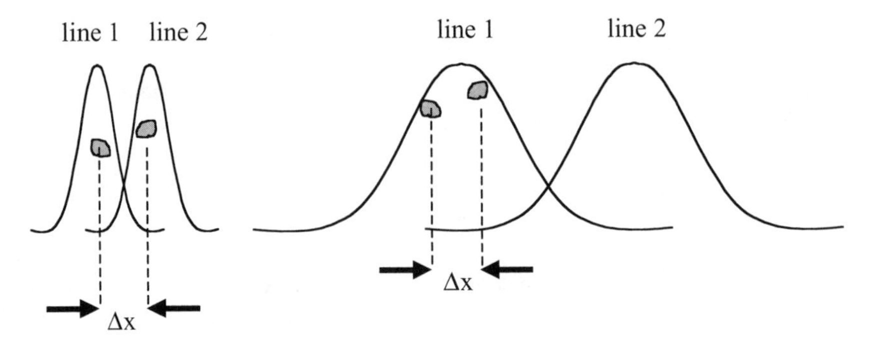

FIGURE 3.8. *The definition of the lateral resolution in terms of the FWHM of the ultrasound beamwidth. (Left) The separation between the two shaded objects Δx is less than the FWHM of the beam. In this case separate echoes are recorded from the two objects, and they can be resolved. (Right) If the beamwidth is wider, then the two objects cannot be resolved because the backscattered echoes from each object are superimposed.*

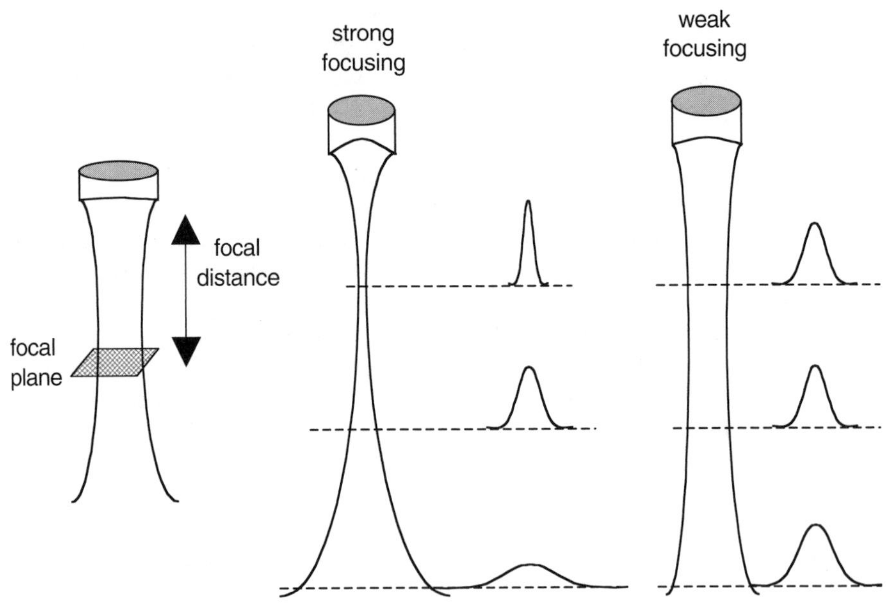

FIGURE 3.9. *(Left) A schematic showing the focal distance and the focal plane of a focused transducer. (Center) A diagram showing the variation in lateral beamwidth as a function of axial distance for a strongly focused transducer. (Right) As for the central diagram, except with a weakly focused transducer.*

that of R by

$$F \approx \frac{R}{1 - 1/f\#} \tag{3.34}$$

Equation (3.34) shows that the focal distance is slightly larger than the radius of curvature of the lens. A transducer is normally referred to as being strongly ($R <$ NFB/4), medium (NFB/4 $< R <$ NFB/2), or weakly ($R >$ NFB/2) focusing.

For a spherical focusing lens, the FWHM at the focal point is given by

$$\text{FWHM} \approx \frac{1.1\lambda R}{2a} \tag{3.35}$$

For a fixed-diameter crystal, therefore, decreasing the radius of curvature will improve the lateral resolution. For a fixed value of the radius of curvature, a larger-diameter crystal has the same effect. The dependence of the FWHM on the ultrasound wavelength arises because the value of the angle θ at which the first side lobe occurs becomes smaller as λ decreases. Therefore, the main beam becomes narrower at these smaller values of the ultrasound wavelength.

The disadvantage of a strongly focused transducer is clear: at locations away from the focal plane the beam diverges much more sharply than for transducers that are focused more weakly. The lateral resolution, therefore, is much poorer away from the focal plane. The on-axis depth of focus (DOF) for a particular transducer is defined to be the distance over which a standard reflector produces an echo reduced in intensity by 50% from that at the focal point. The value of the DOF is given by

$$\text{DOF} = 15\left(1 - 0.01 \sin^{-1} \frac{a}{R}\right) \cdot \text{FWHM} \tag{3.36}$$

By considering equations (3.35) and (3.36), it is clear that a compromise has to be made between lateral resolution and depth of focus. Typical numbers for these parameters at clinical operating frequencies are shown in Table 3.2.

All of the calculations of the values of FWHM and DOF assume a single value of ultrasound wavelength/frequency. As seen previously in Figure 3.6, however, the transducer transmits a broad range of frequencies, and the frequency distribution

TABLE 3.2. Focusing Properties of Various Transducers at 1.5 and 5 MHz

Frequency (MHz)	λ In Tissue (mm)	*R* (cm)	*a* (cm)	*f*-Number	FWHM (mm)	DOF (mm)
1.5	1.0	2	1	1	1.1	11.9
1.5	1.0	3	1	1.5	1.7	20.5
1.5	1.0	5	1	2.5	2.8	37.5
1.5	1.0	10	1	5	5.6	79.8
5	0.31	2	2	1	0.3	3.6
5	0.31	3	2	1.5	0.5	6.1
5	0.31	5	2	2.5	0.8	11.2
5	0.31	10	2	5	1.7	24.0

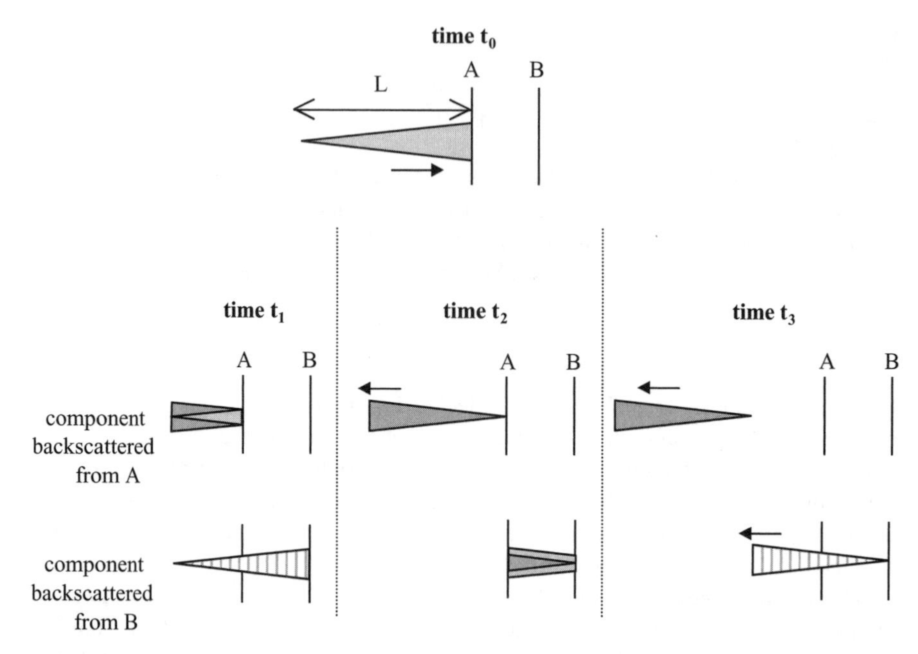

FIGURE 3.10. *An illustration of the principle by which the axial resolution is given by one-half the length of the ultrasound pulse. The damped pulse transmitted from the transducer is represented by the triangle. (Top) At time t_0 the leading edge of the pulse encounters boundary A. A component of the wave is backscattered, with the remaining fraction being transmitted through the boundary. (Bottom) The behavior of the backscattered and transmitted waves at three equally spaced time points: $(t_1 - t_0)$ corresponds to a value given by half the pulse length divided by the speed of sound, $(t_2 - t_1) = (t_1 - t_0)$, and $(t_3 - t_2) = (t_1 - t_0)$. The two waves backscattered from boundaries A and B do not overlap, and thus can be resolved.*

changes as the wave propagates through tissue, with higher frequencies being attenuated more. Therefore, the lateral resolution of an ultrasound image also depends upon the attenuation properties of the tissue through which the beam is passing.

3.5.1.3. Axial Resolution. The spatial resolution along the axis of the transducer is defined as the closest separation, in the direction of the propagating ultrasound wave, of two scatterers that results in resolvable backscattered signals. Figure 3.10 depicts an ultrasound pulse encountering two reflecting boundaries separated by a distance one-half the length of the transmitted ultrasound pulse. This distance was chosen because it is, in fact, the axial resolution, which can be expressed as

$$\text{axial resolution} = \frac{1}{2}(\text{PD})c \tag{3.37}$$

where PD is the pulse duration (in units of seconds). As the ultrasound frequency increases, the pulse length decreases, and so the axial resolution gets better. Typical values of axial resolution are 1.5 mm at a frequency of 1 MHz and 0.3 mm at 5 MHz. The axial resolution can be improved by increasing the degree of transducer damping or using higher operating frequencies. In the latter case, however, attenuation of the ultrasound beam in tissue increases.

3.5.2. Transducer Arrays

There are several problems with using a single crystal for ultrasonic imaging. These include the need for either manual or mechanical steering of the beam to produce a two-dimensional image, the tradeoff between lateral resolution and depth of focus, and the relatively large distance from the face of the transducer to the NFB. One way to circumvent these limitations is to use an array of small piezoelectric crystals, and nowadays almost all commercial imaging transducers consist of such arrays. An array of crystals allows electronic steering of the beam and enables the position of the focal point to be changed easily. During signal reception, dynamic beam forming, covered in Section 3.5.3, can be used to optimize the lateral resolution continuously at different depths. The disadvantage of arrays is the added physical complexity: each piezoelectric element needs to be decoupled electrically from all the other elements, and also connected to separate impedance matching circuits via thin cabling. In addition, the discrete nature of the individual elements of the array results in grating lobes, similar to those produced by an optical diffraction grating.

There are three basic types of array, linear sequential, linear phased, and annular, described in turn in the next sections.

3.5.2.1. Linear Sequential Arrays. A linear sequential array consists of a large number, typically 64–512, of rectangular piezoelectric crystals, each having a width of the order of the ultrasound wavelength. Each crystal is unfocused and physically and electrically isolated from its neighbors. As shown in Figure 3.11, a planar wavefront can be produced by sending a voltage pulse simultaneously to a number of elements, in this case the first three. The width of the ultrasound beam is determined by the number of elements that are excited. After the backscattered echo is received, a second voltage pulse is applied to the second, third, and fourth elements, producing a planar wavefront with a focal point displaced laterally with respect to the first line. The sequential excitation of three separate elements is continued until all such groups have been excited. Then the process can be repeated using simultaneous excitation of an even number of elements, in this case four, which produces focal points at locations between those acquired previously. In this fashion, almost twice as many scan lines as there are transducer elements can be formed. An image is produced with a rectangular FOV, as shown in Figure 3.11. These types of array are used particularly when a large FOV is required close to the surface of the array. The linear sequential array is essentially an unfocused device and, if required, focusing can be introduced by designing a curved array or adding a cylindrical lens.

As mentioned previously, because the array consists of a regularly spaced matrix of individual elements, substantial grating lobes are present. For a rectangular element, the angle ϕ_g with respect to the main beam at which these occur is given by

$$\phi_g = \arcsin\left(\frac{n\lambda}{g}\right) \tag{3.38}$$

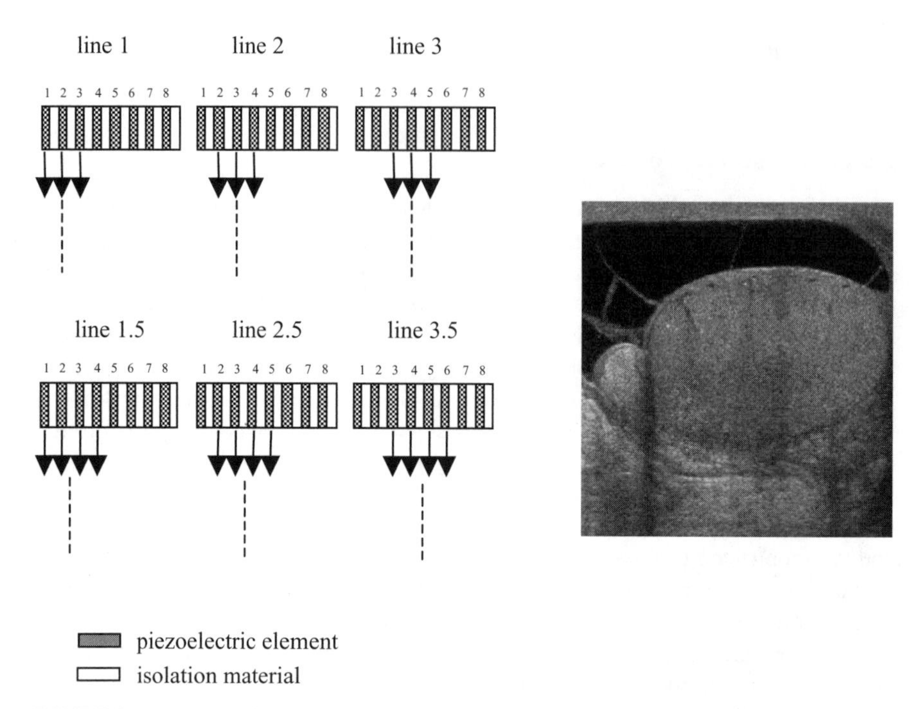

FIGURE 3.11. *(Left) Formation of a rectangular FOV image using a linear sequential array. The dashed line represents the center of the beam. Almost twice the number of image lines as there are transducer elements can be produced. (Right) An image of an enlarged, abnormal testicle obtained using a linear sequential array (©2000 ATL Ultrasound).*

where g is the gap between the elements and $n = \pm 1, \pm 2, \pm 3$, etc. In addition to the grating lobes, there are the normal side lobes (from both the main lobe and grating lobes), and the angle at which the main beam intensity first reaches zero is given by

$$\theta = \arcsin\left(\frac{\lambda}{w}\right) \tag{3.39}$$

where w is the width of the array. The magnitude of the grating lobes can be reduced by introducing small random variations into the spacing between adjacent elements of the array. Alternatively, the spacing between elements can be made so small that the value of ϕ_g is close to 90°, and the first grating lobe falls close to the edge of the FOV of the image.

3.5.2.2. Linear Phased Arrays. The physical layout of a linear phased array is very similar to that of a linear sequential array, but the mode of operation is quite different. In a phased array, a much larger number of elements is excited for each line of the image, rather than just a small subset as for a sequential array. The voltage pulses exciting each element of a phased array are delayed in time with respect to

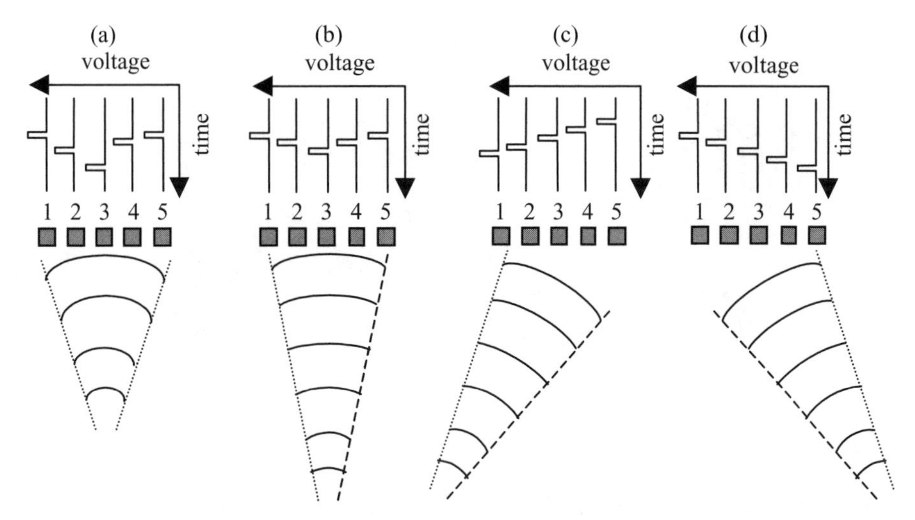

FIGURE 3.12. *An illustration of the operation of a linear phased array transducer. (a) Voltage pulses are applied simultaneously to elements 1 and 5; after a time delay the same pulses are applied to elements 2 and 4, and after a second time delay a voltage pulse is applied to element 3. This sequence of pulses produces a curved wavefront, with a focal distance governed by the values of the time delays. (b) A reduction in the value of the time delays produces a larger focal distance. (c, d) Asymmetric time delays, with respect to the individual elements of the array, are used for beam steering.*

each other, to produce a curved wavefront, similar to that produced by a focused single-crystal transducer. At the focal point, the ultrasound waves from each of the individual elements in the array are all in phase, and so add constructively. Figure 3.12 shows how a simple five-element phased array can be used to steer the ultrasound beam electronically, and also to change the value of the focal distance. Because the individual elements of the array are smaller than the ultrasound wavelength, the focal point lies well beyond the NFB for each of the individual elements of the array, and so the geometry of the wavefront is well-characterized.

The thickness of each crystal is governed by the speed of sound in the particular piezoelectric material and the operational frequency of the transducer array [equation (3.27)]. The elements are usually of rectangular geometry, with a width of one-fourth the ultrasound wavelength or less. The width of each element should be at least 10 times its thickness for the ultrasound to be produced via the desired "thickness" mode. The length of each element defines the "slice thickness" of the image in the third ("elevation") dimension, and is typically between 2 and 5 mm.

A process termed "dynamic focusing" or "dynamic aperture" can be used to optimize the lateral resolution over the entire depth of tissue being imaged. Using a small number of elements to transmit the beam produces a focal point close to the transducer surface. At larger depths, the number of elements necessary to achieve the best lateral resolution increases. Therefore, the number of elements excited is increased dynamically during transmission of the ultrasound beam.

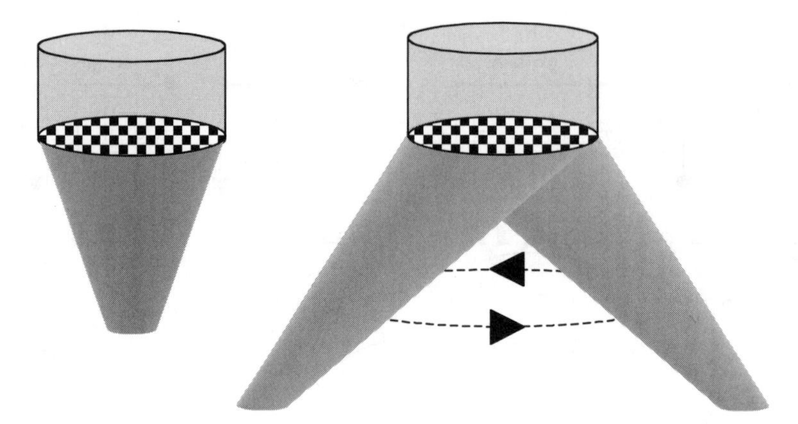

FIGURE 3.13. The operation of a two-dimensional array. The black squares represent the individual crystals in the array. (Left) Two-dimensional focusing can be achieved using appropriate time delays applied symmetrically with respect to the individual elements of the array. (Right) Electronic beam steering can be performed in two dimensions.

3.5.2.3. Multidimensional Arrays. A one-dimensional phased array can only focus and steer in the lateral dimension. Increasing the dimensionality of the array by adding extra rows of crystals allows focusing in the elevation dimension. If a small number of rows is added, typically 3–10, then the array is called a 1.5-dimensional array, and limited focusing in the second direction can be achieved. If a large number of rows is added, up to a value equal to the number of elements in each row, then this geometry constitutes a true two-dimensional array. Representations of such an array, two-dimensional focusing, and two-dimensional steering are all shown in Figure 3.13.

3.5.2.4. Annular Arrays. The third type of array is termed an annular array, and is shown schematically in Figure 3.14. This type of array provides two-dimensional lateral focusing, but the beam cannot be steered, and so the transducer must be moved either mechanically or manually to form an image.

3.5.3. Beam Forming and Time–Gain Compensation

The successive components of the receiving system after the transducer include variable-time-delay elements for beam forming, a time–gain compensation unit, logarithmic compression amplifiers, A/D converters, and finally data storage and display.

Much of the recent improvement in ultrasound image quality has resulted from the introduction of digital beam-forming. Using a phased array transducer, the effective focal length and the aperture of the transducer can be changed dynamically while the signal is being acquired, a process termed beam forming. This process is essentially the reverse of that of dynamic focusing during signal transmission, described in Section 3.5.2.2. During the time required for the backscattered echoes to return, incremental delays are introduced to the voltages recorded by each element of the

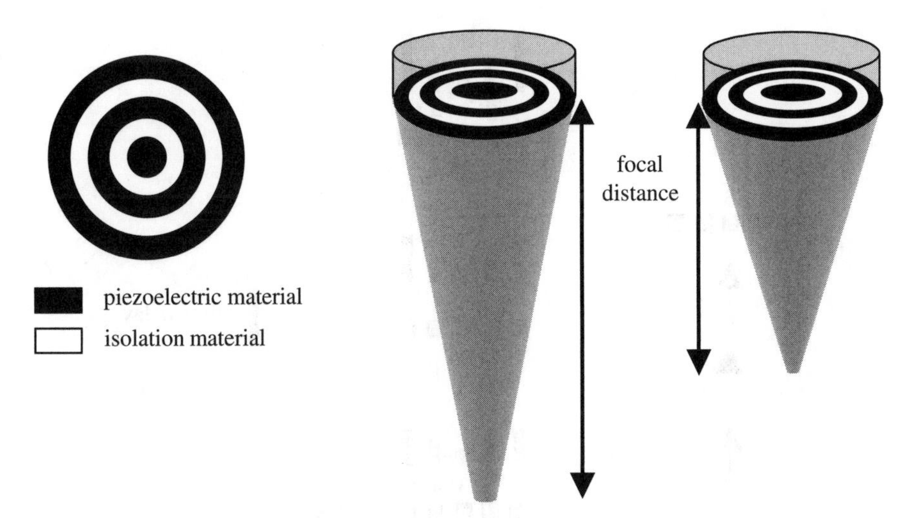

FIGURE 3.14. *(Left) A side view of an annular array transducer. (Right) Two-dimensional lateral focusing can be performed using an annular array, but the focal point always lies along the principal axis of the beam.*

transducer before the signals are passed to the time–gain compensation unit. These delays result in each backscattered signal effectively being "in focus," as shown in Figure 3.15.

The voltages corresponding to the backscattered echoes have a large range of amplitudes: very strong signals appear from reflectors close to the transducer and very weak signals from low concentrations of scatterers deep within the body. The total range of signal amplitudes may be as high as 80–100 dB. Radiofrequency (RF) amplifiers typically cannot amplify signals with a dynamic range greater than about 40–50 dB with a linear gain. Nonlinear amplification would result in the signals from the weaker echoes being attenuated severely. The solution to this problem is to use time–gain compensation (TGC) of the acquired signals, a process in which the amplification factor is increased as a function of time. Signals arising from structures close to the transducer are therefore amplified by a smaller factor than those from greater depths. Various linear or nonlinear functions of gain versus time can be used, and these functions can be chosen on-line by the operator. The net effect of TGC is to compress the dynamic range of the backscattered echoes, as shown in Figure 3.16.

After TGC, the signals pass through a logarithmic compression amplifier, which further reduces the dynamic range to 20–30 dB. Older systems demodulated the signal to very low frequencies before digitization, but recent advances in digital receivers allow direct digitization of the signal at the fundamental frequency, giving a higher image SNR. Dynamic receiver filtering, a process in which there is a progressive reduction in the receiver frequency bandwidth as a function of time after pulse transmission, can also be used. Since the high-frequency content of the backscattered signal decreases with depth due to the greater attenuation in tissue at higher

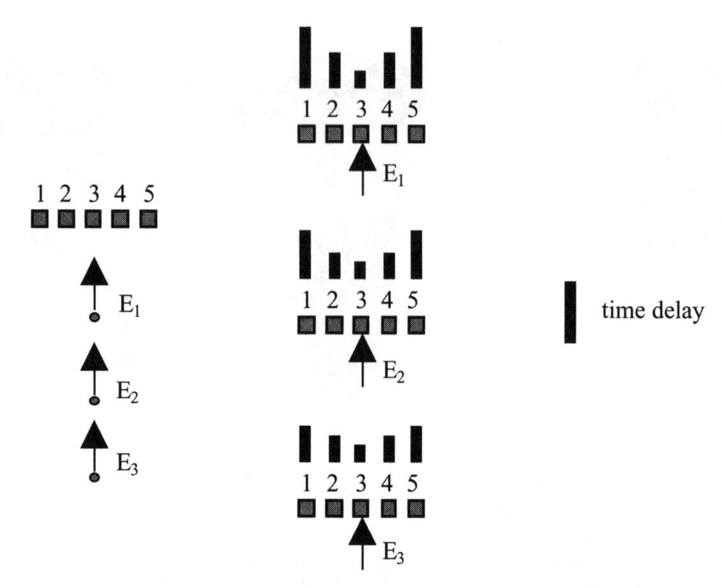

FIGURE 3.15. *The process of dynamic beam forming. (Left) Three backscattered ultrasound waves E_1, E_2, and E_3 arrive at the transducer at surface different times. (Top right) As the first echo (E_1) reaches the transducer, time delays for the voltages from elements 1–5 are introduced to produce the best lateral resolution at the depth at which E_1 was formed. (center and bottom right) Values of the time delays are dynamically varied to optimize the lateral resolution for echoes E_2 and E_3.*

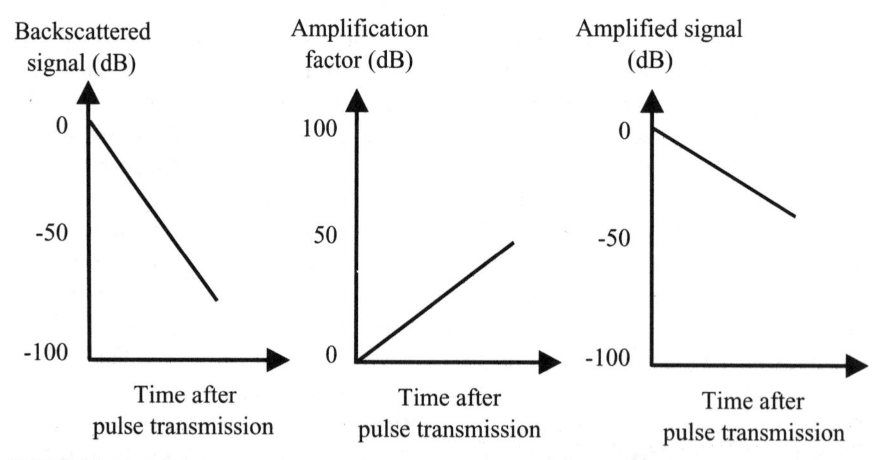

FIGURE 3.16. *The principle of time–gain compensation. (Left) The dynamic range of backscattered echoes is larger than can be amplified linearly. (Center) A time-dependent amplification factor is applied to the backscattered echoes. (Right) The dynamic range of the amplified signals has been reduced to a level appropriate for further processing.*

frequencies, the receiver bandwidth can be reduced accordingly. This results in an improved SNR in the image because the noise level is proportional to the square root of the receiver bandwidth. After the signal has been digitized, it can be processed via envelope detection, edge detection, or whichever algorithm is appropriate for the particular application, and then displayed as a gray-scale image.

3.6. DIAGNOSTIC SCANNING MODES

There are three basic modes of diagnostic "anatomical imaging" using ultrasound: A-mode, M-mode, and B-mode scanning. Depending upon the particular clinical application, one or more of these modes may be used. Recent technical advances include the use of compound imaging and three-dimensional imaging, which are also described in this section. The use of ultrasound to measure blood flow is covered in Section 3.10.

3.6.1. A-Mode, M-Mode, and B-Mode Scans

Amplitude (A)-mode scanning refers to the acquisition of a one-dimensional scan. An A-mode scan simply plots the amplitude of the backscattered echo versus the time after transmission of the ultrasound pulse. Some detectors use the unrectified, rather than rectified, digitized signal because the leading edge is better defined. A-mode scanning is used most often in opthalmology to determine the relative distance between different regions of the eye, and can be used, for example, to detect corneal detachment. High-frequency (>10 MHz) ultrasound is used to produce very high axial resolution. Tissue attenuation, even at this high frequency, is not problematic because the dimensions of the eye are so small.

A motion (M)-mode scan provides information on tissue movement within the body, and essentially displays a continuous series of A-mode scans. The brightness of the displayed signal is proportional to the amplitude of the backscattered echo, with a continuous time ramp being applied to the horizontal axis of the display, as shown in Figure 3.17. The maximum time resolution of the M-mode scan is dictated by how long it takes for the echoes from the deepest tissue to return to the transducer. M-mode scanning is used most commonly to detect motion of the heart valves and heart wall in echocardiography.

Brightness (B)-mode scanning produces a two-dimensional image, such as shown in Figure 3.1, through a cross section of tissue. Each line in the image consists of an A-mode scan with the brightness of the signal being proportional to the amplitude of the backscattered echo. B-mode scanning can be used to study both stationary and moving structures, such as the heart, because complete images can be acquired very rapidly. For example, in the case of an image with a 10-cm depth-of-view, it takes 130 μs after transmission of the ultrasound pulse for the most distant echo to return to the transducer. If the image consists of 120 lines, then the total time to acquire one frame is 15.6 ms and the frame rate is 64 Hz. If the depth-of-view is increased, then the number of lines must be reduced in order to maintain the same frame rate.

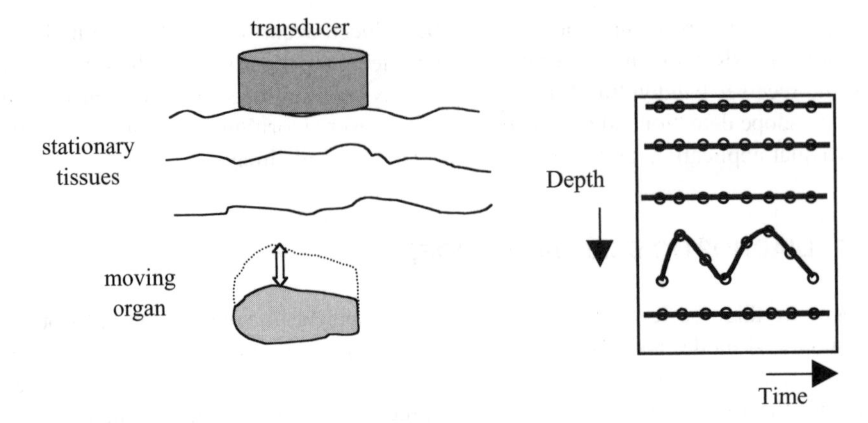

FIGURE 3.17. A schematic of M-mode ultrasound scanning. (Left) A transducer is placed over the area of interest, which consists of several stationary tissues and one that is moving periodically. (Right) The M-mode scan comprises a time series of A-mode scans, allowing the degree of movement of the individual tissues to be seen.

3.6.2. Three-Dimensional Imaging

As with all imaging techniques, the advantages of three-dimensional data acquisition are based on the ability to view a given image volume in a number of different planes. This extra information gives more accurate measures of, for example, tumor volume or tissue malformations. Small pathologies are also more likely to be visualized using three-dimensional volume reconstructions than from two-dimensional scans. Currently, three-dimensional ultrasound scans are produced by mechanically or manually scanning a phased-array transducer in a direction perpendicular to the plane of each B-mode scan. The advent of true two-dimensional phased arrays, as described in Section 3.5.2.3, should significantly improve three-dimensional imaging,

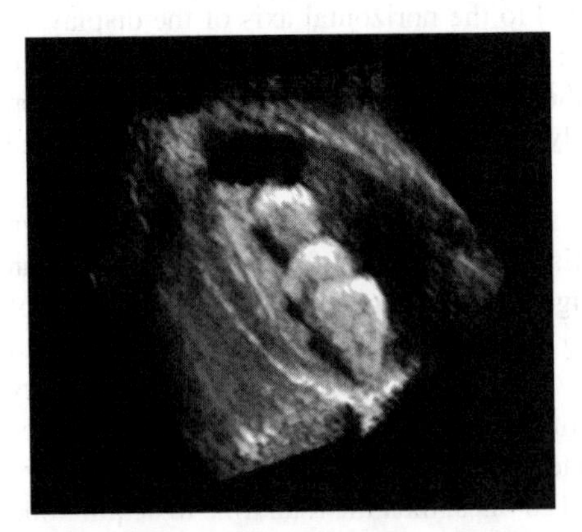

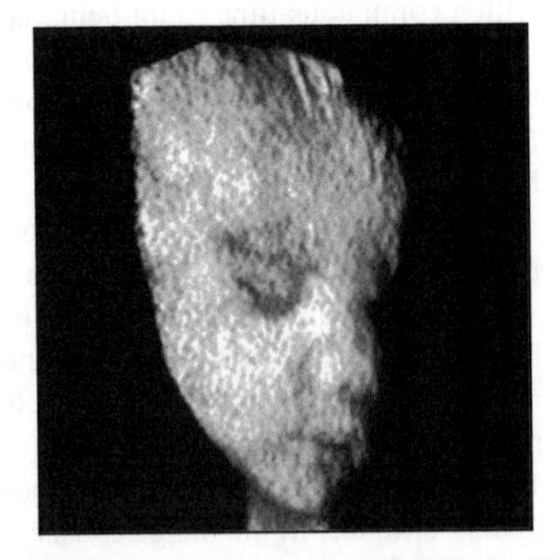

FIGURE 3.18. (Left) A three-dimensional abdominal ultrasonic scan showing individual gall stones. (Right) A three-dimensional image of a fetal head in utero (©2000 ATL Ultrasound).

increasing data acquisition speed and enabling isotropic spatial resolution to be achieved. Although still in its infancy, three-dimensional ultrasonic imaging already has shown promise in several clinical applications including estimation of the dimensions of cardiac valves, the study of fetal and uterine malformations, and the detection of pancreatic, hepatobiliary, and endorectal tumors. Examples of three-dimensional images are shown in Figure 3.18.

3.7. ARTIFACTS IN ULTRASONIC IMAGING

Image artifacts, in which spatial features present in the image do not accurately represent the physical structure of the tissue, can arise from a number of sources. Such artifacts must be recognized to avoid incorrect image interpretation, but once recognized can, in fact, give useful diagnostic information. Image artifacts considered here include the effects of reverberation, acoustic enhancement or shadowing, and refraction.

Reverberations occur if there is a very strong reflector close to the transducer surface. Multiple reflections occur between the surface of the transducer and the reflector, and these reflections appear as a series of repeating lines in the image, as shown on the left of Figure 3.19. These artifacts are relatively simple to detect due to the equidistant nature of the lines. Typically, they occur when ultrasound interacts with either bone or air.

Acoustic shadowing occurs when either a very strong reflector such as a gas/tissue boundary or a highly attenuating medium "shadows" a deeper-lying organ. Acoustic shadowing results in a dark area or "hole" in the image, as shown on the right of Figure 3.19. The opposite phenomenon, known as acoustic enhancement, occurs when a region of low attenuation is present within an otherwise homogeneous medium.

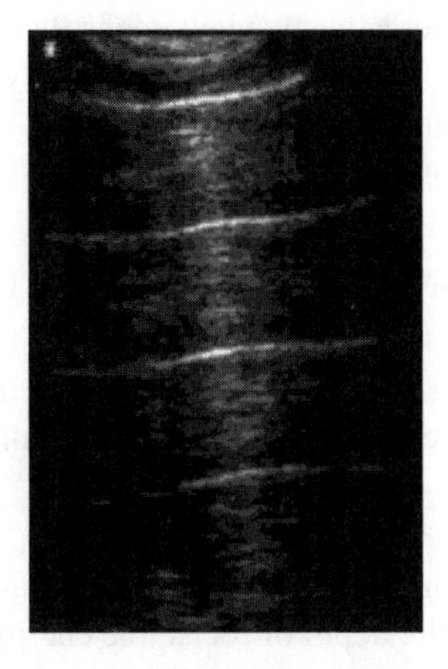

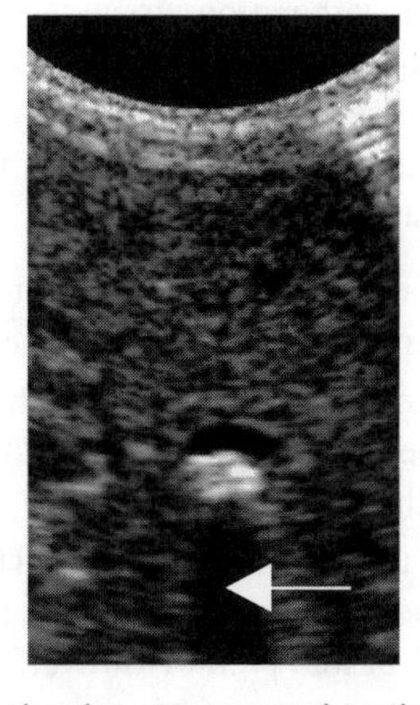

FIGURE 3.19. *(Left) An ultrasonic image of the lung showing strong reverberation artifacts. (Right) An image showing acoustic shadowing (arrow) behind a strongly reflecting gall stone.*

Clinical examples of tissues with low attenuation coefficients are cysts, vessels, and fluid-filled organs such as the gallbladder. The areas behind such tissues have higher than expected intensity, which is a useful diagnostic tool for differentiating between fluid-filled cysts and solid masses, for example tumors in breast imaging, as described in Section 3.13.2.

The refraction of ultrasound at a boundary between two tissues with different characteristic acoustic impedances has already been described (Section 3.3). Refraction is most troublesome at a bone/soft tissue interface, where large angular deviations of up to 20° in the direction of the transmitted wave can occur. At interfaces between different soft tissues the refraction angle is only 1–2° and hence is not very important except when extremely precise measurements of distance are required as, for example, in the eye.

3.8. IMAGE CHARACTERISTICS

Since almost all of the factors that affect the image SNR, spatial resolution, and CNR have been introduced, the following sections represent a brief summary.

3.8.1. Signal-to-Noise Ratio

The noise in ultrasound images has three components. The first arises from the electronics of the detection system. Provided that the backscattered signal has a high enough amplitude and is amplified by a sufficient factor, the contribution of this noise source can be minimized. The second source, speckle, corresponds to coherent wave interference in tissue. Speckle gives a granular appearance to what should appear as a homogeneous tissue, as seen on the right in Figure 3.19. The small particles which give rise to the scattered signal are too small to be visualized directly, but the pattern produced on the ultrasound image is characteristic of particular size distributions. The final term, "clutter," is applied to signal arising from side lobes, grating lobes, multipath reverberation, tissue motion, and other acoustic phenomena that add noise to the ultrasound image. The clutter strength can be reduced significantly by using harmonic imaging methods, covered in Section 3.11.

As outlined in previous sections, the signal intensity of the backscattered ultrasound signals is affected by:

1. The intensity of the ultrasound pulse transmitted by the transducer: The higher the intensity, the higher is the amplitude of the detected signals.
2. The operating frequency of the transducer: The higher the frequency, the greater is the tissue attenuation, and therefore the lower is the SNR, especially at large depths within the body.
3. The type of focusing used: The stronger the focusing at a particular point, the higher is the energy per unit area of the ultrasound wave, and the higher is the SNR at that point. However, outside of the depth of focus, the energy per unit area is very low, as is the image SNR.

4. The degree of transducer damping: The lower the amount of damping, the higher is the intensity of the transmitted pulse at the fundamental frequency of the transducer and the higher is the SNR.

3.8.2. Spatial Resolution

Factors affecting the spatial resolution have also been described in detail and include:

1. The degree of focusing: The stronger the focusing, the higher is the spatial resolution at the focal spot. Using the techniques of dynamic focusing and beam forming with phased array transducers, one can minimize the depth dependence of the lateral resolution.
2. The length of the transmitted ultrasound pulse: The longer the pulse, the poorer is the axial resolution of the image. The pulse length is determined by the degree of damping of the transducer and the operating frequency of the transducer. The higher the degree of damping, or the higher the operating frequency, the shorter is the pulse and the better is the axial resolution.

3.8.3. Contrast-to-Noise Ratio

Factors that affect the SNR also contribute to the image CNR. Noise sources such as clutter and speckle reduce the image CNR, especially for small pathologies within tissue. Although compound imaging can reduce the contribution from speckle, the greatest improvements in the CNR are obtained by using ultrasound contrast agents, tissue harmonic imaging, and pulse inversion techniques, all of which are covered in Section 3.11.

3.9. COMPOUND IMAGING

Compound imaging, also called sonoCT, uses a phased array transducer to acquire multiple coplanar B-mode images at different angles, as shown in Figure 3.20, and combines these multiple views into a single compound image. The effects of speckle and clutter are reduced considerably by the combination of views from different angles because backscattered echoes from each scan add coherently, whereas speckle and clutter only add in a partially coherent manner. The improved SNR of the compound image results in improved visualization of internal structures, enabling, for example, detection of small lesions and calcifications. The greatest improvement in image SNR occurs in the center of the image, where the greatest number of lines overlap. The effects of acoustic shadowing or enhancement are also reduced, but not eliminated. In cases where these artifacts are actually useful diagnostically, the imaging mode can be switched between compound scanning and simple B-mode scanning. An example of a compound image, showing very high SNR, is shown in Figure 3.20.

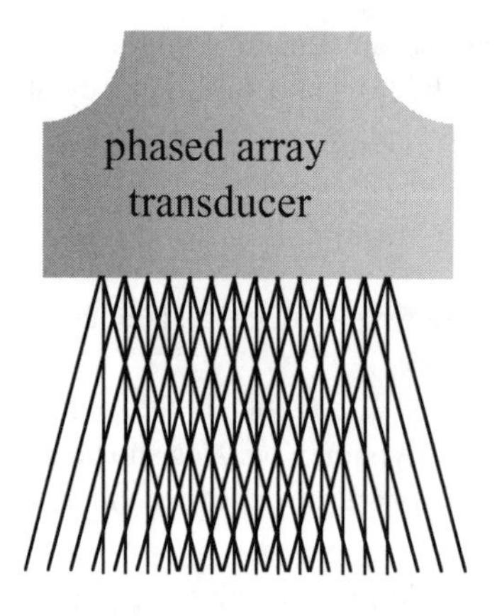

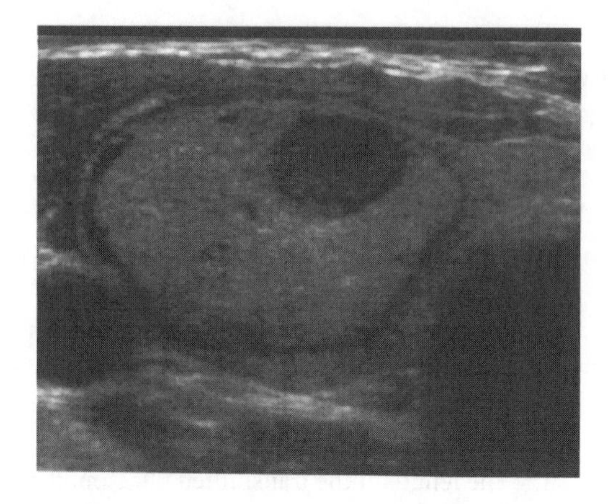

FIGURE 3.20. (Left) An illustration of the intersecting lines used in compound imaging. (Right) A compound image, formed from nine separate scans, of an abnormal thyroid (©2000 ATL Ultrasound).

3.10. BLOOD VELOCITY MEASUREMENTS USING ULTRASOUND

Noninvasive, localized blood velocity measurements are vital in the diagnosis of a number of diseases, and ultrasound is used extensively for this purpose. For example, blood velocity profiles change in areas of stenosis or narrowing of the arteries, conditions which can lead ultimately to cardiac arrest. Children at risk of stroke often display cerebral blood velocities up to three or four times greater than normal, due to lumenal narrowing. Two ultrasound techniques are used to estimate blood velocity: those based on measuring Doppler shifts and those involving time-domain signal correlation. A number of variations on each technique exist: for example, Doppler-based methods can be carried out in CW mode, pulsed mode, or duplex imaging mode, in which acquisition of two-dimensional blood velocity maps is interlaced with high-resolution B-mode scanning.

3.10.1. The Doppler Effect

The Doppler effect is familiar as, for example, the higher pitch of an ambulance siren as it approaches the observer than when it has passed. Similarly, blood flow, either toward or away from the transducer, alters the frequency of the backscattered echoes, as shown in Figure 3.21. Because blood contains a high proportion of red blood cells (RBC), which have a diameter of 7–10 μm, the interaction between ultrasound and blood is a scattering process, as described in Section 3.4.2. The wavelength of the ultrasound is much greater than the dimensions of the scatterer and therefore the wave is scattered in all directions. This means that the backscattered, Doppler-shifted signals have low signal intensities. The signal intensity is proportional to the fourth power of the ultrasound frequency, and so higher operating frequencies are often used for blood velocity measurements.

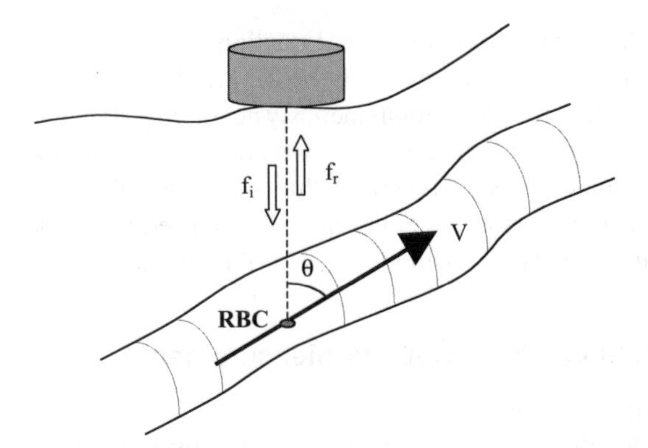

FIGURE 3.21. *An illustration of the Doppler shift in flowing blood. The RBCs scattering the ultrasound beam are traveling at velocity v. Here f_i is the ultrasound frequency transmitted by the transducer and f_r is the frequency of the backscattered echo. The difference in these frequencies is the measured Doppler shift.*

Using the parameters defined in Figure 3.21, the component of the velocity of the RBCs toward the transducer is given by $v \cos\theta$. The "apparent" frequency f_{RBC} of the transmitted ultrasound beam, as seen by the RBC, is given by

$$f_{\mathrm{RBC}} = \frac{c + v\cos\theta}{\lambda} \tag{3.40}$$

The wavelength of the ultrasound is independent of the velocity of the RBC:

$$\lambda = \frac{c}{f_{\mathrm{i}}} \tag{3.41}$$

Therefore the frequency shift Δf_{RBC} due to the Doppler effect can be calculated as

$$\Delta f_{\mathrm{RBC}} = f_{\mathrm{RBC}} - f_{\mathrm{i}} = \frac{f_{\mathrm{i}} v \cos\theta}{c} \tag{3.42}$$

Because the transmission and backscattered paths must both be considered, the overall Doppler shift Δf of the received signal is given by

$$\Delta f = f_{\mathrm{i}} - f_{\mathrm{r}} = \frac{2 f_{\mathrm{i}} v \cos\theta}{c} \tag{3.43}$$

Equation (3.43) shows that the Doppler frequency shift is linearly proportional to the blood velocity. Using values of $f_{\mathrm{i}} = 5$ MHz, $\theta = 45°$, and $v = 50\,\mathrm{cm\,s^{-1}}$ gives a Doppler shift of 2.26 kHz, a frequency within the audio range. The fractional change in frequency $\Delta f / f_{\mathrm{i}}$ is extremely small, in this case less than 0.05%. The Doppler shift can be increased by using higher ultrasound frequencies, but in this case the maximum depth at which vessels can be measured decreases due to increased attenuation of the beam at the higher operating frequencies. Equation (3.43) also shows that an accurate measurement of blood velocity can only be achieved if the angle θ is known. This angle is usually estimated from simultaneously acquired B-mode scans using "duplex imaging" described in Section 3.10.4. A fixed error in the value of θ has the smallest effect when θ is small, and so in practice values of θ of less than 60° are used. Doppler measurements can be performed either in CW or pulsed mode, depending upon the particular application. These methods are described in the next two sections.

3.10.2. Continuous Wave Doppler Measurements

CW Doppler measurements are used when there is no need to localize exactly the source of the Doppler shifts. A continuous pulse of ultrasound is transmitted by one transducer and the backscattered signal is detected by a second one: usually both transducers are housed in the same physical structure. The transducers are fabricated with only a small degree of mechanical damping in order to increase the intensity of the signal transmitted at the fundamental frequency f_0. The region of overlap of the sensitive regions of the two transducers defines the area in which blood flow is detected. This area is often quite large, and problems in interpretation can occur when there is more than one blood vessel within this region. The measured blood velocity is the average value over the entire sensitive region. The advantages of CW Doppler over pulsed Doppler methods, in which exact localization *is* possible, are that the method is neither limited to a maximum depth nor to a maximum measurable velocity. These limitations of the pulsed techniques are covered in Section 3.10.3.

As outlined in the previous section, the Doppler shift is calculated by comparing the frequencies of the transmitted and the received ultrasound waves. This is achieved in practice using the hardware configurations shown in Figure 3.22. The oscillator used

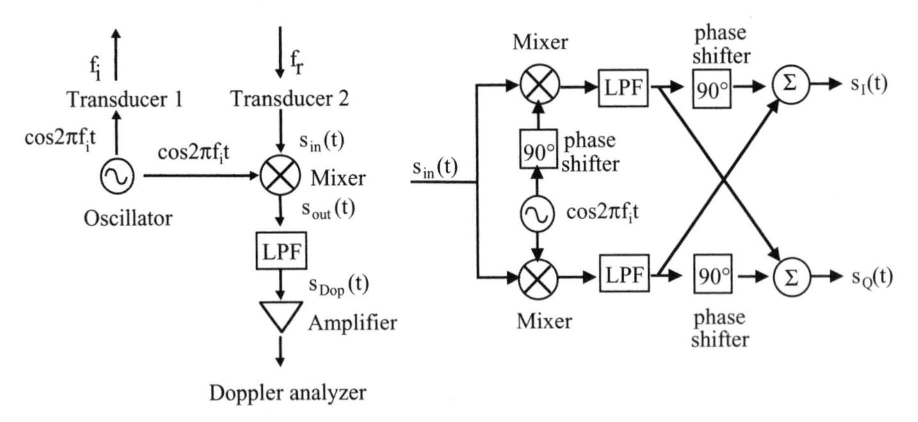

FIGURE 3.22. *(Left) A schematic of a homodyne demodulator used to extract the Doppler frequency in CW measurements. After mixing the received voltage $s_{in}(t)$ with the oscillator voltage, the output signal $s_{out}(t)$ is passed through a low-pass filter (LPF) and amplified. (Right) A schematic of a heterodyne demodulator which can be used to resolve directional ambiguity in the CW Doppler signal.*

to transmit the ultrasound wave from the first transducer is also used to "demodulate" the received signal from the second. The simplest "homodyne" demodulation scheme is shown on the left of Figure 3.22.

The signal detected by the second transducer can be represented as

$$s_{\text{in}}(t) = A\cos[2\pi(f_{\text{i}} + \Delta f)t] \tag{3.44}$$

where A is the amplitude of the backscattered signal and Δf is the Doppler shift (in this case assumed to be positive). After amplification (not shown in Figure 3.22), the signal is mixed with the output of the oscillator used to excite the first transducer. The mixer effectively multiplies the two signals together, and so the output $s_{\text{out}}(t)$ is given by

$$s_{\text{out}}(t) = A\cos[2\pi(f_{\text{i}} + \Delta f)t]\cos(2\pi f_{\text{i}}t) \tag{3.45}$$

Using trigonometric identities, we can re express this as

$$s_{\text{out}}(t) = \frac{1}{2}A\{\cos[2\pi(2f_{\text{i}} + \Delta f)t] + \cos(2\pi\Delta f t)\} \tag{3.46}$$

This signal then passes through a low-pass filter with a cutoff frequency f_{co} given by $\Delta f \ll f_{\text{co}} \ll f_{\text{i}}$. The ouput from this filter $s_{\text{Dop}}(t)$ is

$$s_{\text{Dop}}(t) = \frac{1}{2}A\cos(2\pi\Delta f t) \tag{3.47}$$

Finally, the signal passes through a high-pass filter to remove high-intensity reflected signals from the relatively slow movement of vessel walls during the cardiac cycle. Typical values for the cutoff frequency of the high-pass filter are 50–1000 Hz. The final signal is amplified, digitized, and stored. Fourier transformation of the time-domain signal gives the frequency spectrum, corresponding to the range of blood velocities. CW Doppler measurements are usually displayed as a time series of spectral Doppler plots, as shown in Figure 3.23.

One problem with the homodyne detector, shown on the left of Figure 3.22, is that there is a directional ambiguity in the output signal. Suppose that, instead of blood flowing toward the transducer as in the analysis above, the velocity has the same magnitude, but the flow is away from the transducer. The positive Doppler shift $+\Delta f$ in equation (3.44) is replaced by $-\Delta f$, and the demodulated signal is given by

$$s_{\text{Dop}}(t) = \frac{1}{2}A\cos(-2\pi\Delta f t) \tag{3.48}$$

However, because $\cos(x) = \cos(-x)$, equations (3.47) and (3.48) are equivalent, and there is no way to determine whether blood is flowing toward or away from the transducer.

In order to resolve this ambiguity, a more sophisticated form of demodulation, called quadrature or heterodyne detection, is needed, as shown on the right of

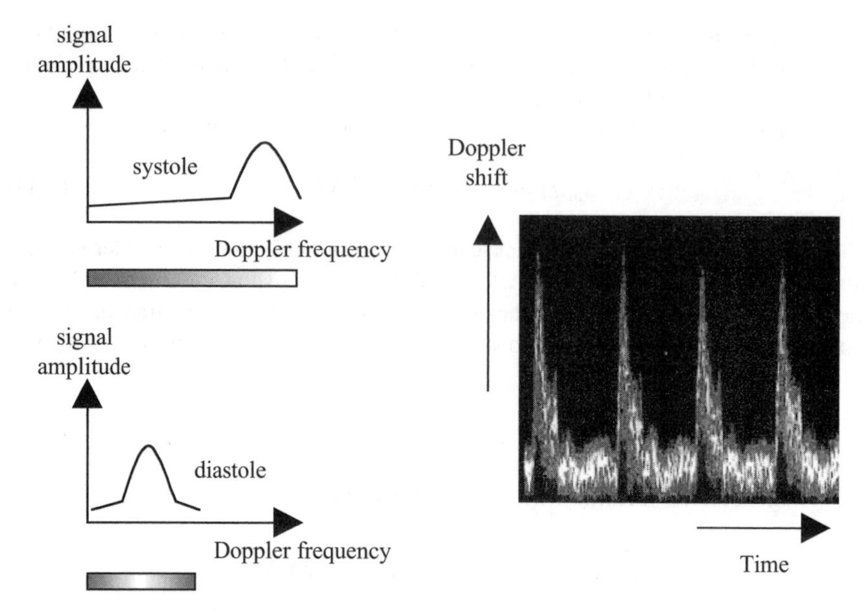

FIGURE 3.23. Spectral Doppler shifts from an area encompassing the carotid artery. Large frequency shifts, corresponding to high blood flow rates, are measured during the systolic part of the heart cycle (top left), with lower frequency shifts measured during diastole (bottom left). At each time point, the two-dimensional amplitude versus Doppler frequency graphs are reduced to a single "spectral dimension," with the length of the "bar" representing the total range of frequencies present and the color representing the amplitude at each frequency (gray to white representing low to high amplitudes, respectively). (Right) A two-dimensional display of spectral Doppler plots (vertical axis) as a function of time over several cardiac cycles.

Figure 3.22. In the case of a positive Doppler shift, the outputs of the heterodyne receiver are $s_{\mathrm{I}}(t) = A\cos(\Delta f t)$ and $s_{\mathrm{Q}} = 0$, and for a negative Doppler shift, $s_{\mathrm{I}}(t) = 0$ and $s_{\mathrm{Q}}(t) = A\cos(\Delta f t)$. Therefore, a heterodyne detector is able to distinguish both the direction and the magnitude of the blood velocity.

3.10.3. Pulsed-Mode Doppler Measurements

In pulsed-mode Doppler systems, only one transducer is used, which transmits pulses and receives backscattered signals a number of times in order to estimate the blood velocity. The major advantage of pulsed-mode over CW Doppler is the ability to measure Doppler shifts in a specific region of interest at a defined depth within the body. This volume can be chosen using the following variables: (1) the transducer diameter and focusing scheme, which define the cross section of the ultrasound beam, (2) the time delay after pulse transmission before acquisition of the backscattered signal is started (defining the minimum depth), and (3) the time for which the signal is acquired (defining the maximum depth). The minimum and the maximum depths can be calculated from

$$\mathrm{depth}_{\min} = \frac{c(t_{\mathrm{d}} - t_{\mathrm{p}})}{2}, \qquad \mathrm{depth}_{\max} = \frac{c(t_{\mathrm{d}} + t_{\mathrm{g}})}{2} \tag{3.49}$$

where t_p is the length of the ultrasound pulse, t_d is the time delay between the end of the transmitted pulse and the receiver gate being opened, and t_g is the time for which the receiver gate is open. For example, suppose that flow information is desired from a vessel that is 4 mm in diameter and lies at a depth of 5 cm below the skin. A train of ultrasound pulses is sent out, each pulse consisting of five cycles of ultrasound at a frequency of 5 MHz, resulting in a 1-μs-long pulse. Assuming an ultrasound velocity of 1540 m/s in tissue, the receiver should be gated on ~65 μs after the end of each transmitted pulse. The time t_g corresponds to the time delay between the return of the leading edge of the pulse from the shallowest depth (5 cm) and the return of the trailing edge of the pulse from the deepest depth (5.4 cm), and has a value of ~4.2 μs.

Calculation of the blood velocity relies on the fact that the time delay between the transmitted pulse and the backscattered signal decreases if blood is flowing toward the transducer and increases if blood is flowing away from the transducer. Figure 3.24 shows a series of backscattered signals acquired after successive pulses in a pulse train: typically 64 or 128 pulses are used in a pulsed-mode Doppler measurement. The amplitudes of the signals corresponding to a particular depth are plotted as a function of time after the initial ultrasound pulse. The Fourier transform of this plot gives the frequency-domain representation of the signal intensities, which can be converted into a velocity spectrum using equation (3.43).

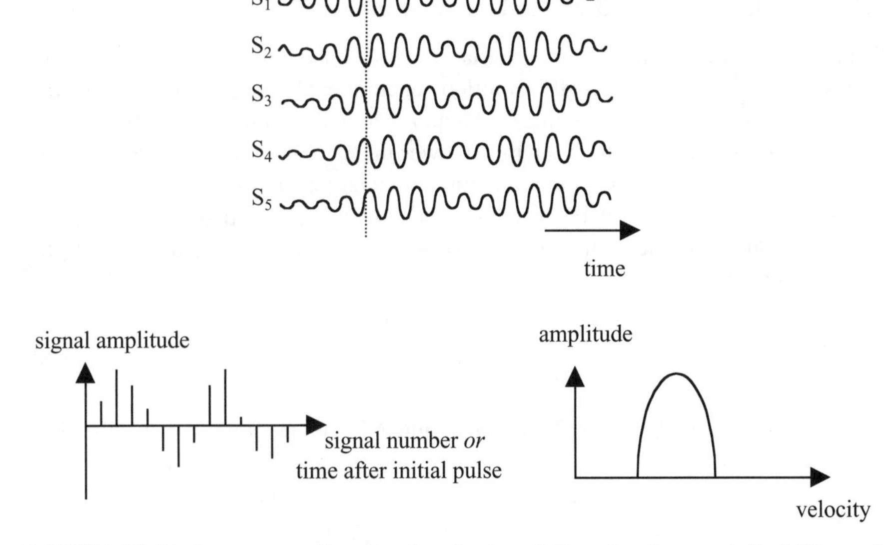

FIGURE 3.24. *The basic processing steps in pulsed-mode Doppler ultrasound. (Top) After each pulse in a pulse train a backscattered signal ($S_1, S_2, \ldots, S_5$) is recorded. (Bottom left) The signal amplitude at a particular depth, corresponding to the dotted line in the top figure, is plotted as a function of the time after the initial pulse. (Bottom right) Fourier transformation of this plot results in the Doppler frequency, and hence blood velocity, distribution at the chosen location.*

One of the disadvantages of pulsed-mode Doppler measurements is that there is a limit to the highest velocity v_{max} that can be measured. The Nyquist theorem states that in order to detect a given frequency component in a waveform, the sampling frequency must be at least twice that of the desired component. The pulse repetition rate (PRR) is defined as the reciprocal of the sampling frequency, and therefore the relationship between the highest measurable Doppler frequency f_{max} and the PRR is given by

$$f_{\mathrm{max}} = \frac{\mathrm{PRR}}{2} \tag{3.50}$$

The corresponding value of v_{max} is given by

$$v_{\mathrm{max}} = \frac{(\mathrm{PRR})c}{4f_{\mathrm{i}}} \tag{3.51}$$

If the Doppler shift has a value greater than f_{max}, then it will "alias," that is, appear as a low frequency. If aliasing is suspected, the machine can be switched to CW mode, which does not suffer from this limitation.

The value of the PRR also determines the maximum depth d_{max} which can be studied, with a value of d_{max} given by $c/2\mathrm{PRR}$. The relationship between d_{max} and v_{max} is therefore given by

$$v_{\mathrm{max}} = \frac{c^2}{8f_{\mathrm{i}}d_{\mathrm{max}}} \tag{3.52}$$

3.10.4. Color Doppler/B-Mode Duplex Imaging

Doppler flow measurements can be interlaced with B-mode imaging in order to superimpose the flow maps onto high-resolution "anatomical" images. This combination is called duplex imaging. Flow imaging requires long ultrasound pulses because the backscattered Doppler signal has a much lower intensity than the B-mode scan. The B-mode scan uses short pulses to maintain high axial resolution.

Only the mean value of the velocity, and not the full velocity distribution, is determined at each pixel. The mean value of the velocity $\bar{v}$ is calculated from the following equation:

$$\bar{v} = \frac{\bar{f}}{f_{\mathrm{i}}}\frac{c}{2\cos\theta} \tag{3.53}$$

where θ is the angle defined in Figure 3.21 and $\bar{f}$ is the mean frequency shift given by

$$\bar{f} = \frac{\displaystyle\int_{-\infty}^{\infty} f\left[S_{\mathrm{I}}^2(f) + S_{\mathrm{Q}}^2(f)\right]df}{\displaystyle\int_{-\infty}^{\infty}\left[S_{\mathrm{I}}^2(f) + S_{\mathrm{Q}}^2(f)\right]df} \tag{3.54}$$

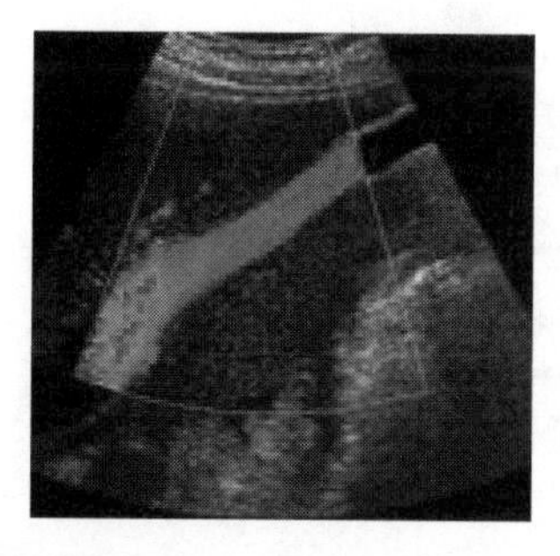

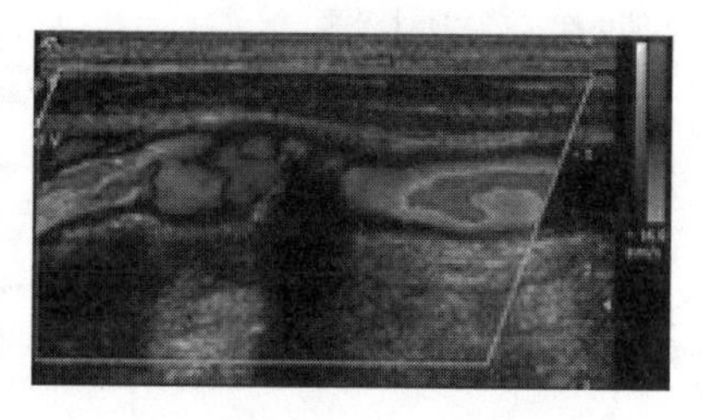

FIGURE 3.25. *(Left) Flow in a recanalized umbilical cord. (Right) Flow inside a carotid artery. A parallelogram-shaped region of interest is needed for vessels that are parallel to the transducer surface (©2000 ATL Ultrasound).*

where $S_I(f)$ and $S_Q(f)$ are the Fourier transforms of the output time-domain signals from the quadrature demodulator. The mean velocity, its sign (positive or negative), and its variance are represented by the hue, the saturation, and the luminance, respectively, of the color plot. Efficient computation of the mean and the variance values is important so that the frame rate can be as high as possible. Practical implementation on commercial machines involves calculating the autocorrelation function between the real and the imaginary signals. Because the Doppler signal is calculated on a pixel-by-pixel basis, as opposed to integrating over the entire volume as in spectral Doppler measurements, this results in a very low SNR in the flow image. Many scans must be averaged to improve the SNR, but this means that the flow imaging is relatively slow compared to the B-mode scan. Examples of duplex images are shown in Figure 3.25.

One of the difficulties in measuring color Doppler shifts occurs when a vessel lies parallel to the face of the phased array transducer. If flow is normal and unidirectional, one-half of the image shows flow toward the transducer and the other shows flow away from the transducer. Directly below the center of the transducer there is a signal void. The angle dependence can be removed by using the so-called "power Doppler" mode. The area under the plot of Doppler frequency versus amplitude is integrated to give the "Doppler power." The Doppler power depends *only* upon the number of RBC scatterers, and is not angle-dependent. Aliasing artifacts at high flow rates are also eliminated because the integral of an aliased signal is the same as that of a nonaliased signal. The major disadvantage with power Doppler is the loss of directional information.

3.10.5. Time-Domain Correlation/Color Velocity Imaging

The second class of methods for estimating blood velocity using ultrasound involves time-domain correlation (TDC) techniques. The basis for TDC methods is that the RBC distribution within a vessel is inhomogeneous, meaning that different-sized groups of RBCs give "signature" signals in the backscattered echo. Over the relatively

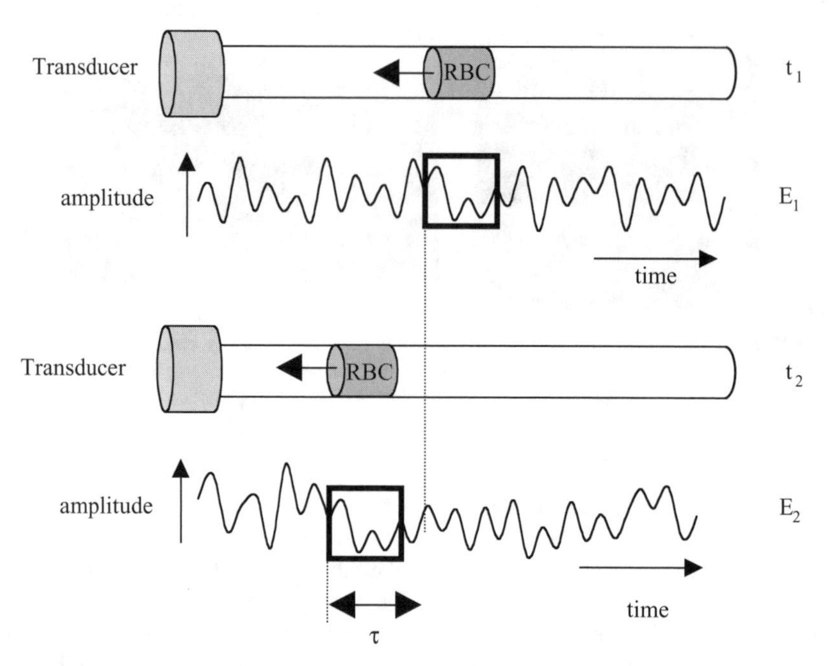

FIGURE 3.26. A diagram showing the basis of time-domain correlation methods for measuring blood velocity. A pulse of ultrasound is transmitted at time t_1 and the backscattered echo E_1 recorded. A second pulse is transmitted at time t_2 and the signature signal from the particular group of RBCs is time-shifted by an amount τ in the corresponding echo E_2. Correlation methods, as described in the text, are used to estimate the value of τ and hence the blood velocity.

short periods of time during which each individual group of RBCs lies within the transducer beam, these signature signals remain correlated. The general principle of velocity estimation is shown in Figure 3.26. The value of the time shift τ is estimated by correlating the two signals E_1 and E_2 with each other and calculating the correlation coefficient $R(s)$, given by

$$R(s) = \int_t E_1[t + s]E_2[t] \tag{3.55}$$

The maximum of $R(s)$ occurs when the value of s equals τ, and having determined the value of τ, one can calculate the velocity v of the RBCs from

$$v = \frac{c\tau}{2(t_2 - t_1)} \tag{3.56}$$

Time-domain methods have several advantages over pulsed Doppler methods. First is the lack of aliasing artifacts arising from the Nyquist sampling criterion: the limit on the maximum blood velocity that can be measured depends only upon the time that the scatterers remain within the ultrasound beam. Second, the direction of flow is automatically measured as a negative or positive time shift without the need for quadrature demodulation. Finally, in situations where the SNR is not very high ($<10:1$) cross-correlation techniques perform significantly better than Doppler methods. Time-domain methods can also be extended to two dimensions and then integrated with B-mode gray-scale scans as in conventional duplex scanners. The algorithm used is simply two-dimensional cross-correlation rather than one-dimensional as described here. This mode is often called color velocity imaging.

3.11. ULTRASOUND CONTRAST AGENTS, HARMONIC IMAGING, AND PULSE INVERSION TECHNIQUES

The detection of blood flow in small vessels deep in tissue is very difficult due to the low SNR of the Doppler signal. In order to carry out these experiments, the backscattered signal from blood must be made larger by somehow increasing the echogenicity of blood. This can be achieved using ultrasound contrast agents, which are injected directly into the bloodstream. These contrast agents usually consist of gas-filled microspheres or microbubbles with diameters less than 10 μm so that they pass through the pulmonary, the cardiac, and the capillary systems. There are two basic mechanisms by which such agents increase significantly the backscattered signal from blood. The first is the large difference in acoustic properties between gas-filled particles and the surrounding blood and tissue. The second mechanism is termed "resonance," in which gas-filled microspheres essentially expand and contract under the influence of the traveling ultrasound wave. Both effects, outlined in more detail below, result in an effective scattering cross section much larger than a correspondingly sized liquid-filled microsphere. The power P_{r} received by a transducer is given by

$$P_{\mathrm{r}} = \frac{I_{\mathrm{i}} N \sigma a^2}{4R^2} \tag{3.57}$$

where R is the distance between the scatterer and transducer, a is the radius of the transducer, N is the number of scatterers, I_{i} is the intensity of the incident ultrasound beam, and σ is the scattering cross section. Therefore, the larger the effective scattering cross section of the microsphere, the larger is the backscattered signal.

In terms of the difference in acoustic properties of the microsphere, equation (3.24) shows that the magnitude of the backscattered signal depends upon the differences in density and compressibility between the contrast agent and the surrounding medium. For a gas-filled microsphere, $\kappa_{\mathrm{s}} \gg \kappa$ and $\rho_{\mathrm{s}} \ll \rho$, resulting in a very high scattering cross section. However, it must be remembered that the concentration of the injected contrast agent in the blood is very low, and without the effect of resonance, described below, use of these contrast agents would not result in a significantly enhanced signal from blood.

The compressibility for a gas-filled microsphere is more than 10,000 times greater than for a correspondingly sized liquid-filled particle, and the size of the microsphere changes appreciably as a result of the applied ultrasound pressure field. Gas-filled microspheres can act as harmonic oscillators, producing increases in scattering cross section three orders of magnitude greater than their actual geometric cross section. The resonance frequency f_0 of a bubble of radius r is given by

$$f_0 = \frac{1}{2\pi r}\sqrt{\frac{3\gamma p_0}{\rho_0}} \tag{3.58}$$

where γ is the adiabatic ideal gas constant, p_0 is the ambient pressure of the surrounding blood, and ρ_0 is the ambient blood density. Gas bubbles are usually stabilized using some form of physical encapsulation, and the resonant frequency of such microspheres is altered by the surface tension σ_{st} of the particular compound used:

$$f_0 = \frac{1}{2\pi r}\sqrt{\frac{3\gamma}{\rho_0}\left(p_0 + \frac{2\sigma_{st}}{r}\right)} \tag{3.59}$$

It is highly fortuitous that the size of microspheres, 1–10 μm, needed to cross capillary beds corresponds to a resonant frequency within the ultrasound diagnostic imaging range.

A number of different contrast agents have been developed, the vast majority based on gas microbubbles or gas-filled microspheres. Levovist is made from a suspension of galactose in water, with air microbubbles sticking to the surface of the solid microcrystals. A small amount of palmitic acid is added as a surfactant and, when injected, the microcrystals dissolve and the gas bubbles, with a diameter of less than 6 μm, enter the blood. These bubbles have a relatively long lifetime in the bloodstream, typically greater than 3 min. Levovist can be used to visualize both the left and the right ventricles in the heart and to calculate the ventricular ejection fraction, which is an important measure of heart function. In addition to air, high-molecular-weight inert gases can be used; these have the advantage that they dissolve more slowly in the blood. Echogen is an emulsion of perfluoropentane, which is a liquid at room temperature when it is prepared, but becomes a gas at body temperature after injection. Other contrast agents are based on encapsulating the gas within a solid shell before injection. These agents have shorter lifetimes in the bloodstream because they are removed very efficiently by the liver and spleen, where they are phagocytosed by the Kuppfer cells. In fact, this allows these agents to be used as "negative" contrast agents for the detection of tumors in the liver because the agent accumulates only in healthy liver tissue and therefore forms a bright ring around the tumor. Examples of these agents include Albunex, which consists of air-filled microspheres with a protein shell made of human serum albumin, and Sonovist, in which the gas is encapsulated in a cyanoacrylate, biodegradable shell. Doppler imaging can also be used for tumor detection with these agents because the tumor periphery typically has a higher vascularity than in the center.

Ultrasound contrast agents are most commonly used in combination with a technique called harmonic imaging. Due to the nonlinear relationship between the volume

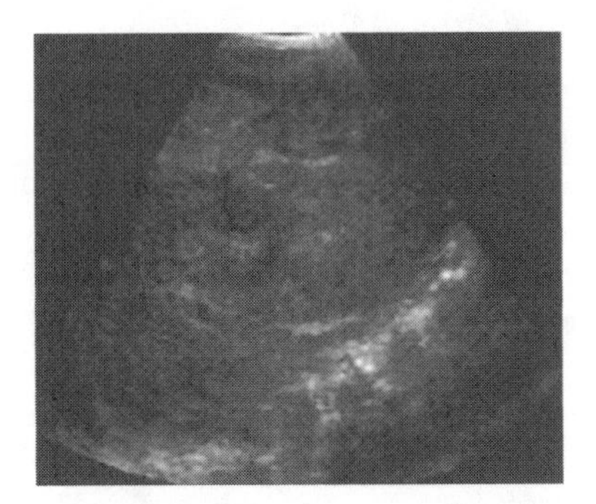
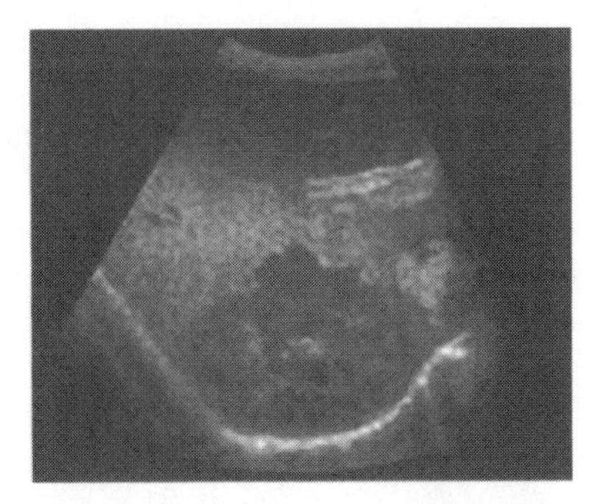

FIGURE 3.27. *(Left) A fundamental mode image of a liver mass using a contrast agent. (Right) The corresponding second harmonic image, showing much clearer delineation of the tumor mass (©2000 ATL Ultrasound).*

of the microbubble and the pressure of the ultrasound wave, the backscattered signal consists not only of the transmitted (fundamental) frequency, but also harmonics and subharmonics of this frequency. These harmonic signals have lower intensities than those at the fundamental frequency, but can actually have a higher SNR because they have very low signal contributions from clutter and tissue motion. The most common implemention of harmonic imaging uses the second harmonic of the fundamental frequency.

The signal component at the fundamental frequency can be almost entirely eliminated by using so-called "pulse inversion techniques" in which the images from two scans are combined. In the first scan, both the returning fundamental signal as well as its harmonic component are stored. In the second scan, an inverted pulse is transmitted. The backscattered fundamental signal is inverted, but the harmonic signal has the same phase as for the first scan. Summation of these two signals therefore results in cancellation of the fundamental signals, with the harmonic components adding constructively, thus producing a pure harmonic signal. A comparison of fundamental and second harmonic mode images, both acquired using contrast agents, is shown in Figure 3.27.

3.12. SAFETY AND BIOEFFECTS IN ULTRASONIC IMAGING

Under normal operating conditions, ultrasonic imaging is extremely safe, with no limit having been set by the FDA on the number of patient examinations over any given period of time. Increasingly sophisticated image acquisition processes such as compound scanning and power color Doppler have, however, increased the amount of energy that is deposited in the body, and there are a number of regulatory guidelines for recommended safety levels. Several measures are used to estimate the safety of an ultrasonic imaging protocol. The average intensity of a CW ultrasound wave was described in equation (3.6). However, as has been described, the majority of ultrasound experiments are carried out in pulsed mode. The "duty cycle" in pulsed ultrasound is defined as the duration of the ultrasound pulse divided by the time between pulses. Temporal-averaged ultrasound intensity is calculated simply by multiplying the average intensity during the pulse by the duty cycle. The Gaussian beam profile can be accounted for by calculating the spatially averaged intensity I_{SA}. Common acronyms used for reporting ultrasound intensities for different procedures use a combination of these terms, for example, spatial average temporal average (SATA), spatial peak temporal average (SPTA), spatial peak pulse average (SPPA), spatial peak temporal peak (SPTP), spatial peak (SP), and spatial average (SA). The American Institute of Ultrasound in Medicine sets guidelines for these values, based on estimations on the tissue heating produced. For example, for fetal imaging, the current FDA regulatory limit for I_{SPTA} is 720 mW/cm^2.

Although outside the scope of this book, it should be noted that ultrasound can be used therapeutically as a method for thermal destruction of tumors. Relatively low intensity ultrasound is used for hyperthermic tumor treatment, in which the tumor is heated to temperatures between 42°C and 45°C in order to accelerate tumor cell destruction. Alternatively, very high intensities of ultrasound can be used for tumor thermoablation, in which the temperature in the tumor is raised rapidly to between 70°C and 90°C for a few seconds. The mechanism for this rapid heating involves cavitation effects, the formation and destruction of small air bubbles within the tumor.

3.13. CLINICAL APPLICATIONS OF ULTRASOUND

The noninvasive, nonionizing nature of ultrasonic imaging, its ability to measure blood velocity, together with real-time image acquisition and easy patient access mean that a very wide range of clinical protocols have ultrasonic imaging as an integral part. The most common use of ultrasound is in the abdomen and pelvis, imaging the gallbladder and renal system, and transabdominal imaging of the uterus and ovaries in women, and the testicles in men. As examples, applications to obstetrics, breast imaging, musculoskeletal damage, and cardiac studies are outlined briefly below.

3.13.1. Obstetrics and Gynecology

Ultrasound is the only imaging technique routinely used for fetal studies. Parameters such as the size of the head and the brain ventricles (for diagnosis of hydrocephalus) and the condition of the spine are measured to assess the health of the fetus. If amniocentesis is necessary to detect disorders such as Down syndrome, then ultrasound is used for needle guidance. Doppler ultrasound is also used to measure fetal blood velocity. The high spatial resolution possible is shown in Figure 3.28.

3.13.2. Breast Imaging

In breast imaging, ultrasound is used in conjunction with the primary technique of X-ray mammography in the diagnosis of breast cancer. If mammography suggests

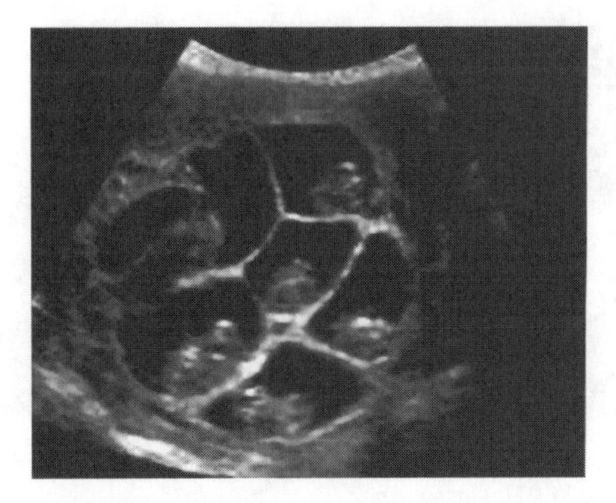

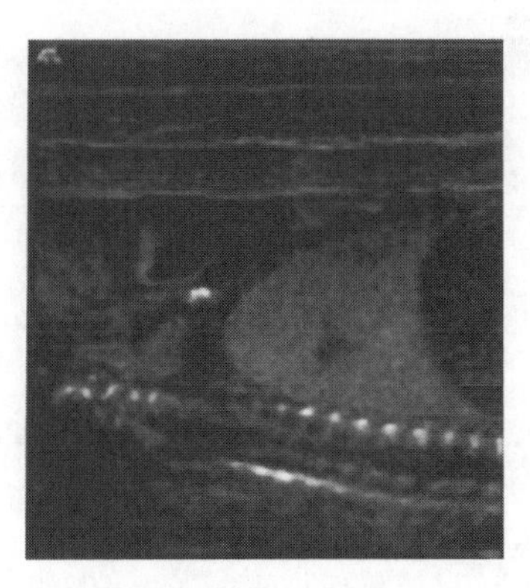

FIGURE 3.28. *(Left) A B-mode image showing sextuplets in utero. (Right) An image of a fetal lung (©2000 ATL Ultrasound).*

that a "lump" is present, then ultrasound can help to determine whether it is a fluid-filled cyst or a solid mass. Cysts typically have a round shape and anechoic interiors, and acoustic enhancement is often seen behind the cyst. Since cysts are fluid-filled, the presence of acoustic streaming (fluid motion arising from the ultrasound pressure, detected using Doppler techniques) is also a useful diagnostic. Ultrasound is particularly valuable in women with dense breast tissue or young women because the tissue is relatively opaque to X-rays. If a needle biopsy is needed in order to determine whether a solid mass is cancerous or not, then real-time B-mode ultrasonic imaging can be used to guide the needle into the tumor. Ultrasound can also be used in the detection of microcalcifications, with spatial compound imaging being particularly useful due to the reduction in speckle. Figure 3.29 shows two images: the first of a breast carcinoma acquired using compound imaging, and the second of a needle biopsy.

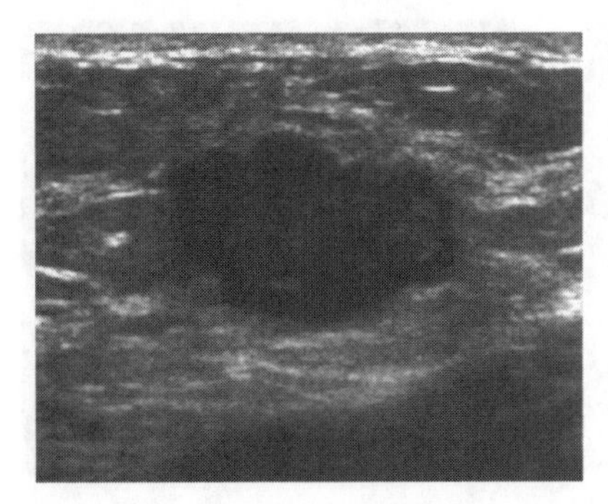

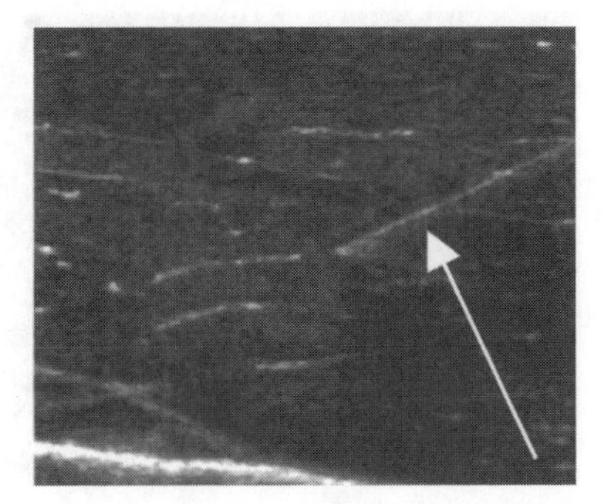

FIGURE 3.29. *(Left) A compound image of a dark mass within the breast. (Right) Tracking a needle biopsy of breast tissue using real-time compound B-mode scanning (©2000 ATL Ultrasound).*

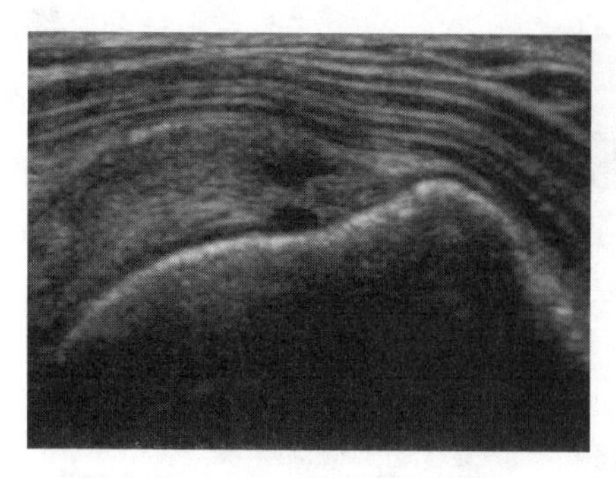
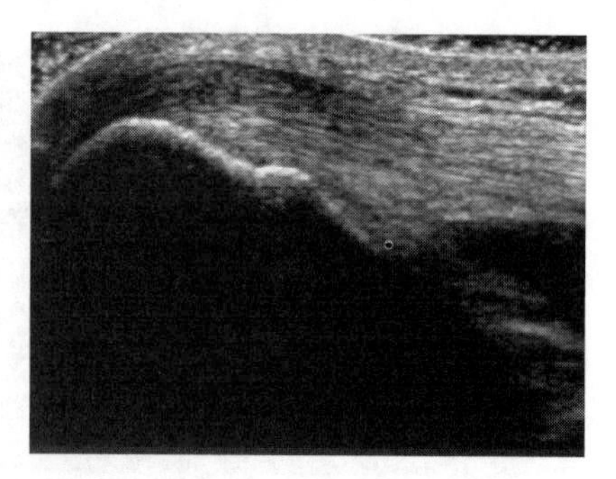

FIGURE 3.30. (Left) A compound B-mode image of a rotator cuff injury. (Right) A similar scan showing tendinitis in the tricep tendon (©2000 ATL Ultrasound).

3.13.3. Musculoskeletal Structure

Musculoskeletal damage can be quickly and effectively diagnosed using ultrasound, again most commonly with compound scanning for images with high spatial resolution and high SNR. Figure 3.30 shows two examples of images acquired for such injuries.

3.13.4. Cardiac Disease

Ultrasonic imaging of the heart can be used to diagnose diseases such as mitral valve stenosis, regurgitation, congenital heart disease, and the presence of cardiac tumors. It can also be used to assess left-ventricular function, often in combination with a stress test. Doppler techniques can be used to measure blood velocity in the arteries and veins in the heart. Contrast agents can be used to produce blood perfusion maps;

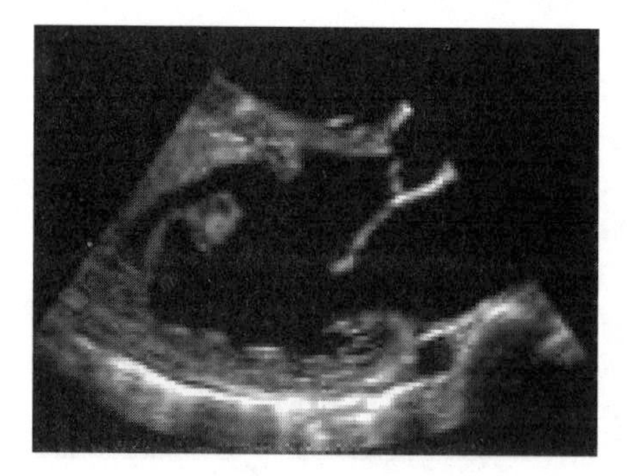
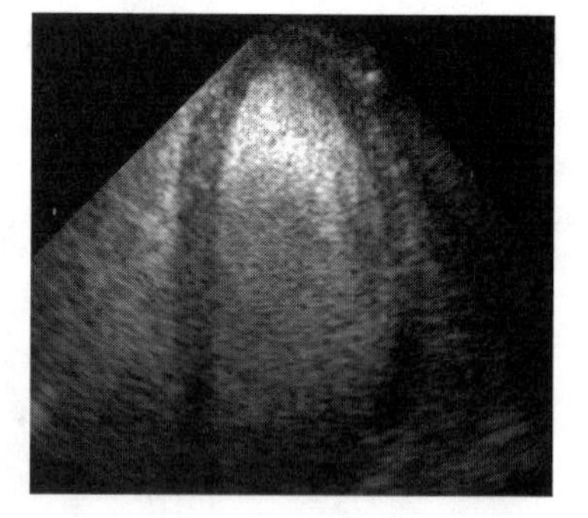

FIGURE 3.31. (Left) A B-mode image of a patient with congenital cardiomyopathy. (Right) A perfusion map of the heart obtained using a pulse inversion harmonic technique (©2000 ATL Ultrasound).

myocardial infarcts often show reduced perfusion compared to areas of healthy tissue. Figure 3.31 shows an example of a patient with congenital cardiomyopathy, and a normal perfusion map of the heart.

EXERCISES

3.1. Calculate the intensity transmission coefficient T_I for the following interfaces, assuming that the ultrasound beam is exactly perpendicular to the interface: muscle/kidney, air/muscle, and bone/muscle. Discuss briefly the implications of these values of T_I for ultrasonic imaging.

3.2. Repeat the calculations in Exercise 3.1 with the angle of incidence of the ultrasound beam now being 60°.

3.3. Within tissue lies a perfect reflector, which backscatters 100% of the intensity of the ultrasound beam. Given a 100-dB receiver dynamic range and an operating frequency of 3 MHz, what is the maximum depth within tissue at which the reflector can be detected?

3.4. Calculate the distance at which the intensity of a 1-MHz and a 5-MHz ultrasound beam will be reduced by half traveling through (a) bone, (b) air, and (c) muscle.

3.5. Plot the transmitted frequency spectrum of an ultrasound beam from a transducer operating at a central frequency of 1.5 MHz. Assume that the transducer is damped. Repeat the plot for the beam returning to the transducer after passing through tissue and being backscattered.

3.6. In order to improve the efficiency of a given transducer, the amount of energy reflected by the skin directly under the transducer must be minimized. A layer of material with an acoustic impedance Z_{ML} is placed between the transducer and the skin. If the acoustic impedance of the skin is denoted by Z_s and that of the transducer crystal Z_c, show mathematically that the value of Z_{ML} that minimizes the energy of the reflected wave is given by $Z_{ML} = \sqrt{Z_c Z_s}$.

3.7. Consider a transducer with a thickness given by equation (3.27). A matching layer (Exercise 3.6) is used to maximize the energy transferred from the transducer to the body. Show that the thickness of this matching layer should be one-fourth of the ultrasound wavelength.

3.8. Consider a focused transducer with a radius of curvature of 10 cm and a diameter of 4 cm. This transducer operates at a frequency of 3.5 MHz and transmits a pulse of duration 0.857 μs. What is the axial and the lateral resolution at the focal point of the transducer?

3.9. Explain why a very fast or very slow tissue relaxation time results in a very small amount of energy being lost due to absorption.

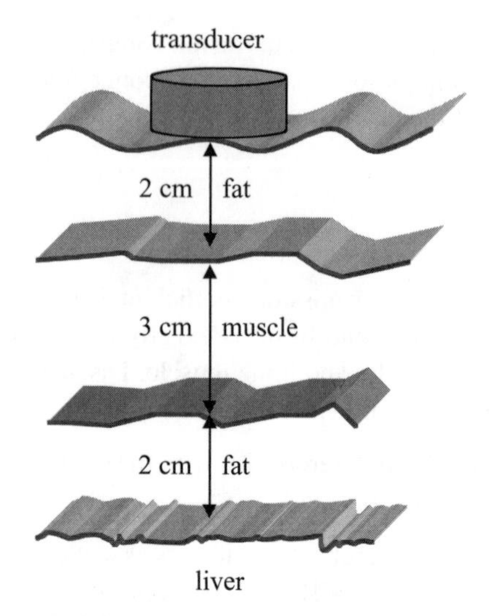

FIGURE 3.32. *Illustration for Exercise 3.10.*

3.10. Use the following data to sketch the A-mode scan from Figure 3.32. The amplitude axis should be on a decibel scale and the time axis in microseconds. Ignore any reflected signal from the transducer/fat interface, and assume that a signal of 0 dB enters the body. At a transducer frequency of 5 MHz, the linear attenuation coefficient for muscle and liver is 5 dB cm^{-1} and for fat is

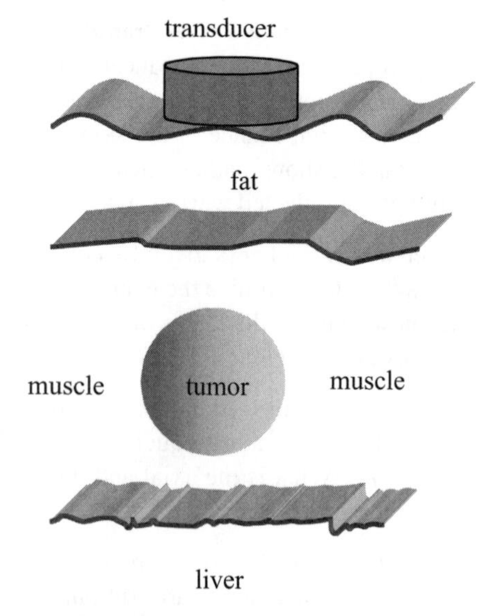

FIGURE 3.33. *Illustration for Exercise 3.11.*

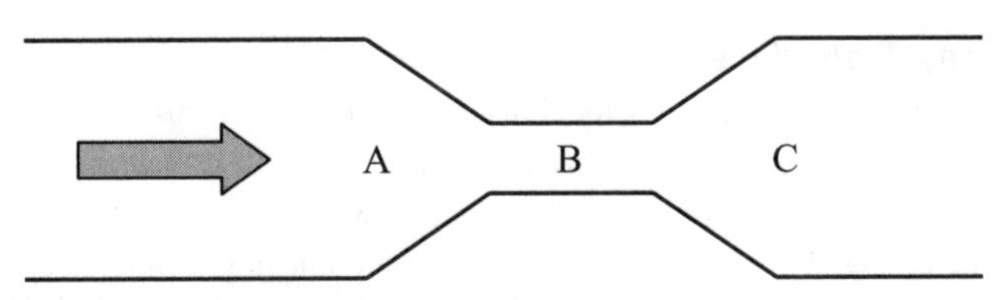

FIGURE 3.34. Illustration for Exercise 3.15.

7 dB cm^{-1}. Relevant values of the characteristic acoustic impedance and speed of sound can be found in Table 3.1.

3.11. Determine and sketch the A-mode scan using the same parameters as in Exercise 3.10, but with a time–gain compensation of 0.8 dB μs^{-1}.

3.12. For the object shown in Figure 3.33, qualitatively sketch the B-mode ultrasound image. Ignore speckle or scatter and only consider signals backscattered from the tissue boundaries. Acoustic impedance: tissue 1.61, tumor 1.52 ($\times 10^5$ g/cm^2 s). Attenuation coefficient: tissue 1.0, tumor 0.4 (dB/cm/MHz). Speed of sound: tissue 1540, tumor 750 (m/s).

3.13. In a particular real-time imaging application the transducer moves through a 90° sector with a frame rate of 30 frames per second, acquiring 128 lines of data per frame. If the image is acquired up to a depth of 20 cm and the lateral resolution of the beam width at this depth is 5 mm, calculate the effect of transducer motion on overall image blurring, that is, is it the dominant factor?

3.14. Sketch the shape of the acoustic shadowing artifact produced from compound scanning.

3.15. Sketch the Doppler spectral patterns at points A, B, and C in the model system of a stenotic artery shown in Figure 3.34.

3.16. Show that the outputs of the quadrature detector covered in Section 3.9.2 allow differentiation between positive and negative blood velocity by deriving the equations for $s_I(t)$ and $s_Q(t)$ in the main text.

FURTHER READING

Original Papers

Early Papers in Medical Ultrasound

J. J. Wild, The use of ultrasonic pulses for the measurement of biologic tissues, and the detection of tissue density changes, *Surgery* **27,** 183–188 (1950).

D. H. Howry and W. R. Bliss, Ultrasonic visualization of soft-tissue structures of the body, *J. Lab. Clin. Med.* **40,** 579–592 (1952).

I. Edler and C. H. Hertz, The use of an ultrasonic reflectoscope for the continuous recording of the movement of heart walls, *Kungl. Fysiogr. Sällskap. Lund Förhandl.* **24,** 1–19 (1954).

Phased Array Transducers

J. C. Somer, Electronic sector scanning for ultrasonic diagnosis, *Ultrasonics* **6,** 153–159 (1968).

N. Bom, C. T. Lancee, J. Honkoop, and P. G. Hugenholtz, Ultrasonic viewer for cross-sectional analysis of moving cardiac structures, *Biomed. Eng.* **6,** 500–508 (1971).

F. L. Thurstone and O. T. von Ramm, A new ultrasonic imaging technique employing two-dimensional electronic beam steering, in *Acoustical Holography,* Vol. 5 (P. S. Green, ed.), pp. 249–259, Plenum Press, New York (1974).

Blood Velocity Measurements

S. Satomura, Ultrasonic Doppler method for the inspection of cardiac functions, *J. Acoust. Soc. Am.* **29,** 1181–1185 (1957).

D. W. Baker, Pulsed ultrasonic Doppler blood-flow sensing, *IEEE Trans. Son. Ultrason.* **SU-17,** 170–185 (1970).

D. Dotti, E. Gatti, V. Svelto, A. Ugge, and P. Vidali, Blood flow measurements by ultrasound correlation techniques, *Energia Nucleare* **23,** 571–575 (1976).

K. Namekawa, C. Kasai, M. Tsukamoto, and A. Koyano, Realtime bloodflow imaging system utilizing autocorrelation techniques, in *Ultrasound '82* (R. Lerski and P. Morley, eds.), pp. 203–208, Pergamon Press, Oxford (1982).

Compound Scanning

D. P. Shattuck and O. T. von Ramm, Compound scanning with a phased array, *Ultrason. Imaging* **4,** 93–107 (1982).

S. K. Jespersen, J. E. Wilhjelm, and H. Sillesen, Multi-angle compound scanning, *Ultrason. Imaging* **20,** 81–102 (1998).

Contrast Agents

R. Gramiak and P. M. Shah, Echocardiography of the aortic root, *Invest. Radiol.* **3,** 355–356 (1968).

T. Fritzsch, M. Schartl, and J. Siegert, Preclinical and clinical results with an ultrasonic contrast agent, *Invest. Radiol.* **23,** S302–5 (1988).

Harmonic Imaging

B. Schrope, V. L. Newhouse, and V. Uhlendorf, Simulated capillary blood flow measurement using a nonlinear ultrasonic contrast agent, *Ultrason. Imaging* **14,** 134–158 (1992).

B. Schrope and V. L. Newhouse, Second harmonic ultrasound blood perfusion measurement, *Ultrasound Med. Biol.* **19,** 567–579 (1993).

Bioeffects

W. J. Fry and F. Dunn, Ultrasound: Analysis and experimental methods in biological research, in *Physical Techniques in Biological Research,* Vol. IV (W. L. Nastuk, ed.), pp. 261–394, Academic Press, New York (1962).

Books

Physical Principles of Acoustics and Ultrasound

W. R. Hedrick, D. L. Hykes, and D. Starchman, *Ultrasound Physics and Instrumentation,* Mosby-Year Book, St. Louis (1995).

J. A. Zagzebski, *Essentials of Ultrasound Physics,* Mosby-Year Book, St. Louis (1996).

L. E. Kinsler, A. R. Frey, A. B. Coppens, and J. V. Sanders, *Fundamentals of Acoustics,* 4th ed., Wiley, New York (1999).

Diagnostic Ultrasonic Imaging

F. W. Kremkau and A. Allen, eds., *Diagnostic Ultrasound: Principles and Instruments,* Saunders, Philadelphia (1998).

S. C. Bushong, *Diagnostic Ultrasound,* McGraw-Hill, New York (1999).

Flow Measurements Using Ultrasound

J. A. Jensen, *Estimation of Blood Velocities Using Ultrasound: A Signal Processing Approach,* Cambridge University Press, Cambridge (1996).

D. H. Evans, W. N. McDicken, and N. McDicken, *Doppler Ultrasound: Physics, Instrumental and Clinical Applications,* 2nd ed. Wiley, New York (2000).

Safety

S. B. Barrett and G. Kossoff, eds., *Safety of Diagnostic Ultrasound,* Parthenon, New York (1998).

Clinical Applications

G. M. Baxter, P. L. P. Allan, and P. Morley, eds., *Clinical Diagnostic Ultrasound,* Blackwell Science, London (1999).

Review Articles

I. A. Hein and W. D. O'Brien, Current time-domain methods for assessing tissue motion by analysis from reflected ultrasound echoes—A review, *IEEE Trans. Ultrason. Ferrelect. Freq. Control* **2,** 84–102 (1993).

B. B. Goldberg, J.-B. Liu, and F. Forsberg, Ultrasound contrast agents: A review, *Ultrasound Med. Biol.* **20,** 319–333 (1994).

T. A. Whittingham, New and future developments in ultrasonic imaging, *Br. J. Radiol.* **70,** S119–S132 (1997).

F. Calliada, R. Campani, O. Bottinelli, A. Bozzini, and M. G. Sommaruga, Ultrasound contrast agents: Basic principles, *Eur. J. Radiology* **27,** S157–S160 (1998).

G. Maresca, V. Summaria, C. Colagrande, R. Manfredi, and F. Calliada, New prospects for ultrasound contrast agents, *Eur. J. Radiol.* **27,** S171–S178 (1998).

T. R. Nelson and D. H. Pretorius, Three-dimensional ultrasonic imaging, *Ultrasound Med. Biol.* **24,** 1243–1270 (1998).

P. N. Wells, Current status and future technical advances of ultrasonic imaging, *IEEE Trans. Eng. Med. Biol.* **19,** 14–20 (2000).

M. Claudon, F. Tranquart, D. H. Evans, F. Lefevre, and M. Correas, Advances in ultrasound, *Eur. Radiology* **12,** 7–18 (2002).

A. Fenster, D. Downey, and H. N. Cardinal, Three-dimensional ultrasonic imaging, *Phys. Med. Biol.* **46,** R67–R99 (2001).

Specialized Journals

European Journal of Ultrasound
IEEE Transactions on Ultrasonics, Ferroelectrics and Frequency Control
Journal of Clinical Ultrasound
Journal of the Acoustical Society of America
Ultrasonic Imaging
Ultrasound in Medicine and Biology
Journal of the American Ultrasound Society

4

Magnetic Resonance Imaging

4.1. GENERAL PRINCIPLES OF MAGNETIC RESONANCE IMAGING

Magnetic resonance imaging (MRI) is a nonionizing technique with full three-dimensional capabilities, excellent soft-tissue contrast, and high spatial resolution ($\sim$1 mm). In general, the temporal resolution is much slower than for ultrasound or computed tomography, with scans typically lasting between 3 and 10 min, and MRI is therefore much more susceptible to patient motion. The cost of MRI scanners is relatively high, with the price of a typical clinical 1.5-T whole-body imager on the order of $1.5 million. The major uses of MRI are in the areas of assessing brain disease, spinal disorders, angiography, cardiac function, and musculoskeletal damage.

The MRI signal arises from protons in the body, primarily water, but also lipid. The patient is placed inside a strong magnet, which produces a static magnetic field typically more than 10,000 times stronger than the earth's magnetic field. Each proton, being a charged particle with angular momentum, can be considered as acting as a small magnet. The protons align in two configurations, with their internal magnetic fields aligned either parallel or antiparallel to the direction of the large static magnetic field, with slightly more found in the parallel state. The protons precess around the direction of the static magnetic field, in an analogous way to a spinning gyroscope under the influence of gravity. The frequency of precession is proportional to the strength of the static magnetic field. Application of a weak radiofrequency (RF) field causes the protons to precess coherently, and the sum of all of the protons precessing is detected as an induced voltage in a tuned detector coil.

Spatial information is encoded into the image using magnetic field gradients. These impose a linear variation in all three dimensions in the magnetic field present within the patient. As a result of these variations, the precessional frequencies of the protons

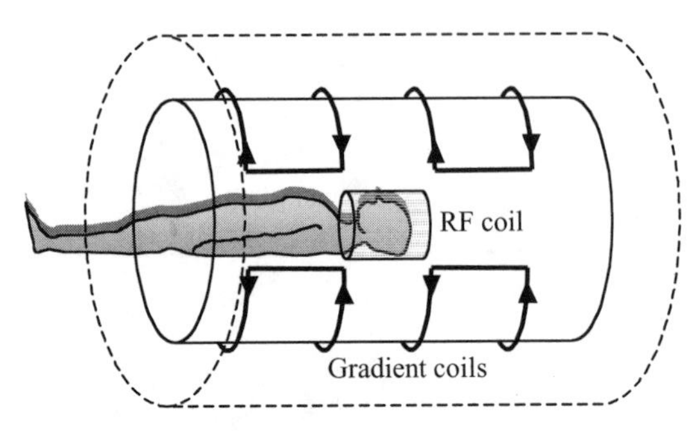

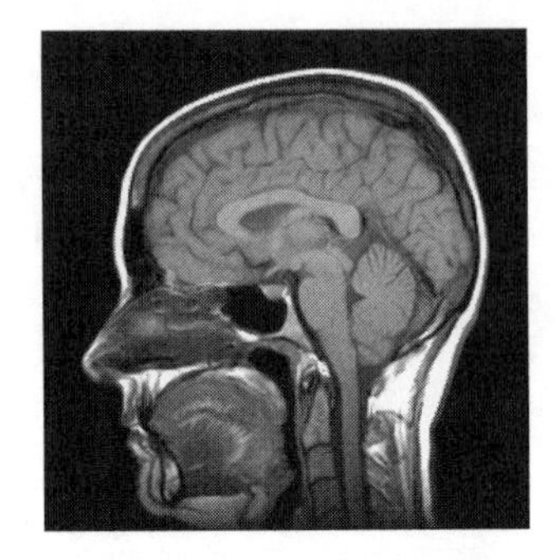

FIGURE 4.1. (Left) The instrumentation involved in MRI consists of a superconducting magnet, three sets of magnetic field gradients (only one is shown), and a radiofrequency coil. (Right) A single-slice MRI of the brain showing excellent soft-tissue contrast between gray and white matter and high spatial resolution.

are also linearly dependent upon their spatial location. The frequency and the phase of the precessing magnetization is measured by the RF coil, and the analog signal is digitized. An inverse two-dimensional Fourier transform is performed to convert the signal into the spatial domain to produce the image. By varying the data acquisition parameters, differential contrast between soft tissues can be introduced, as shown in Figure 4.1.

4.2. NUCLEAR MAGNETISM

In MRI the patient is placed inside a very strong magnet for scanning. A typical value of the magnetic field, denoted B_0, is 1.5 T (15,000 G), which can be compared to the earth's magnetic field of approximately 50 μT (0.5 G). The MRI signal arises from the interaction between the magnetic field and hydrogen nuclei, or protons, which are found primarily as water in tissue and also lipid. This interaction can be described in terms of the nuclear magnetism, either from a quantum mechanical or a classical approach, both of which are described in the following sections.

4.2.1. Quantum Mechanical Description

All nuclei with an odd atomic weight and/or an odd atomic number possess a fundamental quantum mechanical property termed "spin." For MRI the most important nucleus is the hydrogen nucleus, or proton. Although not a rigorously accurate model, the property of spin can be viewed as a proton spinning around an internal axis of rotation giving it a certain value of angular momentum **P.** Because the proton is a charged particle, this rotation gives the proton a magnetic moment $\boldsymbol{\mu}$**.** This magnetic

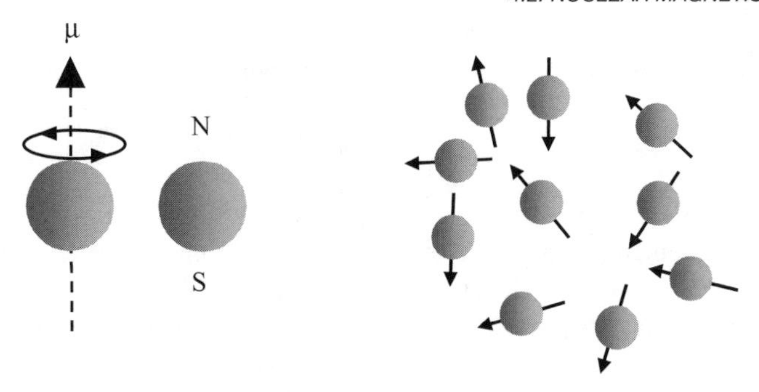

FIGURE 4.2. *(Left) A spinning proton possesses a magnetic moment μ and acts as a small magnet with a north and a south pole. (Right) In the absence of an external, imposed magnetic field, the orientations of the magnetic moments are random. There is therefore zero net magnetic moment in any given direction.*

moment produces an associated magnetic field, which has a configuration similar to that of a bar magnet, as shown in Figure 4.2. In the absence of an external magnetic field the orientation of the individual magnetic moments is random.

The magnitude of the value of **P** of the protons is quantized, that is, it can only take a certain discrete value. This value is determined by another fundamental property of the proton, the spin quantum number I:

$$|\boldsymbol{P}| = \frac{h}{2\pi}\,[I(I+1)]^{1/2} \tag{4.1}$$

where h is Planck's constant (6.63×10^{-34} J s). The value of I depends on the number of protons and neutrons in the nucleus, and is nonzero for nuclei having an odd atomic number, an odd number of neutrons, or both. In the case of protons, the value of I is $1/2$, and so the magnitude of **P** is given by

$$|\mathbf{P}| = \frac{h}{2\pi}\frac{\sqrt{3}}{2} \tag{4.2}$$

The magnitudes of the magnetic moment and the angular momentum of the proton are related by

$$|\boldsymbol{\mu}| = \gamma\,|\mathbf{P}| \tag{4.3}$$

where γ is the gyromagnetic ratio of the nucleus, and has a characteristic value for different nuclei such as protons, phosphorus, or carbon. Because the value of the magnitude of **P** is quantized, so is the value of the magnitude of $\boldsymbol{\mu}$:

$$|\boldsymbol{\mu}| = \gamma\,|\mathbf{P}| = \frac{\gamma h}{2\pi}\,[I(I+1)]^{1/2} \tag{4.4}$$

For the proton the magnitude of the magnetic moment is therefore given by

$$|\mu| = \frac{\gamma h\sqrt{3}}{4\pi} \tag{4.5}$$

The magnetic moment, being a vector, contains three components (μ_x, μ_y, and μ_z), each of which can have any value, provided that equation (4.5) is observed. However, in the presence of a strong magnetic field $\mathbf{B}_0$ the value of μ_z can only have values given by

$$\mu_z = \gamma P_z = \frac{\gamma h}{2\pi} m_I \tag{4.6}$$

where m_I is the nuclear magnetic quantum number, and can take values I, I − 1, ..., −I. So, in the case of a proton, m_I takes two values, +1/2 and −1/2, and the corresponding values of μ_z are $\pm\gamma h/4\pi$. Because the total magnetic moment is given by equation (4.5), it is clear that the magnetic moment is oriented in a direction only partially aligned with (parallel) or against (antiparallel) the main magnetic field, as shown in Figure 4.3.

One point which requires clarification is the representation of the direction of the $\mathbf{B}_0$ field as being vertical, which is common to all texts and descriptions of NMR. This is because historically all of the early NMR experiments were performed on high-resolution spectroscopy magnets in which the direction of the $\mathbf{B}_0$ field is vertical: such is indeed the situation today for high-resolution NMR spectroscopy. However,

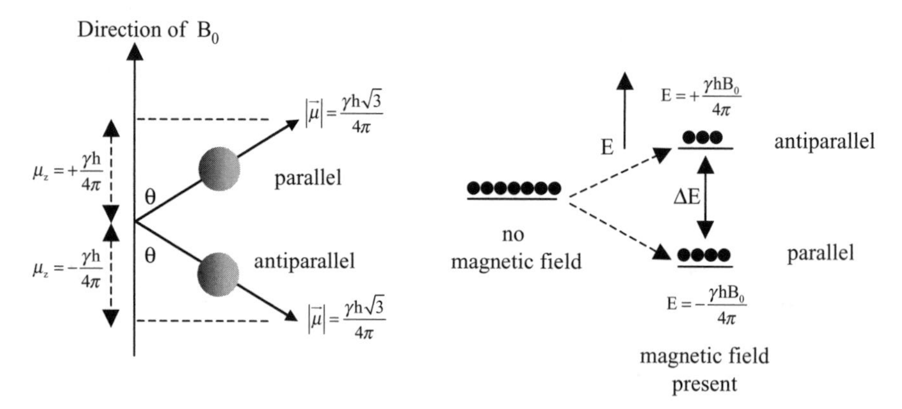

FIGURE 4.3. *(Left) The quantization of the magnitude of the z component of a proton's angular momentum means that the proton's magnetic moment has two possible physical orientations, parallel and antiparallel, with respect to the direction of the main magnetic field. The value of the angle θ is 54.7°. (Right) In the absence of an external magnetic field, there is only one energy level. When the external magnetic field is applied, Zeeman splitting results in two energy levels, with more protons occupying the lower energy level, corresponding to the proton magnetic moments being aligned parallel to the main magnetic field, than the higher energy level, corresponding to an antiparallel alignment.*

most imaging magnets are oriented horizontally such that the direction of the $\mathbf{B}_0$ field is actually horizontal. The important thing to note is that the z direction is always defined as the direction of the $\mathbf{B}_0$ field, irrespective of the actual magnet orientation.

The relative number of protons in the parallel and the antiparallel configurations can be calculated by considering the interaction energy E of a magnetic moment with the magnetic field. The magnetic field only interacts with the z component of the magnetic moment, and the value of E is given by

$$E = -\mu_z \mathbf{B}_0 \tag{4.7}$$

where $\mathbf{B}_0$ was defined previously as the strength of the magnetic field. So, from equations (4.6) and (4.7)

$$E = \mp \frac{\gamma h \mathbf{B}_0}{4\pi} \tag{4.8}$$

The two possible interaction energies correspond to the protons being in the parallel configuration (E is negative, implying a lower interaction energy) and the antiparallel configuration (E is positive, a higher interaction energy). The energy difference between the two states is shown in Figure 4.3 and is given by

$$\Delta E = \frac{\gamma h \mathbf{B}_0}{2\pi} \tag{4.9}$$

The Boltzmann equation can now be used to calculate the relative number of nuclei in each configuration:

$$\frac{N_{\text{antiparallel}}}{N_{\text{parallel}}} = \exp\left(-\frac{\Delta E}{kT}\right) = \exp\left(-\frac{\gamma h \mathbf{B}_0}{2\pi kT}\right) \tag{4.10}$$

where k is the Boltzmann coefficient, with a value of 1.38×10^{-23} J/K, and T is the temperature measured in kelvins. A first-order approximation can be made ($e^{-x} \approx 1 - x$):

$$\frac{N_{\text{antiparallel}}}{N_{\text{parallel}}} = 1 - \frac{\gamma h \mathbf{B}_0}{2\pi kT} \tag{4.11}$$

The magnitude of the MRI signal is proportional to the difference in populations between the two energy levels:

$$N_{\text{parallel}} - N_{\text{antiparallel}} = N_{\text{s}} \frac{\gamma h \mathbf{B}_0}{4\pi kT} \tag{4.12}$$

where N_{s} is the total number of protons in the body. At an operating magnetic field of 1.5 T, equation (4.12) shows that for every one million protons, there is only a

TABLE 4.1. Properties of Nuclei Found at High Abudance in the Body

Nucleus	Atomic Number	Atomic Mass	I	$\gamma/2\pi$(MHz/T)	MRI Signal
Proton	1	1	1/2	42.58	Yes
Phosphorus	15	31	1/2	17.24	Yes
Carbon	6	12	0	—	No
Oxygen	8	16	0	—	No
Sodium	11	23	3/2	11.26	Yes

population difference of five protons between the parallel and the antiparallel orientations. MRI is often referred to as an intrinsically insensitive technique because it can detect only the small excess of protons aligned with magnetic field, rather than each proton individually.

Finally, it should be noted from equation (4.1) that if $I = 0$ for a particular nucleus, then it has no angular momentum and no magnetic moment, and cannot be detected using MRI. Shown in Table 4.1 are the values of γ and I for naturally occurring nuclei within the body. Neither of the major isotopes of carbon (^{12}C) nor oxygen (^{16}O), both abundant in the body, gives an MRI signal. It is possible to detect these elements, but only the isotopes ^{13}C and ^{17}O, which exist in very low natural abundance, 1.1% and 0.048%, respectively.

4.2.2. Classical Description

The quantum mechanical model describes the basics of nuclear magnetism, but becomes cumbersome when analyzing complicated MRI pulse sequences. A more intuitive approach is to consider the interactions of protons with magnetic fields purely in terms of classical mechanics. As derived in the previous section, the proton magnetic moment $\boldsymbol{\mu}$ is aligned at an angle of 54.7° to the axis of the external magnetic field $\mathbf{B}_0$. This magnetic field attempts to align the proton magnetic moment parallel to the direction of $\mathbf{B}_0$, and this action creates a torque $\mathbf{C}$ given by

$$\mathbf{C} = \boldsymbol{\mu} \times \mathbf{B}_0 = i_N \, |\mu| \, |B_0| \sin\theta \tag{4.13}$$

where i_N is a unit vector normal to both $\boldsymbol{\mu}$ and $\mathbf{B}_0$. The direction of the torque, shown in Figure 4.4, is out of the plane of the page at right angles to the direction of $\boldsymbol{\mu}$. The result of the torque is that the proton precesses around the axis of the magnetic field, keeping a constant angle between $\boldsymbol{\mu}$ and $\mathbf{B}_0$. This is exactly analogous to the behavior of a spinning gyroscope, also shown in Figure 4.4.

In order to calculate the frequency at which the protons precess, consider that the torque is defined as the time rate of change of the total angular momentum of the proton:

$$\mathbf{C} = \frac{d\mathbf{P}}{dt} = \boldsymbol{\mu} \times \mathbf{B}_0 \tag{4.14}$$

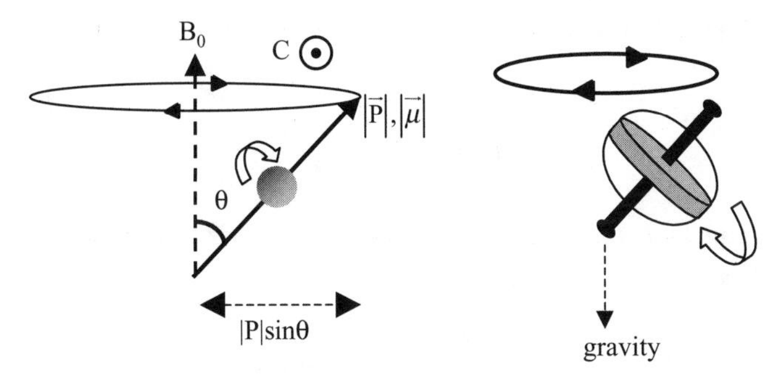

FIGURE 4.4. *(Left) Classically, the action of B_0 trying to align the proton magnetic moment along the direction of B_0 produces a torque C, the direction of which is out of the plane of the figure. (Right) An analogous situation of a spinning gyroscope precessing under the effect of gravity.*

From Figure 4.4, the magnitude of the component of the angular momentum that is precessing in the plane perpendicular to $\mathbf{B}_0$ is given by $|\mathbf{P}|\sin\theta$. In a short time dt, the magnetic moment precesses through an angle $d\phi$ producing a change $d\mathbf{P}$ in the angular momentum. Simple trigonometry gives

$$\sin(d\phi) = \frac{d\mathbf{P}}{|\mathbf{P}|\sin\theta} = \frac{\mathbf{C}\,dt}{|\mathbf{P}|\sin\theta} \tag{4.15}$$

If $d\phi$ is small, then $\sin(d\phi) \sim d\phi$. The angular precessional frequency ω is given by $d\phi/dt$ and so can be evaluated as

$$\omega = \frac{d\phi}{dt} = \frac{\mathbf{C}}{|\mathbf{P}|\sin\theta} = \frac{\boldsymbol{\mu}\times\mathbf{B}_0}{|\mathbf{P}|\sin\theta} = \frac{\gamma\mathbf{P}\times\mathbf{B}_0}{|\mathbf{P}|\sin\theta} \tag{4.16}$$

Expanding the cross product gives

$$\omega = \frac{\gamma\,|\mathbf{P}|\,|\mathbf{B}_0|\sin\theta}{|\mathbf{P}|\sin\theta} = \gamma B_0 \tag{4.17}$$

where $\mathbf{B}_0$ is universally, and henceforward, used to represent $|\mathbf{B}_0|$. Classical mechanics, therefore, shows that the effect of placing a proton in an magnetic field is that it precesses around the axis of that field at a frequency proportional to the strength of the magnetic field. This frequency is termed the Larmor frequency.

4.2.3. Radiofrequency Pulses and the Rotating Reference Frame

In order to obtain an MRI signal, transitions must be induced between the protons in the parallel and the antiparallel energy levels. The energy required to do this is supplied by an oscillating electromagnetic field, as covered further in Section 4.4.3. Because there is a specific energy gap ΔE in equation (4.9) between the two energy levels, the electromagnetic field must be applied at a specific frequency, called the resonance frequency. The frequency f of this electromagnetic field can be calculated from

$$hf = \Delta E = \frac{\gamma h B_0}{2\pi} \tag{4.18}$$

resulting in equations for the resonant frequency in hertz (f) or radians per second (ω):

$$f = \frac{\gamma B_0}{2\pi}, \qquad \omega = \gamma B_0 \tag{4.19}$$

The value of f for a 1.5-T clinical scanner is approximately 63.9 MHz. By comparing equations (4.17) and (4.19) it can be seen that the Larmor precession frequency is identical to the frequency of the electromagnetic field that must be applied for transitions to occur between the parallel and the antiparallel energy levels in the quantum mechanical model.

The electromagnetic energy is supplied to the system as a single pulse or series of pulses commonly referred to as radiofrequency (RF) pulses. The most common method used to analyze the effects of a given sequence of pulses is the "vector model." The starting point is to consider the net effect of all of the protons in the body, rather than single nuclei that have been considered until now. The net magnetization of the sample is defined as M_0, where

$$M_0 = \sum_{n=1}^{N_s} \mu_{z,n} = \frac{\gamma h}{4\pi}\left(N_{\text{parallel}} - N_{\text{antiparallel}}\right) = \frac{\gamma^2 h^2 B_0 N_s}{16\pi^2 kT} \tag{4.20}$$

When the patient is placed in the magnetic field, this net magnetization can be considered as the vector sum of all of the individual proton magnetic moments. These magnetic moments precess around B_0, and are randomly distributed around a "precession cone" as shown in Figure 4.5. The net magnetization only has a z component because the vector sum of the components in the x and y axes is zero:

$$M_z = M_0, \qquad M_y = 0, \qquad M_x = 0 \tag{4.21}$$

As explained later in this section, a detectable signal can only be produced by M_x and M_y components of magnetization, and not by the M_z component. In order to create M_x and M_y components, it is necessary to rotate the net magnetization from the z axis into the xy, or transverse, plane. In direct analogy with the classical interaction between B_0 and the proton magnetic moments, application of a second magnetic field at a 90° angle to the z axis produces a second torque, which rotates the magnetization toward the xy plane.

This second magnetic field, termed the B_1 field, oscillates at the Larmor frequency, and is created from an RF coil, designs of which are described in Section 4.4.3. The net magnetization precesses around the axis of the applied B_1 field at an angular frequency

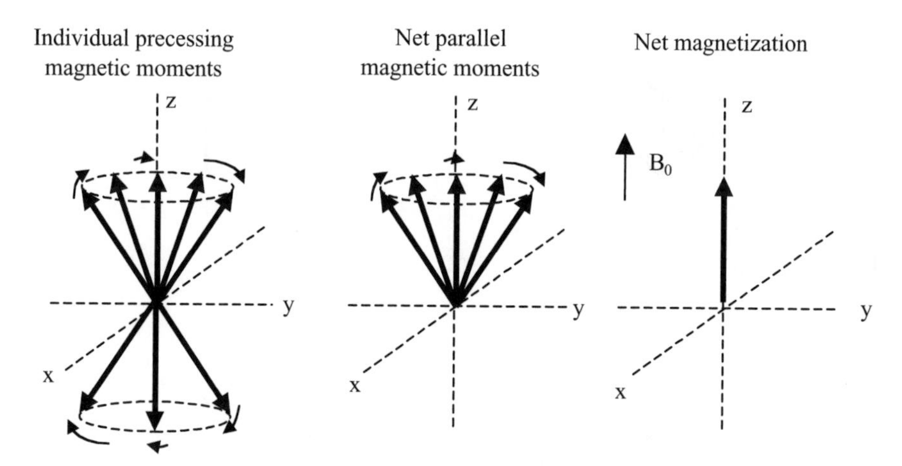

FIGURE 4.5. *(Left) The magnetic moments of each proton precess around the z axis with a frequency $\omega = \gamma B_0$ and at an angle of 54.7° to this axis. (Center) The magnetic moments corresponding to the slightly greater number aligned parallel to the magnetic field than antiparallel. (Right) The vector sum of all of the magnetic moments only has a z (longitudinal) component, with no component in the xy (transverse) plane.*

$\omega_1 = \gamma B_1$ and around the B_0 field at angular frequency $\omega = \gamma B_0$: this complicated motion of precession about two orthogonal axes is known as nutation. Because the magnitude of the B_1 field is very much smaller than that of B_0, precession around the RF field is correspondingly slower. If the B_1 field is applied along the x axis, the cone of magnetic moment vectors is tipped toward the y axis. This is shown in Figure 4.6 using the vector model.

The effect of applying the B_1 field about the x axis is to create a component of magnetization M_y in the y direction. The nuclei are now said to be "phase coherent" because all of the vectors are pointing in the same direction. The "tip angle" α is defined as the angle through which the net magnetization is rotated by the action of the B_1 field. This angle is proportional to the product of the strength of the applied RF field and the time τ_{B1} for which it is applied:

$$\alpha = \gamma B_1 \tau_{B1} \tag{4.22}$$

A tip angle of 90° results in the maximum value of the M_y component, whereas one of 180° produces no transverse magnetization, converting $+M_z$ into $-M_z$. Because the B_1 field is applied for a fixed duration, it is usually referred to as an RF pulse; one producing a tip angle of 90° is termed a 90° pulse.

In order to simplify visualization of the evolution of the net magnetization over time, the concept of a "rotating reference frame" (x', y', z') can be introduced into the vector model. In this frame the z' axis is identical to that of the "stationary" or "laboratory" frame (x, y, z) used previously, but the $x'y'$ axis rotates around the z' axis at the Larmor frequency. This effectively removes the need to consider nuclear

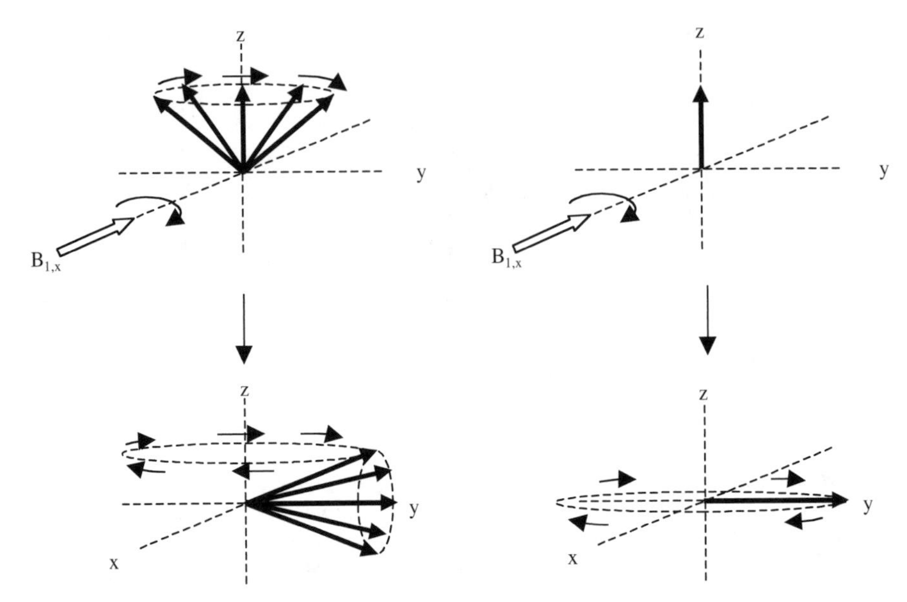

FIGURE 4.6. *(Top left) Application of a B_1 field ($B_{1,x}$) along the x axis rotates the individual proton magnetic moments around the x axis toward the y axis. (Bottom left) After applying the B_1 field for a certain time duration, the "cone" of magnetic moments has been rotated by 90°. The magnetic moments continue to precess around the B_0 axis. (Top and bottom right). The vector model representations of the effect of the B_1 field. The initial longitudinal magnetization (M_z) has been rotated into the transverse plane and has been converted into transverse magnetization (M_y) along the y axis.*

precession around the z axis in the vector model using the laboratory frame. The simplified rotation of the magnetization is shown in Figure 4.7 using the vector model in the rotating frame. It must be emphasized that the rotating reference frame is only a convenient model. In reality, of course, protons aligned parallel and antiparallel all continually precess around B_0, and also around B_1 for the time for which it is applied.

Signal detection involves placing an RF coil close to the patient. In its simplest form this coil is a single loop of wire. Faraday's law states that, when the magnetic flux enclosed by a loop of wire changes with time, a current is produced in the loop and a voltage is induced across the ends of the loop. The induced voltage E is proportional to the negative of the time rate of change of the magnetic flux ($d\phi/dt$):

$$E \propto -\frac{d\phi}{dt} \tag{4.23}$$

The time-varying magnetic field produced by the precession of the magnetization vectors results in a voltage being induced in the RF coil. The requirement for a

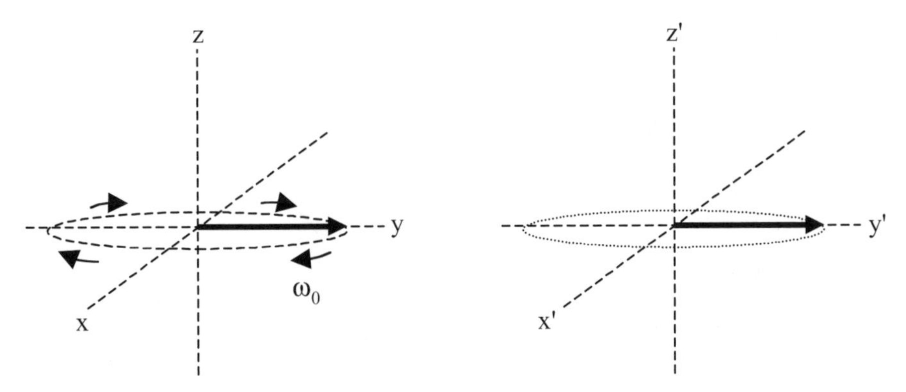

FIGURE 4.7. An illustration of the evolution of magnetization in the rotating reference frame. (Left) In the "laboratory frame," the net magnetization precesses around the z axis at the Larmor frequency. (Right) In the rotating reference frame, the x′y′ plane rotates around the z′ axis at the Larmor frequency, and therefore the net magnetization is static.

time-varying magnetic flux is the reason why only precessing magnetization in the xy plane gives rise to a nuclear magnetic resonance (NMR) signal: the z component does not precess and therefore produces no voltage. At higher strengths of the B_0 field, the protons precess at a higher frequency, and so the value of $d\phi/dt$ increases. So higher magnetic fields produce higher signal not only due to greater nuclear polarizations, equation (4.12), but also due to the higher voltage induced in the RF coil.

4.2.4. Spin–Lattice and Spin–Spin Relaxation

The effect of an RF pulse is to transfer energy from the transmitting coil to the protons. This excess energy results in a non-Boltzmann distribution of the populations of the parallel and the antiparallel energy states. In the vector model, the M_z component has been reduced from its equilibrium value of M_0, and the M_x and/or M_y components have a nonzero value. Each of the magnetization components M_z, M_x, and M_y must return to its thermal equilibrum value over time. The time evolutions of M_z, M_x, and M_y are characterized by differential equations, known as the Bloch equations:

$$\begin{aligned}
\frac{dM_x}{dt} &= \gamma M_y\left(B_0 - \frac{\omega}{\gamma}\right) - \frac{M_x}{T_2} \\
\frac{dM_y}{dt} &= \gamma M_z B_1 - \gamma M_x\left(B_0 - \frac{\omega}{\gamma}\right) - \frac{M_y}{T_2} \\
\frac{dM_z}{dt} &= -\gamma M_y B_1 - \frac{M_z - M_0}{T_1}
\end{aligned} \tag{4.24}$$

The return of M_z to its equilibrium value of M_0 is governed by the spin–lattice (T_1) relaxation time. Immediately after an RF pulse of arbitrary tip angle α, the M_z

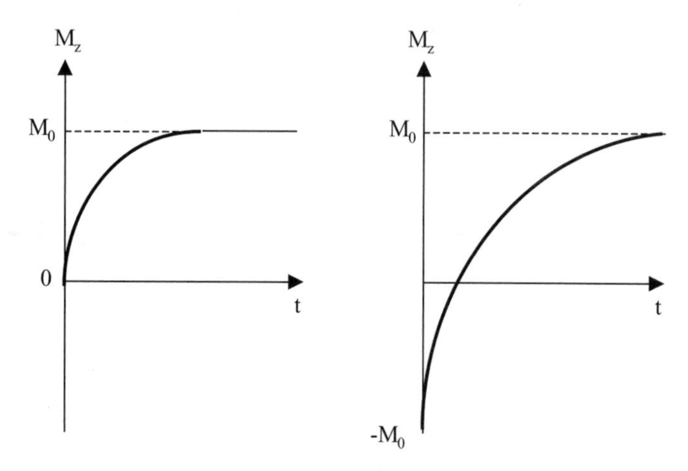

FIGURE 4.8. *Plots of M_z versus time after (left) a 90° pulse and (right) a 180° pulse.*

component is given by $M_0 \cos\alpha$. The value of M_z at a time t after the RF pulse is given by

$$M_z(t) = M_0 \cos\alpha + (M_0 - M_0 \cos\alpha)\left(1 - e^{-t/T_1}\right) \tag{4.25}$$

For example, after a 90° pulse the value of M_z is given by

$$M_z(t) = M_0\left(1 - e^{-t/T_1}\right) \tag{4.26}$$

Figure 4.8 shows the time dependence of the M_z magnetization for two commonly encountered situations, after a 90° pulse and a 180° pulse, respectively.

The physical basis for T_1 relaxation involves the protons losing their energy to the surrounding lattice, hence the name spin–lattice relaxation. Different tissues have different values of T_1, and this difference forms one basis for introducing tissue contrast into the MR image. Some values of the T_1 of commonly imaged tissues at a magnetic field strength of 1.5 T are shown in Table 4.2. The values of T_1 depend upon the magnetic field strength, a topic covered more fully in Section 4.5.2.

The M_x and M_y components of magnetization relax back to their thermal equilibrium values of zero with a time constant termed the spin–spin (T_2) relaxation time:

$$\frac{dM_x}{dt} = -\frac{M_x}{T_2}, \qquad \frac{dM_y}{dt} = -\frac{M_y}{T_2} \tag{4.27}$$

If an RF pulse of arbitrary tip angle α is applied along the x axis, then immediately after the pulse there is no M_x component of magnetization, and the M_y component is given by $M_0 \sin\alpha$. The value of M_y at time t after the RF pulse is given by

$$M_y(t) = M_0 \sin\alpha\, e^{-t/T_2} \tag{4.28}$$

TABLE 4.2. Tissue Relaxation Times at 1.5 T

Tissue	T_1 (ms)	T_2 (ms)
Fat	260	80
Muscle	870	45
Brain (gray matter)	900	100
Brain (white matter)	780	90
Liver	500	40
Cerebrospinal fluid	2400	160

The physical basis of the decay of transverse magnetization is different from that of the T_1 relaxation process. T_2 relaxation involves the loss of "phase coherence" between the protons precessing in the transverse plane. The concept of phase coherence can be thought of as the maintenance of a constant phase relationship between the magnetic moments of the individual protons. Even in a perfectly homogeneous B_0 magnetic field, the magnetic moments of different protons precess at slightly different frequencies due to variations in their interactions with neighboring nuclei. As a result, the net magnetization decreases as a function of time. The effect is shown in Figure 4.9, using the vector model in the rotating frame.

As is the case for T_1 relaxation times, different tissues in the body have different values of T_2, and these can also be used to differentiate between soft tissues in clinical images. Once again, the values depend on the strength of the magnetic field, and Table 4.2 shows typical values at 1.5 T.

In fact, the loss in phase coherence of the transverse magnetization arises from two different mechanisms. The first is the "pure" T_2 decay outlined above. The second arises from spatial variations in the strength of the magnetic field within the body. There are two major sources for these variations. The first is the intrinsic magnet design, that is, it is impossible to design a magnet producing a perfectly uniform magnetic field over the entire patient. The second source is local variations in magnetic field due to the different magnetic susceptibilities of different tissues: this effect is particularly pronounced at air/tissue and bone/tissue boundaries. Together, these factors produce loss of phase coherence, which is characterized by a relaxation time T_2^+. The overall relaxation time that governs the decay of transverse magnetization is a combination of signal loss due to T_2 and T_2^+ effects, and is designated by T_2^*, the value of which is given by

$$\frac{1}{T_2^*} = \frac{1}{T_2^+} + \frac{1}{T_2} \tag{4.29}$$

In the field of high-resolution NMR spectroscopy for chemical analysis, the value of T_2^+ is very small (because the sample is small and spatially homogeneous) and so the value of T_2^* is well approximated by T_2, and equation (4.28) is valid for describing the decay of transverse magnetization after an RF pulse. However, in MRI the value of T_2^+ can be up to 10–100 times shorter than T_2, and then the value of T_2^* should be substituted for T_2 in equation (4.28).

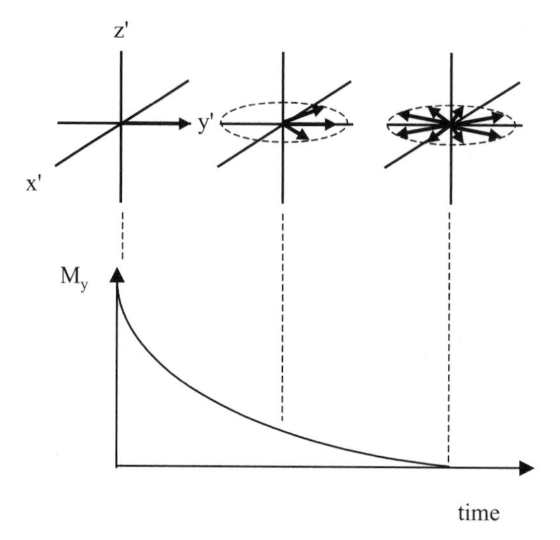

FIGURE 4.9. (Top) After a 90° pulse, the individual magnetic moments precess at different frequencies because they experience slightly different magnetic fields. (Bottom) The M_y component of magnetization decreases over time, and when the individual vectors are randomly distributed in the transverse plane, there is no net magnetic moment, and no signal is detected.

4.2.5. Measurement of T_1 and T_2: Inversion Recovery and Spin-Echo Sequences

Because valuable information about the physiological state of tissue can be obtained from both T_1 and T_2 relaxation times, and knowledge of these values allows sequences to be designed to give maximum image contrast, it is important to be able to measure T_1 and T_2 values for different tissues. The pulse sequences used for measurement are extremely simple, each consisting of two pulses.

The value of T_1 is measured using an inversion recovery sequence, which consists of a 180° pulse, a variable delay τ, and a 90° pulse followed immediately by data acquisition. This sequence is repeated n times, each time with a different value of the variable delay. From equation (4.25) the detected signal $S(\tau_n)$ is given by

$$S(\tau_n) = M_0(1 - 2e^{-\tau_n/T_1}) \tag{4.30}$$

A plot of ln $[S(\tau_n)]$ versus τ_n gives a straight line with a slope of $-T_1$.

Measuring the value of T_2 requires the use of a spin-echo experiment, shown schematically in Figure 4.10, where a 90° pulse is applied, followed by a variable delay τ, a 180° pulse, an identical delay τ, and then signal acquisition. Figure 4.10 also shows the evolution of the magnetization using the vector model and the total integrated M_y intensity.

In order to see how the spin-echo sequence works, consider a single proton, which, due to spatial inhomogeneities in the main magnetic field, resonates at a frequency $\Delta\omega$ less than the nominal Larmor frequency. Immediately succeeding the 90° pulse, the M_y component is M_0 and the M_x component is zero. At time τ after the 90° pulse, the

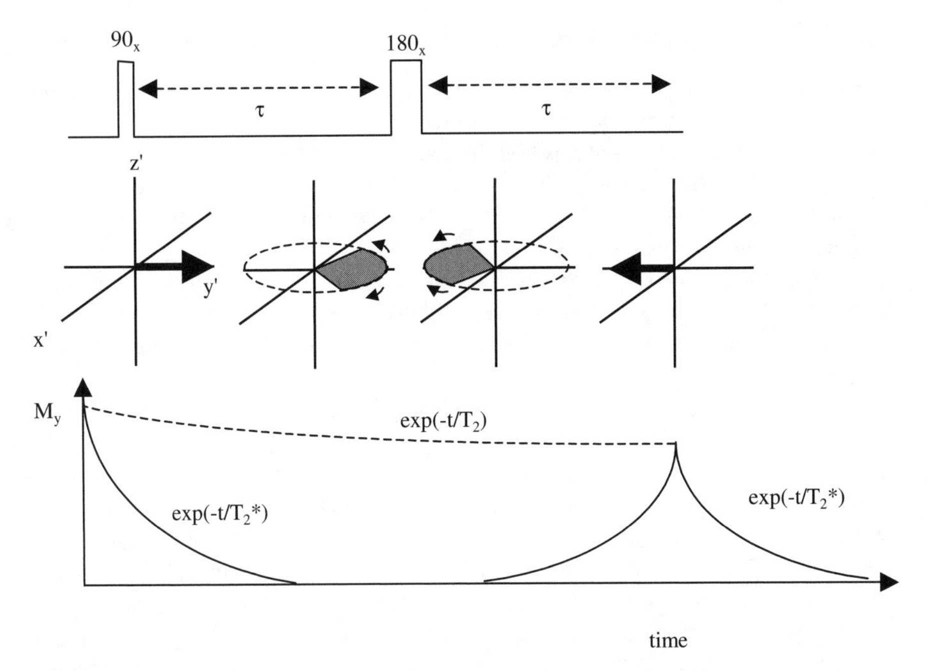

FIGURE 4.10. *A schematic of a spin-echo sequence. The 90° pulse tips the magnetization onto the y axis, where it decays with a time constant T_2^*. The effect of the 180° pulse is to "refocus" the magnetization such that at time τ after the 180° pulse, the individual vectors add constructively, and the signal reaches a peak.*

precessing magnetization has accumulated a phase ϕ given by $\phi = (\Delta\omega)\tau$. This phase can also be represented in terms of the M_y and M_x components of magnetization:

$$\phi = \arctan\left(\frac{M_x}{M_y}\right) \tag{4.31}$$

The 180° pulse applied about the x axis does not affect the M_x component of magnetization, but converts the M_y component into $-M_y$. The effect, therefore, is to convert the accumulated phase of the magnetization from $+\phi$ to $-\phi$. During the second τ interval, the precessing magnetization accumulates a further phase $+\phi$. So the net effect at time 2τ after the 90° pulse is that the precessing magnetization has zero phase, that is, the M_x component is zero and the vector lies along the $-y$ axis. Because the rephasing of the vectors does not depend upon the value of $\Delta\omega$, the effects of T_2^+ are canceled for all protons, leaving only the effects of pure T_2 relaxation. If n different values of τ are used, in the same way as for the measurement of the T_1 value, then

$$S(\tau_n) = M_0 e^{-2\tau_n/T_2} \tag{4.32}$$

A graph of $\ln[S(\tau_n)]$ versus $2\tau_n$ is plotted, giving a straight line with slope $-1/T_2$.

4.2.6. Signal Demodulation, Digitization, and Fourier Transformation

The oscillating voltage induced in the receiver coil using a standard 1.5-T scanner has a magnitude between several tens of microvolts and a few millivolts. Because it is difficult to digitize a signal at this high frequency, 63.9 MHz, using a high-dynamic-range A/D converter, the signal must be "demodulated" to a lower frequency before it can be digitized. A schematic for the typical components of a receiver used in magnetic resonance is shown in Figure 4.11.

The voltage induced in the RF coil first passes through a low-noise preamplifier, with a typical gain factor of 100 and noise figure of ~0.6 dB. If the signal from only the water protons is considered initially, then the induced voltage $s(t)$ is given by

$$s(t) \propto M_0 e^{-j\omega_0 t} e^{-t/T_2^*} \tag{4.33}$$

The first demodulation step uses a mixer to reduce the frequency of the signal from the Larmor frequency ω_0 to an intermediate frequency ω_{IF}, where the value of ω_{IF} is typically 67.2×10^6 rad s^{-1} (10.7 MHz). A simple circuit for the demodulator is shown in Figure 4.12, where the mixer effectively acts as a multiplier. This signal is then fed into a quadrature mixer, which is shown schematically in Figure 4.12.

The quadrature mixer first splits the input signal into two equal-magnitude components and mixes the real channel with a function $\cos \omega_{\mathrm{IF}} t$ and the imaginary channel with a function $\sin \omega_{\mathrm{IF}} t$. The output of each channel is low-pass-filtered to give the signals $s_{\mathrm{R}}(t)$ and $s_{\mathrm{I}}(t)$. As shown in Figure 4.11, these two signals are then amplified and digitized using (usually) two separate A/D converters. The time-domain signals $s_{\mathrm{R}}(t)$ and $s_{\mathrm{I}}(t)$ are collectively referred to as the free induction decay (FID) because they correspond to magnetization precessing freely, (not under the influence of an RF pulse) which induces an exponentially decaying voltage in the RF coil. After the signals are digitized and stored in the computer memory, they are displayed in the frequency domain after complex Fourier transformation:

$$S(\omega) = \int_{-\infty}^{\infty} [s_{\mathrm{R}}(t) + j s_{\mathrm{I}}(t)]\, e^{-j\omega t} \mathrm{d}t \propto M_0 \left[\frac{T_2^*}{1 + (T_2^*\omega)^2} - j \frac{(T_2^*)^2 \omega}{1 + (T_2^*\omega)^2} \right] \tag{4.34}$$

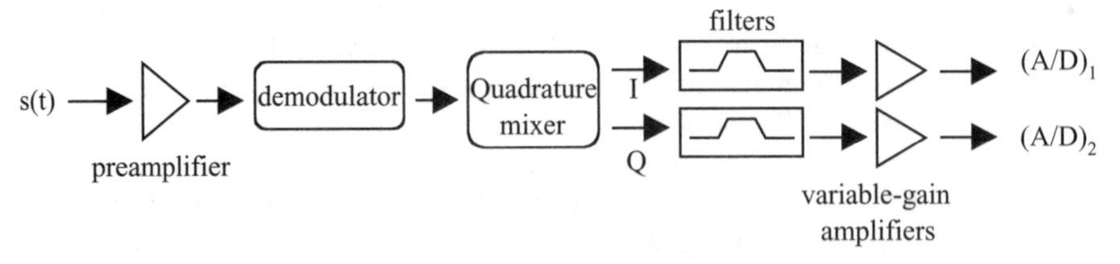

FIGURE 4.11. A block diagram of the receiver used in NMR and MRI systems. The demodulator reduces the frequency of the signal from the Larmor frequency to an intermediate frequency, typically 10.7 MHz. The quadrature mixer separates the real and the imaginary components of the signal, demodulated to the "baseband" frequency. These components are bandpass-filtered, amplified, and fed into two A/D converters.

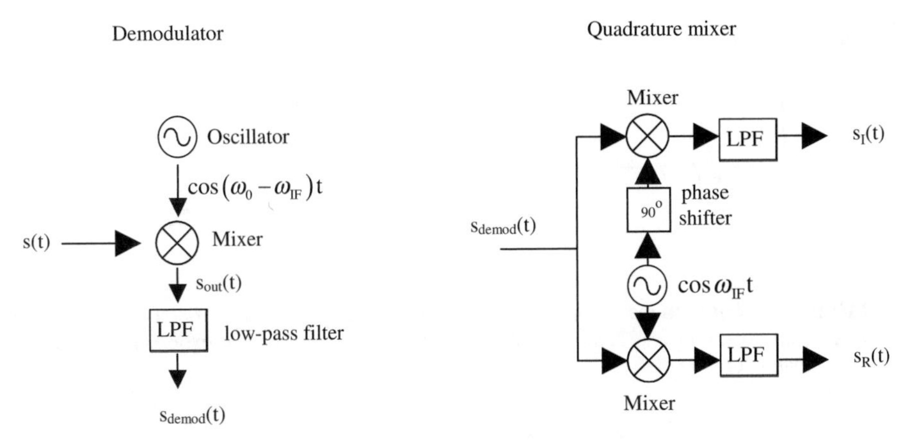

FIGURE 4.12. *(Left) A circuit diagram for a demodulator which takes the signal s(t) at the Larmor frequency and outputs a signal $s_{demod}(t)$ at an intermediate frequency ω_{IF}. (Right) A circuit for a quadrature demodulator which outputs the real and the imaginary components of the signal at baseband frequency.*

The real part of the frequency-domains signal $S_R(\omega)$ is a Lorentzian function with a FWHM given by $(\pi T_2{}^*)^{-1}$. The time-domain data and corresponding frequency-domain spectrum are both displayed in Figure 4.13.

Of course, not all of the protons in the body are water. There is a substantial number of protons in fat as well. The resonant frequencies of protons in fat are different from those in water because the exact value of the magnetic field at the nucleus

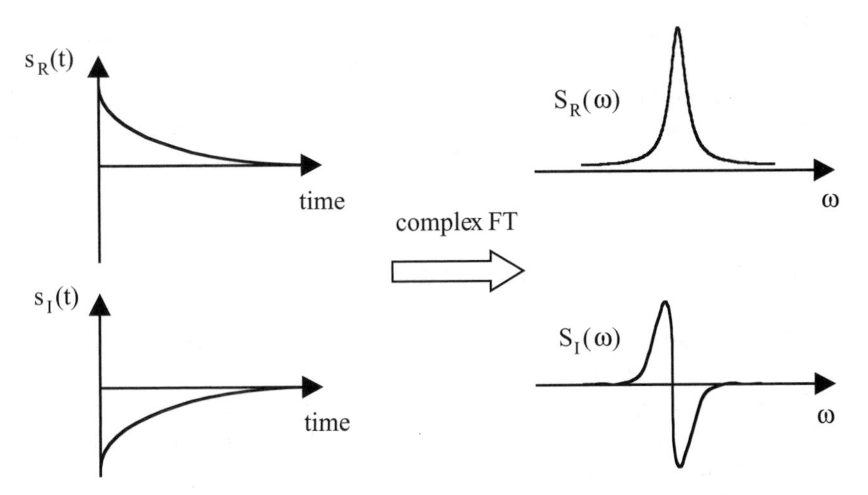

FIGURE 4.13. *Complex Fourier transformation of the real and the imaginary time-domain signals gives the corresponding real and imaginary components of the frequency-domain NMR spectrum.*

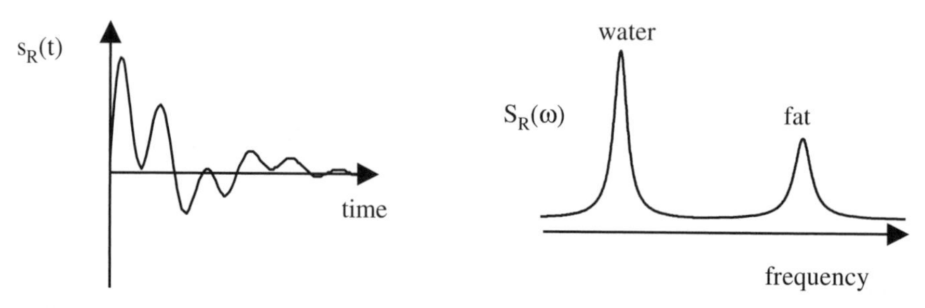

FIGURE 4.14. (Left) The real component of the time-domain signal corresponding to the proton signals from water and fat. (Right) The real component of the NMR spectrum obtained by Fourier transformation of the time-domain signal.

contains contributions from electrons orbiting around the nucleus. The electron spin has an electronic magnetic moment which produces a small magnetic field. This field is opposite in polarity to the main magnetic field B_0 and so reduces the effective magnetic field B_{eff}, at the nucleus:

$$B_{\text{eff}} = B_0(1 - \sigma) \tag{4.35}$$

where σ is called the shielding constant, and is related to the electronic environment surrounding the nucleus. Because fat ($-CH_2-$) and water (H_2O) have different electron distributions around the protons, due in part to the different electronegativities of the oxygen and carbon atoms, these protons resonate at slightly different frequencies. The values of σ for fat and water are $\sim 1.3 \times 10^{-6}$ (commonly referred to as 1.3 ppm, where ppm stands for parts per million) and 4.5 ppm, respectively. At 1.5 T the difference in resonance frequencies between the protons in fat and water, $\Delta\omega$, is roughly 1257 rad s^{-1}. Figure 4.14 shows the real component of the digitized time-domain signal acquired from the whole body at 1.5 T and the corresponding real component of the frequency-domain spectrum. Two peaks are apparent in the latter, one each from the protons in water and fat, with a frequency difference of $\Delta\omega$. The FWHM "linewidths" of each peak are inversely proportional to their respective values of $T_2{}^*$, as discussed earlier.

4.3. MAGNETIC RESONANCE IMAGING

The NMR signal described so far is simply the sum of the individual signals from each proton: there is nothing to distinguish between the signals from protons located at different spatial locations. The development of MRI resulted from the realization by Paul Lauterbur in 1973 that a magnetic field gradient, that is, a spatial variation in the magnetic field across a sample, would result in a range of proton resonant frequencies, each dependent upon the position of the particular proton within the body. The creation of such a magnetic field gradient requires additional hardware, namely "gradient coils," described in Section 4.4.2. Three separate gradient coils are required to encode unambiguously the three spatial dimensions. Because only the z component of the magnetic field interacts with the proton magnetic moments, it is the spatial variation in the z component of the magnetic field that is important. Image reconstruction is simplified considerably if the magnetic field gradients are linear over the region to be imaged, that is,

$$\frac{\partial B_z}{\partial z} = G_z, \qquad \frac{\partial B_z}{\partial x} = G_x, \qquad \frac{\partial B_z}{\partial y} = G_y \tag{4.36}$$

Because MRI uses almost exclusively horizontal superconducting magnets with the geometry shown in Figure 4.1, it is important to note the change in coordinate system used in MRI. These magnets produce a main magnetic field that is oriented in a horizontal direction, and the direction of B_0 is in the head-to-foot direction for the patient lying in a horizontal magnet, as shown in Figure 4.15. In the vector model, therefore, the z direction also lies along the head-to-foot axis. By convention, the y axis corresponds to the vertical (spine-to-abdomen) direction and the x axis from side-to-side (right-to-left).

The gradient coils are designed such that there is no additional contribution to the magnetic field at the isocenter ($z = 0$, $y = 0$, $x = 0$) of the magnet, which means that the magnetic field at this position is simply B_0. Figure 4.15 shows a plot of magnetic field versus spatial position for a gradient applied along the z axis.

The magnetic field B_z experienced by all nuclei with a common coordinate z is

$$B_z = B_0 + zG_z \tag{4.37}$$

where G_z has units of tesla (T) per meter or gauss (G) per centimeter, where 1 T is equivalent to 10,000 G. From the graph shown in Figure 4.15, at position $z = 0$, $B_z = B_0$; for all positions $z > 0$, $B_z > B_0$; and for positions $z < 0$, $B_z < B_0$. The

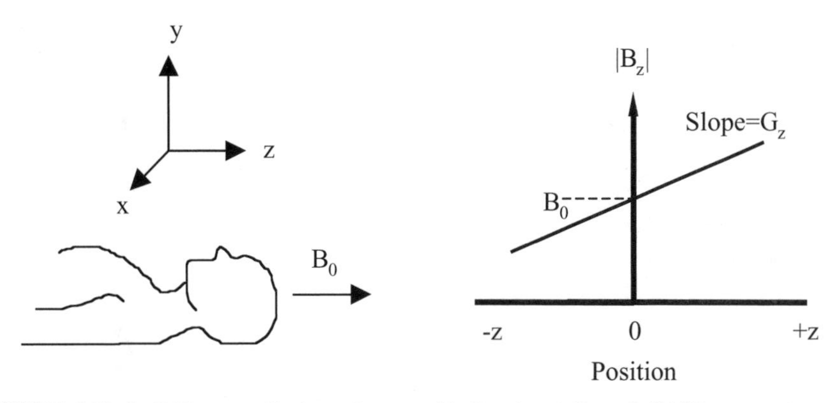

FIGURE 4.15. *(Left) The coordinate system used in the description of all MRI sequences and instrumentation. (Right) A linear magnetic field gradient applied in the z direction produces a linear spatial dependence of the effective magnetic field B_z.*

corresponding precessional frequencies ω_z of the protons as a function of their position in z is given by

$$\omega_z = \gamma B_z = \gamma(B_0 + zG_z) \tag{4.38}$$

In the rotating reference frame the precessional frequency is

$$\omega_z = \gamma z G_z \tag{4.39}$$

Analogous expressions can be obtained for the spatial dependence of the resonant frequencies in the presence of the x and y gradients.

The process of image formation can be broken down into three components: slice selection, phase-encoding, and frequency-encoding, covered in the following sections.

4.3.1. Slice Selection

Most clinical MRI studies acquire a series of slices through the anatomical area of interest, each slice having a well-defined orientation and thickness. Slice selection is accomplished using a frequency-selective RF pulse applied simultaneously with one of the magnetic field gradients, denoted here by G_{slice}. The choice of the slice-select direction dictates the orientation—coronal, axial, or sagittal—of the image, corresponding to slice selection in the y, the z, or the x directions, respectively, as shown in Figure 4.16. If an oblique slice angle is required, then two of the gradients can

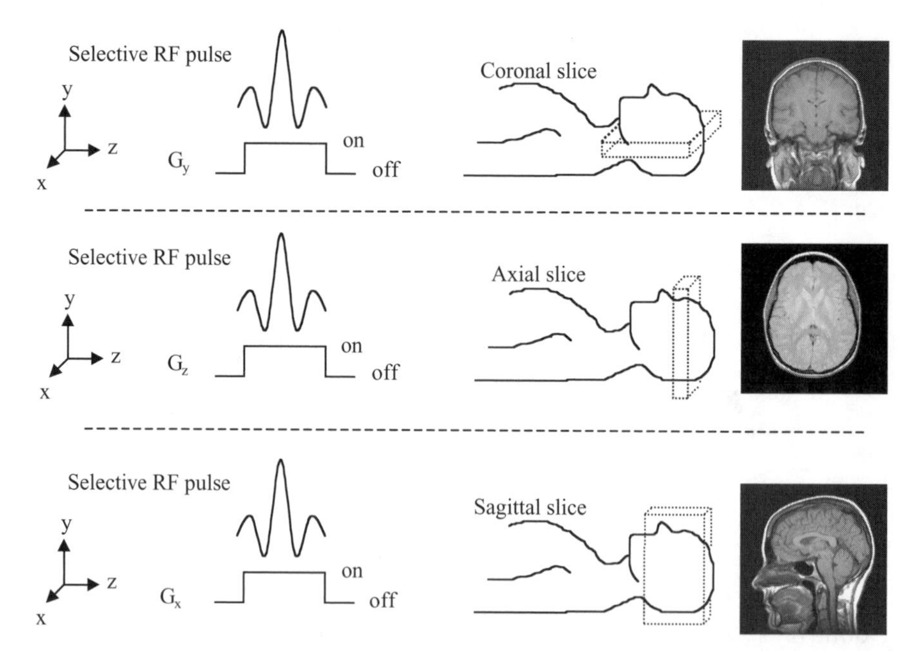

FIGURE 4.16. A schematic of slice selection in MRI. By using a frequency-selective pulse in combination with the y, z, or x gradient, a coronal, axial, or sagittal slice, respectively, can be chosen.

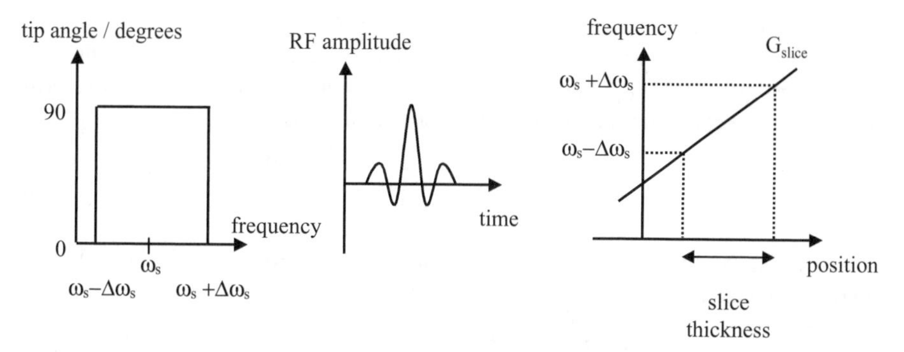

FIGURE 4.17. *(Left) The ideal pulse tips the magnetization precessing at a frequency between $\omega_S - \Delta\omega_S$ and $\omega_S + \Delta\omega_S$ by 90°, leaving the magnetization outside this frequency range completely undisturbed. (Center) A typical shape of an RF pulse used for slice selection. (Right) The relationship between the frequency bandwidth of the pulse, the strength of the slice-select gradient, and the slice thickness of the image.*

be applied, with appropriately weighted strengths, simultaneously with the frequency-selective pulse.

If the selective RF pulse is applied at a frequency ω_s with an excitation bandwidth of $\pm\Delta\omega_S$, then protons precessing at frequencies between $\omega_s + \Delta\omega_s$ and $\omega_s - \Delta\omega_s$ are rotated into the transverse plane; those with resonant frequencies outside this range are not affected and remain in the z direction. The thickness T of the slice corresponding to protons that are affected by the RF pulse is determined by the combination of the frequency bandwidth $2\Delta\omega_s$ of the RF pulse and the value of the slice-select gradient:

$$T = \frac{2\Delta\omega_s}{\gamma G_{\text{slice}}} \tag{4.40}$$

The slice thickness can therefore be increased either by decreasing the strength of G_{slice} or increasing the frequency bandwidth of the excitation pulse. The ideal frequency excitation profile of the RF pulse is a rectangular shape, shown in Figure 4.17, where an equal tip angle is applied to all of the protons within the slice and zero tip angle to protons outside the slice. Because the frequency response of an RF pulse can be reasonably well approximated by its Fourier transform, a sinc-shaped RF pulse, typically with a length of 1–5 ms, is often used to produce a square-shaped frequency excitation profile. From the properties of the Fourier transform, a longer RF pulse results in a narrower frequency spectrum, and therefore a thinner slice for a given value of G_{slice}. By changing the center frequency ω_s of the RF pulse, the slice can be moved to different parts of the patient. Many slices, each offset from one another, can also be acquired, as outlined in Section 4.5.3.

Due to the fact that the RF pulse is relatively long, nuclei within the slice precess around B_0 during the RF pulse and accumulate different phases ϕ_{sl} depending on their position within the slice. If the direction of G_{slice} is denoted by z, then

$$\phi_{\text{sl}}(z) = \gamma G_z z \frac{\tau}{2} \tag{4.41}$$

where τ is the duration of the pulse and z is the proton position within the slice. In order to overcome this undesired loss of phase coherence, a rephasing gradient of the opposite polarity G_z^{ref} is applied for a time τ^{ref}. Assuming that the gradient waveforms are perfectly rectangular, complete refocusing occurs when

$$G_z^{\text{ref}}\tau^{\text{ref}} = \frac{\tau}{2}G_z \tag{4.42}$$

Mathematically, the signal from the precessing magnetization after slice selection can be represented as

$$S \propto \int_{\text{slice}}\int_{\text{slice}} \rho(x, y)\, dx\, dy \tag{4.43}$$

where $\rho(x, y)$ is the number of protons at positions (x, y) within the body, and is called the proton density.

4.3.2. Phase-Encoding

Having selected a slice, the other two-dimensions must be encoded to produce a two-dimensional image. One of these directions is encoded by imposing a spatially dependent phase on the signal from the precessing protons, and the other by creating a spatially dependent precessional frequency during signal acquisition. The difference between the two encoding schemes is that the phase is encoded by a gradient turned on and off *before* data acquisition begins, and a number (N_p) of different values of this phase-encoding gradient G_{phase} must be used. In contrast, the frequency-encoding gradient G_{freq} is turned on *during* data acquisition. The basic imaging sequence is shown schematically in Figure 4.18.

After the slice selection pulse, the phase-encoding gradient G_{phase} is applied for a period τ_{pe} and then switched off before data acquisition begins. If the direction of G_{phase} is denoted by y, during τ_{pe} the protons precess at a frequency $\omega_y = \gamma G_y y$. The net effect of G_{phase} is to introduce a spatially dependent phase shift $\phi(G_y, \tau_{\text{pe}})$ into the acquired signal, with a value given by

$$\phi(G_y, \tau_{\text{pe}}) = \omega_y \tau_{\text{pe}} = \gamma G_y y \tau_{\text{pe}} \tag{4.44}$$

The total signal from the excited slice, after the phase-encoding gradient has been switched off, is given by

$$S(G_y, \tau_{\text{pe}}) = \int_{\text{slice}}\int_{\text{slice}} \rho(x, y)e^{-j\gamma G_y y \tau_{\text{pe}}} dx\, dy \tag{4.45}$$

4.3.3. Frequency-Encoding

The frequency-encoding, also called read, direction is encoded by the nuclei precessing at different frequencies under the influence of a gradient G_{freq}, which is applied

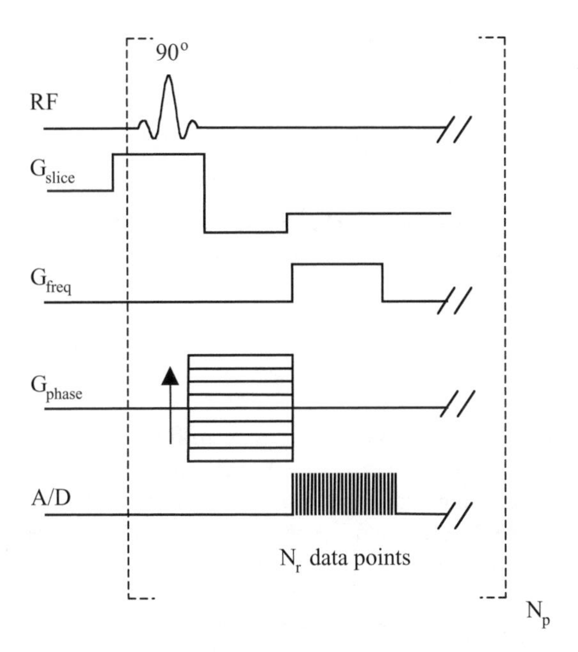

FIGURE 4.18. *A basic imaging sequence using phase- and frequency-encoding gradients. The arrow indicates that the phase-encoding gradient strength is incremented N_p times to form a two-dimensional dataset, which has size $N_r \times N_p$.*

during data acquisition. Assuming that G_{freq} is applied in the x direction, and considering only the effect of this frequency-encoding gradient, the acquired signal is given by

$$s\,(G_x, t) \propto \int_{\text{slice}} \int_{\text{slice}} \rho\,(x, y)\, e^{-j\omega_x t} dx\, dy = \int_{\text{slice}} \int_{\text{slice}} \rho\,(x, y)\, e^{-j\gamma G_x x t} dx\, dy \tag{4.46}$$

The combined effect of the phase-encoding and frequency-encoding gradients, therefore, gives a signal

$$s(G_y, \tau_{\text{pe}}, G_x, t) \propto \int_{\text{slice}} \int_{\text{slice}} \rho\,(x, y)\, e^{-j\gamma G_x x t} e^{-j\gamma G_y y \tau_{\text{pe}}} dx\, dy \tag{4.47}$$

The time between acquisition of successive data points in the frequency-encoding dimension is referred to as the dwell time t_{dw}, which is the reciprocal of the acquisition bandwidth.

4.3.4. The *k*-Space Formalism

A very useful model for understanding exactly how the acquired $N_{\text{r}} \times N_{\text{p}}$ data matrix is transformed into the final image is the "k-space" formalism developed by Ljunggren.

If two variables k_x and k_y are defined as

$$k_x = \frac{\gamma}{2\pi} G_x t, \qquad k_y = \frac{\gamma}{2\pi} G_y \tau_{\mathrm{pe}} \tag{4.48}$$

with x and y being the frequency- and phase-encoding directions, respectively, then equation (4.47) can be expressed in terms of these two variables:

$$S(k_x, k_y) \propto \int_{\mathrm{slice}} \int_{\mathrm{slice}} \rho(x, y) e^{-jk_x x} e^{-jk_y y} dx\, dy \tag{4.49}$$

The $N_r \times N_p$ data matrix can be visualized as a two-dimensional data set in k-space. Consider the N_r data points collected when the maximum negative value of the phase-encoding gradient G_y is applied. From equation (4.48) the value of k_y for all N_r data points corresponds to its maximum negative value. When the frequency-encoding gradient is switched on, the first data point collected corresponds to a small positive value of k_x, the second data point to a slightly more positive value of k_x, and so forth, and so the N_r data points correspond to one "line" in k-space, shown as line 1 in Figure 4.19. The second line in k-space corresponds to the next value of the phase-encoding gradient, and so on. The spacing between the k-space points is dictated by

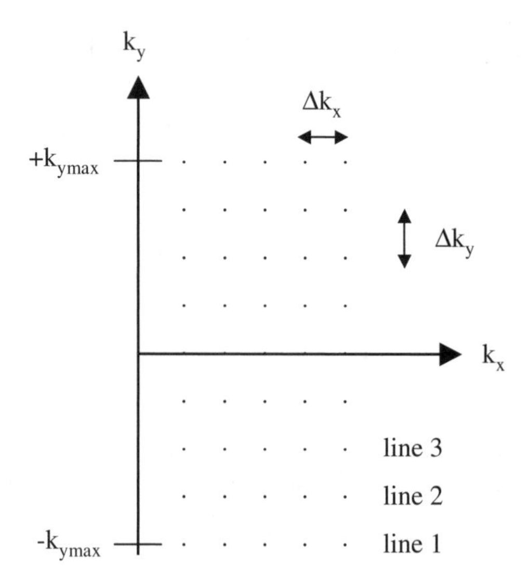

FIGURE 4.19. *The k-space coverage corresponding to the imaging sequence shown in Figure 4.18. Line 1 is acquired using the maximum negative value of the phase-encoding gradient. Subsequent lines are acquired with the value of the phase-encoding gradient increasing in a positive direction.*

the required FOV of the image. It is relatively simple to derive the respective equations for the FOV in the x and the y directions:

$$\begin{aligned} \mathrm{FOV}_x &= \tfrac{1}{\Delta k_x} = \frac{2\pi}{\gamma G_x t_{\mathrm{dw}}} \\ \mathrm{FOV}_y &= \tfrac{1}{\Delta k_y} = \frac{2\pi}{\gamma \Delta G_y t_{\mathrm{pe}}} \end{aligned} \tag{4.50}$$

From equation (4.49) and equation (A.6) in Appendix A, it can be seen that a two-dimensional inverse Fourier transform of the k-space data $S(k_x, k_y)$ gives an estimate of $\rho(x, y)$, that is, an image corresponding to the spatial variation in proton density. This simple relationship between the image and the data acquired in k-space is a major reason why the k-space representation of MRI data acquisition is particularly useful.

The data acquired using the sequence in Figure 4.18 cover k-space from the maximum negative value of k_y to the maximum positive value, but in the k_x direction only data corresponding to positive values of k_x are obtained. Effectively, therefore, only one-half of k-space has been acquired. If full k-space coverage could be achieved, then the SNR of the reconstructed image would be increased, as would the spatial resolution, which is determined in the respective dimensions by the maximum values of k_x and k_y. From equation (4.48) it is clear that negative values of k_x must correspond to negative values of G_x (because t cannot be negative). In practice, an echo, rather than an FID signal, must be acquired. The sequence in Figure 4.18 can be adapted to give such an echo-based sequence, shown in Figure 4.20, which covers k_x-space symmetrically with respect to positive and negative values. A negative gradient

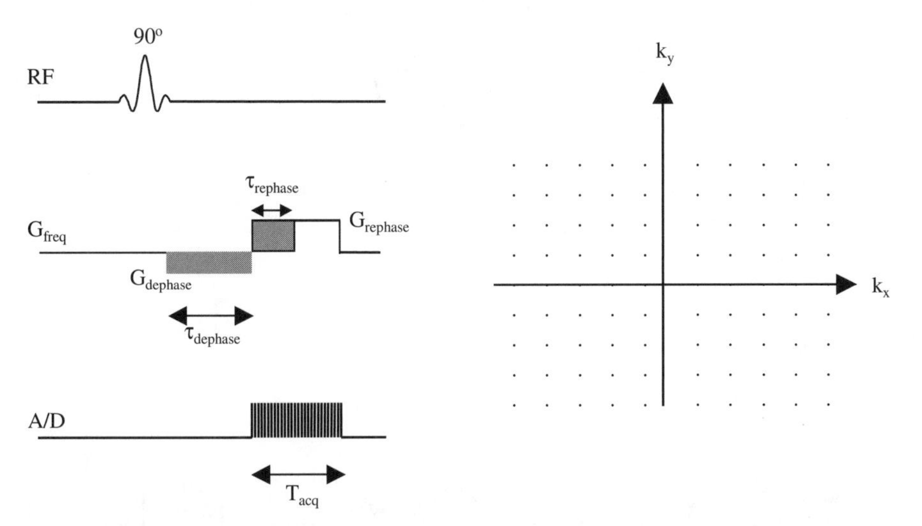

FIGURE 4.20. *(Left) A gradient-echo imaging sequence with dephasing and rephasing frequency-encoding gradients (the phase and slice selection gradients have been omitted for clarity and are identical to those in Figure 4.18). The areas of the two shaded gradients are equal, as expressed in equation (4.51). (Right) The "full" k-space coverage resulting from data acquisition using the sequence on the left, with an incremental phase-encoding gradient.*

G_{dephase} is applied for a time τ_{dephase} before data acquisition, with values given by

$$G_{\text{dephase}}\tau_{\text{dephase}} = \tau_{\text{rephase}}G_{\text{rephase}} = \frac{T_{\text{acq}}}{2}G_{\text{rephase}} \tag{4.51}$$

4.4. INSTRUMENTATION

Three basic components make up the MRI scanner: the magnet, three magnetic field gradient coils, and an RF coil. The magnet polarizes the protons in the patient, the magnetic field gradient coils impose a linear variation on the proton Larmor frequency as a function of position, and the RF coil produces the oscillating magnetic field necessary for creating phase coherence between protons, and also receives the MRI signal via Faraday induction. The physical arrangement of these three components is shown in Figure 4.1. Each MRI system has a number of different-sized RF coils, used according to the particular part of the body being imaged, which are placed on or around the patient. The gradient coils are fixed permanently inside the bore of the superconducting magnet.

In addition to these three elements there is a series of electronic components used to turn the gradients on and off, to pulse the B_1 field, and to amplify and digitize the signal. A simplified block diagram of a system is shown in Figure 4.21. Various components are discussed further in the following sections.

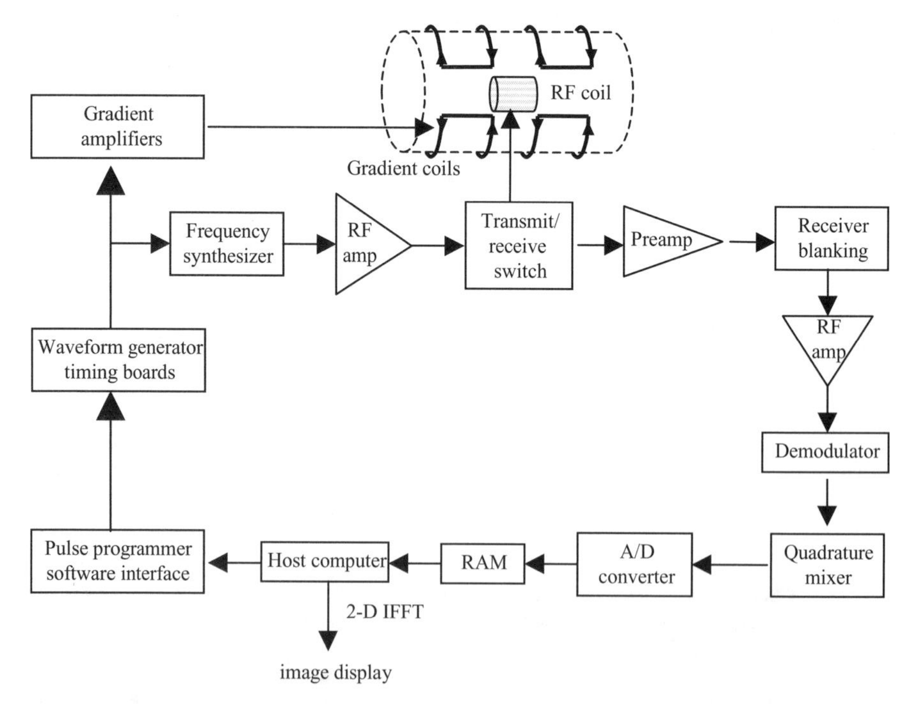

FIGURE 4.21. *A block diagram of the electronic and computer components making up an MRI system.*

4.4.1. Magnet Design

The purpose of the magnet is to produce a strong, temporally stable, and homogeneous magnetic field within the patient. A strong magnetic field increases the amplitude of the MRI signal, a homogeneous magnetic field is required so that the tissue T_2^* value is not too short and images are not distorted by B_0 inhomogeneities, and high stability is necessary to avoid introducing unwanted artifacts into the image. There are three basic types of magnet: permanent, resistive, and superconducting.

For magnetic fields of approximately 0.35 T or less, either resistive or permanent magnets can be used. Permanent magnet systems are usually constructed of rare earth alloys such as cobalt–samarium. Their advantages include relatively low cost, ease of siting due to very limited stray magnetic fields present outside the magnet, the lack of a requirement for cooling the magnet, and a reduced susceptibility to patient claustrophobia due to their open nature, as can be seen in Figure 4.22. Permanent magnet systems are used widely for interventional MRI, in which surgical procedures are carried out in the magnet simultaneously with imaging. The disadvantages of permanent magnets are the very large weight of such magnets and the fact that the field homogeneity and temporal stability are highly temperature-dependent, meaning that sophisticated thermal regulation must be used.

In resistive magnets, the magnetic field is created by the passage of a constant current through a conductor such as copper. The strength of the magnetic field is directly proportional to the magnitude of the current, and thus high currents are

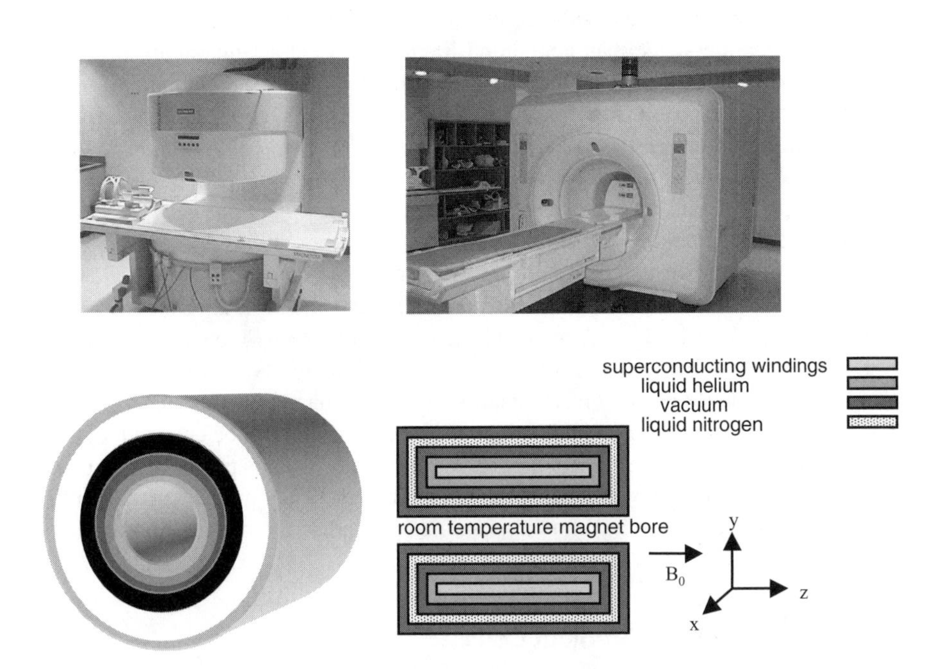

FIGURE 4.22. (Top left) An open "C-arm" permanent magnet operating at 0.3 T. The magnet has two pole pieces, one above and one below the patient bed, an arrangement that allows easy access to the patient. (Top right) A clinical superconducting MRI magnet operating at a magnetic field strength of 1.5 T. (Bottom) A schematic of the construction of a superconducting magnet.

necessary to create high magnetic fields. However, the amount of power dissipated in the wire is proportional to the resistance of the conductor and the square of the current. Because the power is dissipated in the form of heat, cooling the conductors is a major problem, and ultimately limits the maximum current, and therefore magnetic field strength, that can be achieved with a resistive magnet. As with permanent magnets, the field homogeneity and the temporal stability of resistive magnets are highly temperature-dependent.

The solution to the problem of conductor heating is to minimize the resistance of the conductor by using the phenomenon of superconductivity, in which the resistance of many conductors becomes zero at very low temperatures. In order to create high static magnetic fields, it is still necessary for the conductor to carry a large current when it is superconducting, and this capability is only possessed by certain alloys, particularly those made from niobium–titanium. Below a critical temperature (9 K) and critical magnetic field (10 T), once current has been fed into such an alloy, this current will run through the wire with constant magnitude essentially indefinitely. Superconducting magnets are used for most systems above 0.35 T. The most common field for clinical scanning is 1.5 T, although 3 T systems are becoming increasingly common, particularly for brain scanning, and experimental systems operating at 7 and 8 T now exist for human study. Figure 4.21 shows a typical clinical 1.5 T scanner, with a moveable bed used to position the patient at the center of the magnet.

The superconducting alloy is usually fashioned into multistranded filaments within a conducting matrix because this arrangement can support a higher critical current than a single, larger-diameter superconducting wire. This superconducting matrix is housed in a stainless steel can containing liquid helium at a temperature of 4.2 K, as shown in Figure 4.22. This can is surrounded by a series of radiation shields and vacuum vessels to minimize the boil-off of the liquid helium. Finally, an outer container of liquid nitrogen is used to cool the outside of the vacuum chamber and the radiation shields. Because heat losses cannot be completely contained, liquid nitrogen and liquid helium must be replenished on a regular basis.

The exact placement of the superconducting filaments within the magnet is designed to give the maximum B_0 homogeneity over the patient region. The basic design consists of a number of solenoids of different diameters and separations, each wound along the major axis of the magnet. Slight errors in positioning the wires can lead to large variations in the field uniformity, and so additional coils of wire are added in series with the main coil as "correction coils." After the magnet has been energized by passing current into the major filament windings, the current can be changed in these correction coils to improve the homogeneity. Final fine tuning is performed by using a series of independently wired coils, termed shim coils. The operator can adjust the current in these coils for each clinical examination, and so the magnet homogeneity can be optimized for individual patients.

4.4.2. Magnetic Field Gradient Coils

As described in Section 4.3, the basic principle of MRI requires the generation of magnetic field gradients, in addition to the static magnetic field, so that the proton resonant frequencies within the patient are spatially dependent. Such gradients are achieved using "magnetic field gradient coils," a term usually shortened to simply "gradient coils." Three separate gradient coils are required to encode the x, y, and z dimensions of the image. The requirements for gradient coil design are that the gradients are linear over the region being imaged, that they are efficient in terms of producing high gradient strengths per unit current, and that they have fast switching times for use in rapid imaging techniques.

As in the case of magnet design, a magnetic field gradient is produced by the passage of current through conducting wires. Unlike the design of the magnet, however, the geometry of the conductors for the three gradient coils must be optimized to produce a linear gradient, rather than a uniform field. The value of the gradient is relatively small compared to the strength of the main magnetic field, with typical values of 4 G/cm for clinical scanners. Copper at room temperature can therefore be used as the conductor, with chilled-water cooling being sufficient to remove the heat generated by the current. Because the gradient coils fit directly inside the bore of the cylindrical magnet, the geometrical design is usually cylindrical. The simplest configuration for the coil producing a gradient in the z direction is a "Maxwell pair," shown in Figure 4.23, which consists of two separate loops consisting of multiple turns of wire. The two loops are wound in opposite directions around a cylindrical former, and the loops are spaced by a separation of $\sqrt{3}$ times the radius of the loop. The magnetic field produced by this gradient coil is zero at the center of the coil, and is linearly dependent upon position in the z direction over about one-third of the

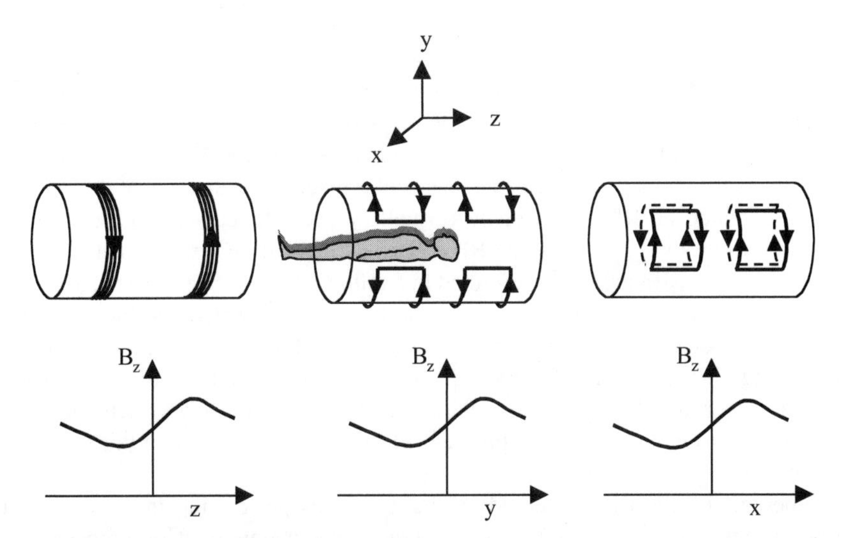

FIGURE 4.23. *The basic design of magnetic field gradient coils used for MRI. The arrows indicate the direction of current flow. (Left) A z-gradient coil, (center) a y-gradient coil, and (right) an x-gradient coil. Each coil consists of multiple turns of wire, which for clarity are only shown for the z-gradient coil. The useable region of the magnet effectively corresponds to the volume over which the gradients are linear.*

separation of the two loops. The gradient strength is proportional to the square of the number of turns.

The x- and y-gradient coils are completely independent from the z-gradient coils, and each gradient coil is connected to a separate gradient amplifier, as shown in Figure 4.20. From symmetry considerations the same basic design can be used for coils producing gradients in the x and y directions with the geometries simply rotated by 90°. The most common configuration is the "saddle coil" arrangement, with four arcs, as shown in Figure 4.23. Each arc subtends an angle of 120°, the separation between the arcs along the z axis is 0.8 times the radius of the gradient coil, and the length of each arc is 2.57 times the radius.

A second design criterion is that the current in the gradient coils should be switched on and off in the shortest possible time. This reduces the time which must be allowed for gradient stabilization in imaging sequences. This criterion is achieved by minimizing the inductance of the gradient coils. A related issue is achieving high efficiency, that is, a high gradient per unit current, which corresponds to minimizing the resistance of the gradient coils. When the gradients are switched rapidly, they induce eddy currents in nearby conducting surfaces such as the radiation shield in the magnet. These currents, in turn, produce additional unwanted gradients, which may decay only very slowly, even after the original gradients have been switched off. All gradient coils in commercial MRI systems are now "actively shielded" to reduce the effects of eddy currents. Active shielding uses a second set of coils placed outside the main gradient coils, the effect of which is to minimize the stray gradient fields.

4.4.3. Radiofrequency Coils

As described previously, in order to produce an MRI signal, magnetic energy must be supplied to the protons at the Larmor frequency in order to stimulate transitions between the parallel and the antiparallel nuclear energy levels, thus creating precessing transverse magnetization. The particular piece of hardware that delivers this energy is called an RF coil, which is usually placed directly around, or next to, the tissue to be imaged. The same RF coil is also usually used to detect the NMR signal via Faraday induction, as outlined in Section 4.2.3. The power needed to generate the RF pulses for clinical systems can be many kilowatts, and the receiver is designed to detect signals only on the order of 1–10 V. Therefore, it is important that during signal transmission there is no possibility of signal "leaking" through to the receiver and damaging the electronics. A transmit/receive switch and active receiver blanking, both shown in Figure 4.21, are used to ensure that this leakage is minimized.

Superficially, the RF coil could be thought of as performing in a similar way to a conventional radio antenna, but there are several important differences in its function and design. An antenna is designed to radiate a large fraction of its input power into the far field. An RF coil, on the other hand, should be designed to store as much of its magnetic energy as possible in the near-field region, that is, within the patient. The most efficient coil design is based on resonant electric circuits, in which

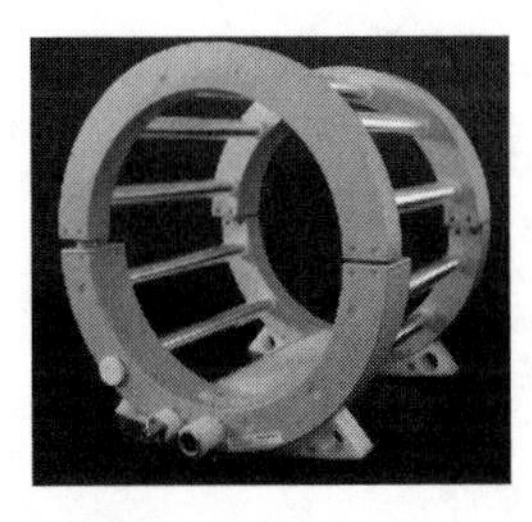
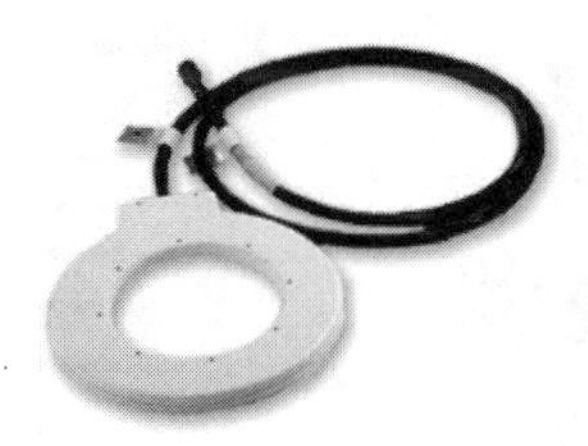
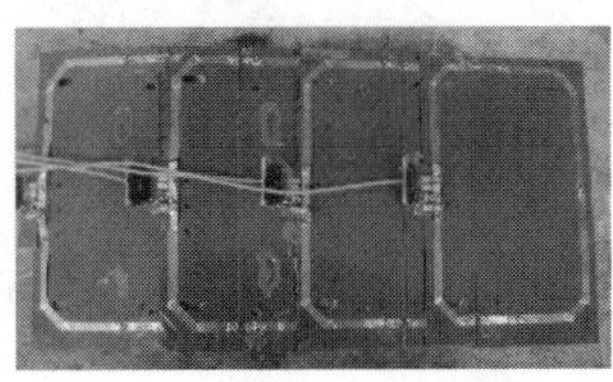

***FIGURE 4.24.** Three RF coils used for magnetic resonance imaging. (Left) a birdcage coil used for brain imaging, (center) a surface coil used for imaging close to the surface of the body, (right) a phased array used for spine imaging.*

there is a resonant frequency ω_r at which the magnetic energy stored in the coil is a maximum.

In terms of the electrical properties of the coil, this frequency is given by

$$\omega_r = \frac{1}{\sqrt{LC}} \tag{4.52}$$

where L is the inductance of the RF coil. The value of C represents both the intrinsic capacitance of the coil and also the capacitance that is added, in the form of discrete capacitors, to the circuit for tuning the resonance to ω_r, and also matching the input impedance to 50 Ω for maximum operational efficiency. A well-designed coil efficiently converts power from a frequency source and RF amplifier into an oscillating magnetic field, thereby minimizing the power deposited in the patient. It also detects the precessing nuclear magnetization efficiently, resulting in a high image SNR.

Examples of RF coil geometries for imaging different body parts are shown in Figure 4.24. The "birdcage" coil, shown on the left, is a "volume coil" designed to give a spatially uniform magnetic field over the entire volume of the coil. It is typically used for brain, abdominal, and knee studies. The circular loop coil, shown in the center, is a "surface" coil, used to image objects at the surface of the body with high sensitivity. The third type of coil, shown on the right, is a "phased array," which consists of a series of surface coils. These coils are typically used to image large structures such as the spine. A phased array maintains the high sensitivity of a small coil, but, by using a large number of coils, the FOV can be made much larger than for a single coil. A phased array needs a system with multiple receiver channels, one for each coil.

The design of volume coils aims to produce a spatially uniform B_1 field across, for example, the entire volume of the head. From electromagnetic theory, a perfectly homogeneous B_1 field transverse to the cylindrical axis can be generated in an infinitely long cylinder by surface currents running parallel to the axis of the cylinder. The required current density is proportional to the sine of the azimuthal angle ϕ, as shown in Figure 4.25. A practical realization of this theoretical result is the "birdcage coil," shown schematically in Figure 4.25, which uses a large number of parallel conductors, typically between 16 and 32.

Many clinical studies only need to look at tissues close to the surface of the body. In this case, the best RF coil design is a surface coil. The simplest design is

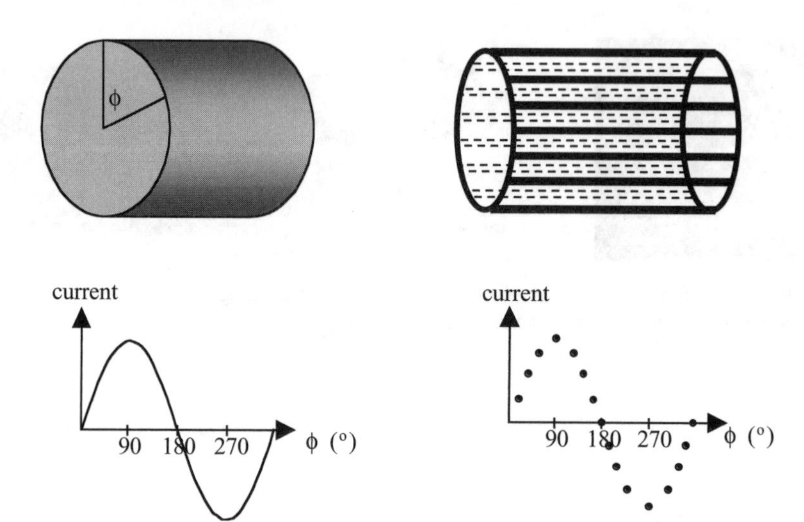

FIGURE 4.25. *(Left) The ideal current density needed to produce a spatially uniform B_1 field across a sample placed in the cylindrical coil. (Right) A practical realization of the theoretical model is the birdcage design with multiple parallel conductors.*

basically a loop of wire, with additional capacitance added to resonate the coil at the required frequency. This coil has very high efficiency close to the coil, but suffers from extremely poor B_1 homogeneity due to its geometry, as shown in Figure 4.26. The normal mode of operation is that the RF pulses are applied by a large volume coil surrounding the patient, and the signal is received from the surface coil. Crossed

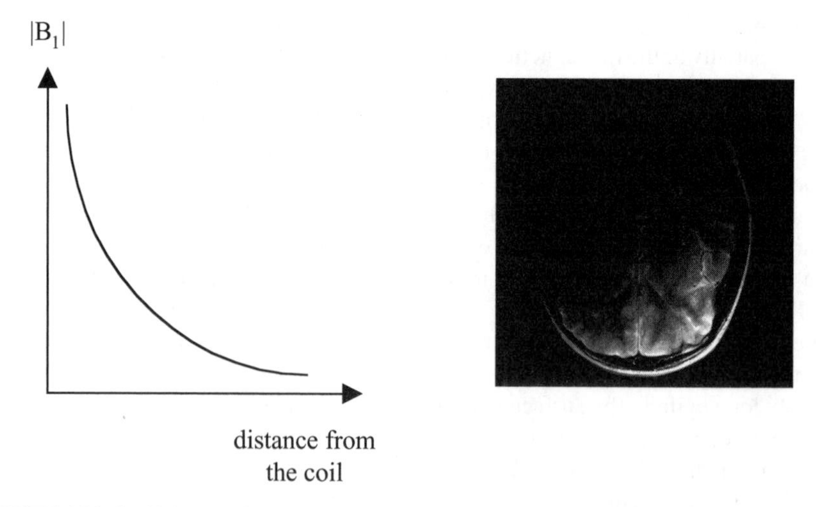

FIGURE 4.26. *(Left) A plot of the magnitude of the B_1 field versus distance from the coil for a surface coil. Very high signal can be obtained close to the coil, but the signal from tissues deep in the patient is very low. (Right) An image obtained using a surface coil placed close to the back of the head.*

diodes are included in the coil networks to decouple the two coils during signal transmission and reception.

4.5. IMAGING SEQUENCES

There are a number of imaging sequences used for different clinical applications. All of these sequences are based on either spin-echo or gradient-echo data acquisition. First, the pulse and gradient waveforms for a spin-echo sequence are analyzed.

4.5.1. Spin-Echo Imaging Sequences

The spin-echo imaging sequence, shown in Figure 4.27, can be considered as an imaging version of the spin-echo spectroscopic sequence used to measure tissue T_2 values. Compared to gradient-echo-based sequences, such as the one shown in Figure 4.18, the spin-echo method has the advantage of refocusing T_2^+ effects, so that the magnitude of the signal detected is governed by the T_2, rather than the T_2^*, value of tissue.

Two RF pulses are used: the first 90° pulse creates components of precessing transverse magnetization, and the 180° pulse refocuses the effects of T_2^+ relaxation. The 90° pulse is applied simultaneously with G_{slice} to select the desired slice, and the 180° pulse is also a frequency-selective pulse applied simultaneously with G_{slice} so that multislice imaging, covered in Section 4.5.3, can be performed. Phase-encoding is carried out exactly as described previously, with the number of incremental steps defining the spatial resolution in this dimension. The time between successive phase-encoding increments is termed TR, and can be set by the operator.

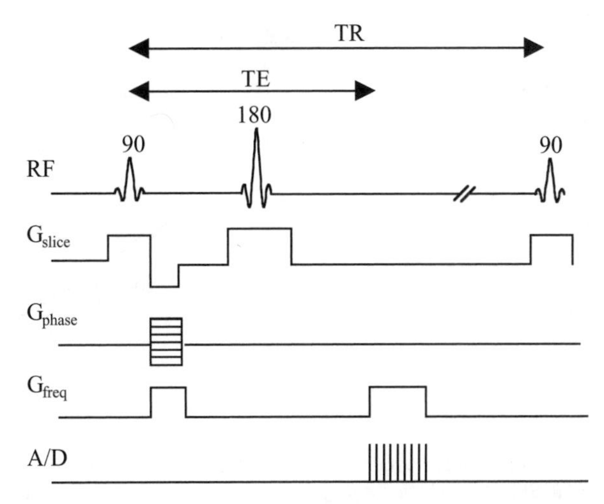

FIGURE 4.27. *The basic spin-echo imaging sequence. The values of the echo time (TE) and the repetition time (TR) between successive increments of the phase-encoding gradient can be adjusted to maximize tissue contrast.*

Instead of applying a negative dephasing gradient followed by a positive rephasing gradient, as for the gradient-echo sequence in Figure 4.20, the dephasing gradient in a spin-echo sequence is usually applied between the 90° and 180° pulses with a positive polarity. As in the spectroscopic sequence used to measure T_2, the 180° pulse reverses the phase accumulated by the protons from, in this case, the two positive-polarity gradients.

There are time periods in the imaging sequence when no gradients or pulses are applied. These delays are introduced to give certain values to the TR and TE in order to introduce corresponding T_1- and T_2-contrast weighting into the image, as discussed in the next section.

4.5.2. T_1- and T_2-Weighted Imaging Sequences

The intensity of an axial image acquired using a spin-echo sequence is given by

$$I(x, y) \propto \rho(x, y)\left(1 - e^{-\mathrm{TR}/T_1}\right) e^{-\mathrm{TE}/T_2} \tag{4.53}$$

where $I(x, y)$ is the pixel intensity at each point (x, y) and $\rho(x, y)$ is the "proton density," the number of protons at each point (x, y). The term $1 - \exp(-\mathrm{TR}/T_1)$ determines the "T_1-weighting" of the sequence, that is, the extent to which the image intensity is governed by the different T_1 values of the tissues. The value of TR can be set by the operator from the imaging console, and this value is chosen to give the best CNR between, for example, tumor and healthy tissue. If the value of TR is set to a value much greater than the T_1 of any of the tissues, then the image has no T_1-weighting because the term $1 - \exp(-\mathrm{TR}/T_1)$ is very close to unity for all tissues. If the value of TR is set closer to the tissue T_1 values, then the image becomes more T_1-weighted. The concept of T_1-weighting is shown in Figure 4.28, using values of T_1 from Table 4.2 for

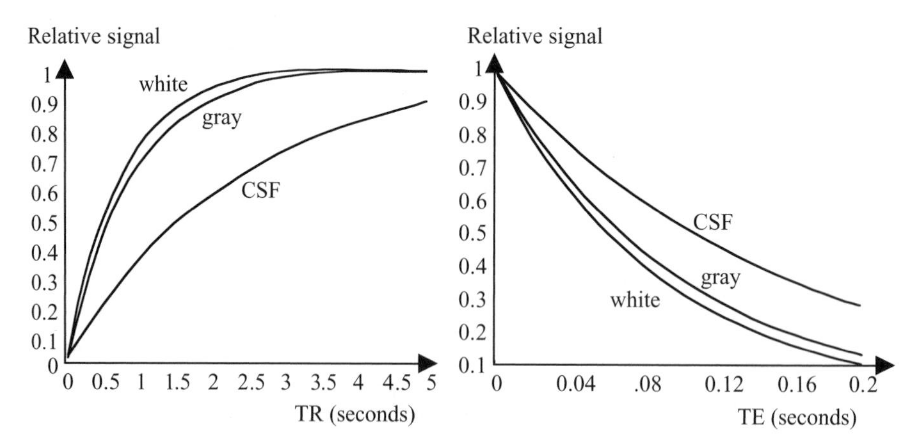

FIGURE 4.28. *The effect of data acquisition parameters on the relative signal intensities from cerebrospinal fluid (CSF), white matter, and gray matter in the brain. (Left) The relationship between signal intensity and TR, showing increased T_1-weighting at shorter TR values. As TR becomes very long, the difference in the relative signals becomes smaller. (Right) A graph showing the corresponding relationship between signal intensity and TE. The highest T_2-weighting occurs at long values of TE, but the image intensities are low.*

cerebrospinal fluid (CSF), white matter, and gray matter. There is clearly an optimal value of TR that maximizes the contrast between CSF and gray matter, and a different optimal value that maximizes the contrast between white and gray matter. As the value of TR becomes smaller, the image SNR decreases. However, the total imaging time is given by $N_p \cdot$ TR, and so reducing the value of TR also decreases the imaging time. There is clearly a tradeoff between the total imaging time and image SNR. Most clinical protocols use acquisition parameters that minimize the imaging time, while maintaining sufficient SNR for accurate diagnosis.

The same types of considerations apply to the term $\exp(-TE/T_2)$ in equation (4.53), which determines the degree of "T_2-weighting" in the sequence. If the value of TE is set to be much shorter than the tissue T_2 values, then no T_2 contrast is present in the image. If the value of TE is too long, then the contrast is high, but the SNR of the image is low. The optimum value of TE results in the highest image CNR.

Images can also be acquired with mixed T_1- and T_2-weighting, or with "proton-density weighting." This last case corresponds to using a TR value much longer than the tissue T_1 and a TE value much smaller than the tissue T_2. The contrast in the image then corresponds mainly to differences in the number of protons in each pixel. Figure 4.29 shows a series of brain images with different contrast weightings.

One obvious question is: Which physical properties of tissue dictate the values of the T_1 and T_2 relaxation times, that is, why are both the T_1 and T_2 values of CSF much longer than those of brain tissue? The mechanism of T_1 relaxation involves the protons losing their excess energy via interactions with oscillating magnetic fields,

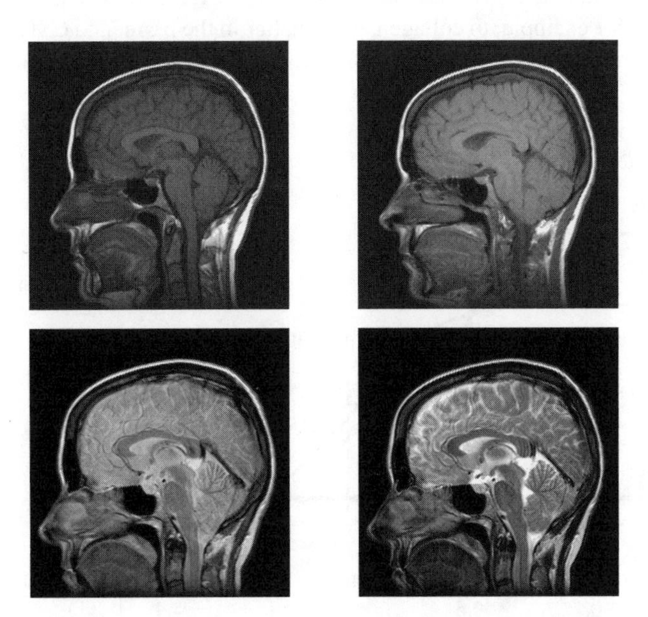

FIGURE 4.29. *Axial images of the brain acquired at 1.5 T. (Top left) A short value of TR (300 ms) gives high T_1-weighting. (Top right) Increasing the TR value to 800 ms reduces the T_1-weighting. (Bottom left) A T_2-weighted image acquired using a TE of 34 ms. (Bottom right) An image with increased T_2-weighting using a TE of 102 ms.*

which are produced by the magnetic moments of nuclei in surrounding molecules as they execute random Brownian motion. These randomly fluctuating magnetic fields contain components at many different frequencies. The component at the Larmor frequency can stimulate transitions between the upper and the lower energy states of the protons, and thereby cause the M_z component of magnetization to return to its equilibrium value of M_0. Slowly moving molecules in a highly viscous, low-mobility environment exhibit only low motional frequencies, producing magnetic fields which fluctuate at low frequencies, and so their contribution to T_1 relaxation occurs at low magnetic field strengths. In contrast, rapidly moving molecules in mobile liquids produce fluctuating magnetic fields over a much larger frequency range. Figure 4.30 plots the spectral density $J(\omega)$ of the magnetic field fluctuations versus frequency, where the value of $J(\omega)$ is defined as

$$J(\omega) \propto \frac{\tau_c}{1 + \omega^2 \tau_c^2} \tag{4.54}$$

The term τ_c is the correlation time of the molecule, and is defined as the time taken by a molecule to diffuse a distance equal to its diameter. $J(\omega)$ can effectively be considered as a measure of the number of nuclei in the surrounding lattice that produce magnetic fields with components oscillating at a frequency ω. The greater the number of nuclei, the larger is the value of $J(\omega)$ and the more effective is the T_1 relaxation.

As an example, consider proton relaxation in three different types of tissue with high, intermediate, and low viscosity, as shown in Figure 4.30. These tissues might correspond, for example, to collagen, gray matter in the brain, and CSF, respectively. At low magnetic fields, for example, 0.15 T, protons in the most viscous tissue have

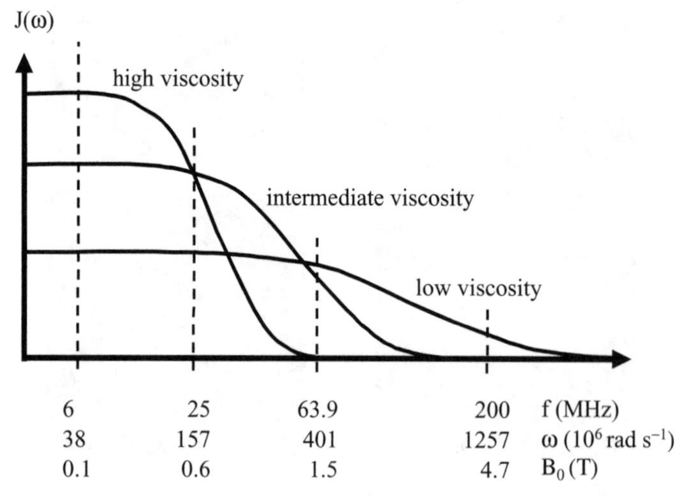

FIGURE 4.30. *A plot of spectral density $J(\omega)$ versus frequency and the corresponding magnetic field strength for tissues with three different viscosities.*

the highest value of $J(\omega)$, T_1 relaxation is the most efficient, and the value of T_1 is the shortest of all the tissues. The protons in the least viscous tissue have the lowest value of $J(\omega)$ at this field strength, and therefore the longest T_1 relaxation time. As can be inferred from Figure 4.30, the relative values of T_1 of the tissues depend strongly upon the magnetic field strength. For example, at 4.7 T the protons in the least viscous tissue have the shortest T_1 value.

Figure 4.30 also shows that the highest contrast between tissues with different viscosities occurs at low magnetic field strengths, and that at very high magnetic fields all tissues have essentially the same value of T_1. There is, therefore, a tradeoff between image contrast and SNR with respect to the strength of the magnet used. Although low magnetic fields give good contrast, the image SNR is also low, as shown by equations (4.20) and (4.23).

Many of the mechanisms that cause T_1 relaxation also give rise to T_2 relaxation. However, there is also an extra contribution that only causes T_2 relaxation. This mechanism is caused by local magnetic field fluctuations that occur at near-zero frequencies. The net result of this additional mechanism is that the value of T_2 can never be as long as that of T_1, and the value of T_2 only approaches T_1 in very mobile liquids where the contribution of this low-frequency component is smallest. Referring to Figure 4.30, at a magnetic field strength of 0.6 T the T_1 values of the tissues with high and intermediate viscosities are the same, but the T_2 value of the viscous material is lower, that is, relaxation is faster and more efficient, due to the greater number of molecules with low-frequency components.

4.5.3. Multislice Imaging

Unlike most other imaging modalities, MRI can acquire multiple slices in essentially the same data acquisition time as for a single slice. The acquisition of multiple slices is advantageous because it allows a larger volume of tissue to be investigated. In a single-slice sequence, the protons in the selected slice undergo T_1 relaxation during the time TR−TE. In multislice imaging, this time can be used to acquire images from adjacent slices, as shown in Figure 4.31. The position of the slice can be moved simply by changing the center frequency of the RF pulses. As can be seen from Figure 4.31, the maximum number of slices is limited by the ratio of TR/TE. In practice, the order in which the slices are acquired is odd-numbered followed by even-numbered. The reason is that the nonideal frequency profile of the RF pulses results in partial excitation of the slices either side of the selected slice. By waiting to acquire these adjacent slices, the magnetization within these slices has time to return to its full equilibrium value.

4.5.4. Rapid Gradient-Echo Sequences and Three-Dimensional Imaging

Spin-echo sequences generally result in images with a high CNR and SNR, but typically take many minutes to acquire. For example, an image with a matrix size

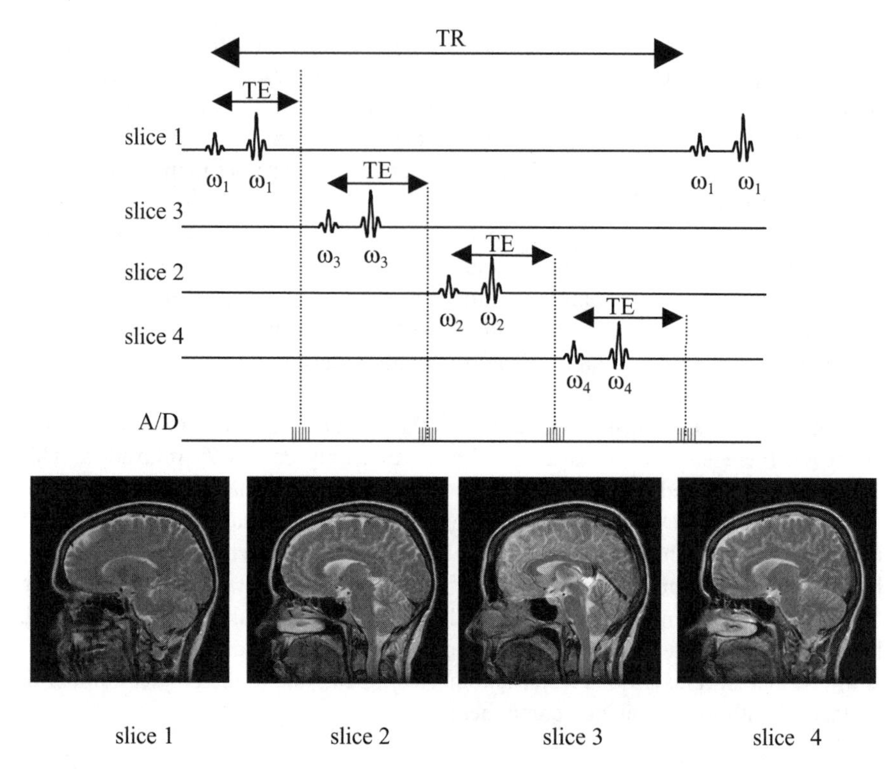

FIGURE 4.31. *(Top) A spin-echo multislice imaging sequence. The slices are acquired from different positions by adjusting the frequency offset ω_n of the RF pulses. Only the RF waveforms are shown; the slice, phase phase-, and frequency-encoding gradient waveforms are identical to those in Figure 4.27. In this example, four slices can be acquired in each TR interval. (Bottom) Four sagittal slices acquired using the multislice sequence.*

of 256 × 256, using a TR of 2 s, requires over 8 min to acquire. There are many applications which require much faster imaging times. One example is abdominal imaging, in which the image should ideally be acquired within a single breath-hold to avoid motion artifacts. This corresponds to a total imaging time between 5 and 25 s, depending upon the health of the patient. The major time constraint in spin-echo imaging is the long TR delay necessary for T_1 relaxation. As described previously, gradient-echo sequences have no 180° refocusing pulse, and this allows shorter TE and TR values to be used. However, signal decay during the TE interval is determined by the T_2^* value of tissue, which is typically of the order of 1–10 ms, and therefore the value of TE should generally be kept as short as possible. In order to image rapidly, the tip angle α of the RF pulse is reduced to a value considerably smaller than 90°. There are many variations on the basic gradient-echo sequence. Common examples include fast low-angle shot (FLASH), fast imaging with steady precession (FISP), gradient-refocused acquisition in the steady state (GRASS), and steady-state free precession (SSFP). In the FLASH sequence, which is essentially that shown in Figure 4.20, the signal intensity is given by

$$I(x, y) \propto \frac{\rho(x, y)\left(1 - e^{-\mathrm{TR}/T_1}\right) e^{-\mathrm{TE}/T_2{}^*}}{1 - e^{-\mathrm{TR}/T_1} \cos\alpha} \tag{4.55}$$

For a given value of TR, the value of α that maximizes the SNR is referred to as the Ernst angle, with a value given by

$$\alpha_{\mathrm{Ernst}} = \cos^{-1} e^{-\mathrm{TR}/T_1} \tag{4.56}$$

So for a TR time equal to the tissue T_1 value, the tip angle should be set to 68°. In order to image faster, the TR must be made much shorter than the T_1 value, and α becomes correspondingly smaller. For example, if TR is reduced to $0.05T_1$, then the optimum value of α is only 8°. Using these parameters, images can be acquired in a few seconds with acceptable SNR, contrast, and spatial resolution.

Rapid gradient-echo imaging also makes it possible to acquire true three-dimensional images within time scales commensurate with clinical practice. Applications of three-dimensional imaging include producing full anatomical maps of structures such as the knee as an aid to surgical procedures. Three-dimensional imaging uses a conventional frequency-encoding gradient, but two incremental

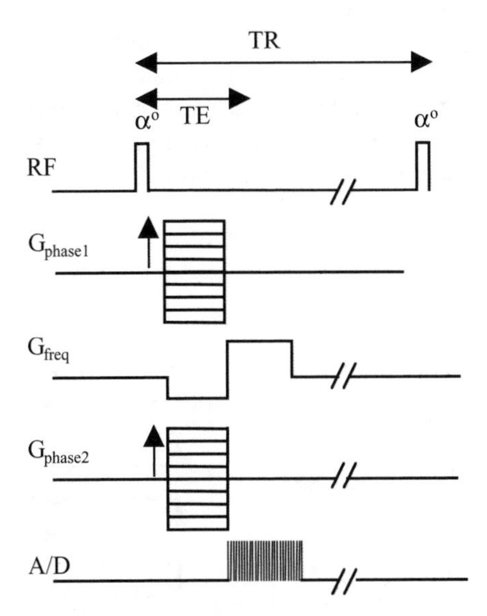

FIGURE 4.32. *A three-dimensional gradient-echo imaging sequence, with two phase-encoding gradients. The RF pulses are not frequency-selective, and so are relatively short in duration compared to those used for slice-selective imaging.*

phase-encoding gradients, as shown in Figure 4.32. Image reconstruction uses a three-dimensional inverse Fourier transform:

$$\rho(x, y, z) = \int_{-\infty}^{\infty} \int_{-\infty}^{\infty} \int_{-\infty}^{\infty} S\left(k_x, k_y, k_z\right) e^{+j2\pi\left(k_x x + k_y y + k_z z\right)} dk_x\, dk_y\, dk_z \tag{4.57}$$

4.5.5. Echo-Planar Imaging

Despite the very rapid image acquisition times possible using the gradient-echo sequences described in the previous section, there is a growing need for even faster imaging sequences. There are a number of clinical applications that require subsecond imaging capability. Examples include many forms of cardiac studies, imaging the dynamic distribution of contrast agents injected into the blood stream, and diffusion- and perfusion-weighted imaging of the brain. In the area of functional MRI, covered in Section 4.11, an entire multislice dataset of the brain has to be acquired within a few seconds.

The fastest type of imaging sequence uses a single RF pulse to excite the protons in the chosen slice, followed by full k-space sampling in a single echo train. These types of sequences are termed "single-shot" because only a single excitation of the spin system is used to acquire the entire image. The most common sequence is called "echo-planar" imaging (EPI). With recent improvements in commercial hardware, clinical scanners are able to obtain single-shot EPI scans in less than 100 ms. The simplest version of the EPI sequence is shown in Figure 4.33, together with the corresponding k-space trajectory.

The EPI sequence can introduce an unacceptable level of image blurring, due to the broad point spread function (PSF), which arises from T_2^* relaxation during the sequence. In order to overcome this effect while maintaining high imaging speed, the EPI sequence is often run in "segmented mode." Segmented EPI involves acquiring, for example, only every fourth data point in k-space and then repeating the

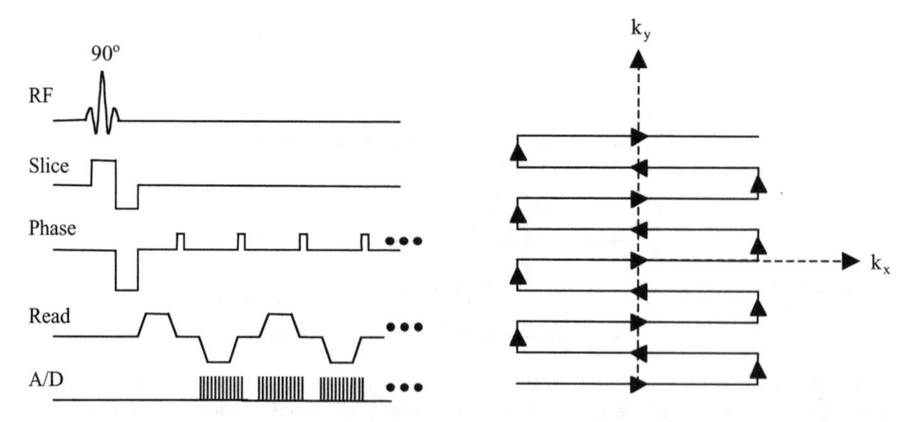

FIGURE 4.33. (Left) One form of an EPI imaging sequence used for very rapid data acquisition. (Right) The corresponding k-space trajectory.

sequence four times to acquire the full k-space matrix. In this way, the T_2^* relaxation during each of the four, interleaved acquisitions is much less than in the single-shot implementation, and the image blurring effect is reduced considerably. There is a large number of other fast imaging sequences, details of which can be found in the specialized books listed in Further Reading at the end of this chapter.

4.5.6. Spiral Imaging

The majority of imaging sequences sample k-space as a rectangular grid with equidistant k-space sampling in each of the two directions k_x and k_y. By acquiring data in this fashion, high and low spatial frequencies are sampled equally, and image reconstruction consists of a simple two-dimensional inverse Fourier transform. There are, however, advantages in acquiring data using nonrectangular k-space trajectories, the most common form of which is "spiral imaging." The pulse sequence and the k-space trajectory for this type of imaging are shown in Figure 4.34.

There are two basic advantages of the particular k-space trajectory traversed in spiral scanning. The first is that the low spatial frequencies are sampled more densely because the spiral is tightest close to the origin of the k-space axes. This results in a higher image SNR and also an inherent degree of compensation for patient motion. The second advantage is that the gradient "slew rate," that is, the rate at which the gradient strength has to be changed, is much lower for spiral scanning than for sequences such as echo-planar imaging. This can be appreciated by considering the smooth gradient patterns shown on the left of Figure 4.34. The first step in image reconstruction involves interpolation of the spiral k-space matrix onto a rectangular grid. After this regridding process, a two-dimensional inverse Fourier transform is applied to give the image. As for EPI and other fast imaging techniques, spiral scanning is most often used in segmented mode, with typically four to eight spirals being used to cover k-space.

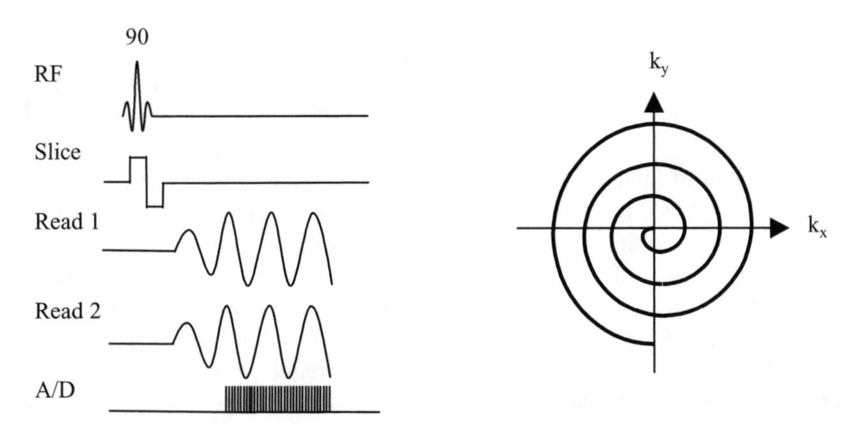

FIGURE 4.34. (Left) The basic sequence for single-shot spiral imaging. (Right) The k-space trajectory corresponding to the imaging sequence. Because k-space is not sampled equidistantly, data interpolation onto a rectangular grid must be performed prior to two-dimensional inverse Fourier transformation to form the image.

4.6. IMAGE CHARACTERISTICS

As for all the imaging modalities covered in this book, there are tradeoffs among the three basic measures of image quality: the SNR, spatial resolution, and the CNR. The factors which affect each of these parameters are summarized in the following sections.

4.6.1. Signal-to-Noise Ratio

Several factors which affect the image SNR have already been covered.

1. The higher the value of B_0, the greater is the nuclear polarization, equation (4.20), and the higher is the SNR; also the larger is the voltage induced in the coil by the precessing magnetization, equation (4.23), and the higher is the SNR. However, the higher the value of B_0, the larger is the value of T_1, and the smaller is the steady-state magnetization for a given value of TR.

2. The dependence of the image SNR on tissue relaxation times and the values of the sequence TE and TR is covered by equations (4.53) and (4.55) for spin-echo and gradient-echo sequences, respectively.

3. In terms of the hardware used to acquire and record the MRI signal, the SNR is proportional also to the sensitivity of the receiving RF coil, which is defined as the B_1 field produced per unit current passed through the coil. The noise contribution from the RF coil arises from random voltage fluctuations in the copper conductor. There is also a noise contribution from the patient because humans are conducting! The overall noise voltage V_{noise} is given by

$$V_{\text{noise}} = \sqrt{4kT(R_{\text{coil}} + R_{\text{patient}})\Delta f} \tag{4.58}$$

where R_{coil} is the coil resistance, R_{patient} is the effective resistance of the patient, T the absolute temperature in degrees kelvin, and Δf is the bandwidth of the received signal. For almost all coil designs at clinical field strengths, R_{patient} is the dominant source of noise. The value of R_{patient} increases with magnetic field. The overall dependence of SNR on magnetic field strength is generally between the $3/2$ and $7/4$ power.

4. A number of images, acquired using identical parameters, can be coadded to increase the SNR. Because the MRI signal is coherent, but the noise is incoherent, the SNR increases as the square root of the number of signal averages (Section 5.3.2).

5. For a given FOV, if the number of phase encoding steps N_p is doubled, then the image SNR is reduced by a factor of two. The total imaging time is doubled, and the digital resolution in this dimension is improved by a factor of two.

6. If the number of points N_r, acquired in the frequency-encoding direction is doubled for a given FOV, the noise increases by a factor of two.

7. If the dwell time t_{dw} between points in the frequency dimension is doubled, then the bandwidth of the image is halved, and the strength of the frequency encoding gradient is also halved to keep a constant FOV in the spatial domain. The reduction in the bandwidth results in an increase in SNR by a factor of two. The disadvantage of the increased value of t_{dw} is that the minimum value of TE is increased.

8. An increase in the slice thickness gives a proportional increase in the image SNR.

4.6.2. Spatial Resolution

The image PSF depends on the particular sequence used to acquire the data, and is generally different in all three spatial dimensions. In the slice-select direction, the PSF is simply related to the frequency response of the slice-selective RF pulse. In the frequency- and phase-encoding directions, three factors affect the PSF: digital resolution, data truncation, and relaxation while the data are being acquired.

1. The digital resolution is determined simply by dividing the FOV of the image in each dimension by the corresponding number of data points acquired. In terms of k-space coverage, the further out in k-space that data are acquired, the higher is the spatial resolution.
2. Because only a finite number of frequency- and phase-encoding data points is taken, the data are effectively truncated, and the corresponding PSF is a sinc function. The width of the sinc function in each dimension is inversely proportional to the number of frequency-encoded data points and phase-encoding steps acquired, respectively.
3. The final factor is related to the degree of T_2^* relaxation during data acquisition. This exponential decay corresponds to a Lorentzian PSF in the spatial domain, with a FWHM given by

$$\mathrm{PSF}_{\mathrm{Lorentz}} = \frac{1}{\pi T_2^* G_{\mathrm{freq}}} \tag{4.59}$$

4.6.3. Contrast-to-Noise Ratio

Image contrast between tissues is primarily affected by the difference in relaxation times and the proton density and the values of the TR and TE parameters used in the imaging sequence. As seen in Section 4.5.2, the intrinsic T_1 contrast between tissues is greater at lower values of the main magnetic field B_0. The dependence of T_2 of different tissues on magnetic field is more complicated, being highly tissue specific, and no general rule applies as to whether T_2 contrast between tissues is increased or decreased as a function of magnetic field. Because the CNR between two tissues depends on the respective values of tissue SNR, the CNR is governed by the same factors as are outlined in Section 4.6.1.

4.7. MRI CONTRAST AGENTS

In many clinical diagnoses, there is a sufficiently high CNR on the appropriately T_1-, T_2-, or proton density-weighted image in order to distinguish pathological from healthy tissue. However, in certain situations, such as the detection of very small lesions, where the signal from the lesion is effectively averaged with that of healthy tissue within the slice, the CNR can be low. In this case, MRI contrast agents can be used to increase the CNR between healthy and diseased tissue. There are two basic classes of MRI contrast agent: paramagnetic agents and superparamagnetic, also called ferromagnetic, agents. Paramagnetic agents primarily shorten the T_1 of the tissue in which they accumulate. Rapid T_1-weighted sequences are used in order to minimize the total imaging time, with tissue in which the agent accumulates appearing bright on the image. Superparamagnetic agents accumulate primarily in healthy rather than pathological tissue, and shorten the T_2 and T_2^* values of the tissue. Therefore, a tumor, for example, can be detected as an area of high signal intensity using a T_2- or T_2^*-weighted sequence.

4.7.1. Paramagnetic Agents

Paramagnetic contrast agents are based on metal ions, such as gadolinium, manganese, or europium, that have a large number of unpaired electrons. Because the magnetic moment of an electron is approximately 660 times as large as that of a proton, these unpaired electrons result in the metal ion having a very large magnetic moment. Most clinical paramagnetic contrast agents contain the Gd^{3+} ion because this has seven unpaired electrons, the maximum number possible. Because the metal ion itself is toxic, it must be contained within a "chemical cage," or chelate, which has a very strong binding constant. The most commonly used clinical paramagnetic contrast agent is gadolinium diethylenetriaminepentaacetic acid (Gd-DTPA; trade name Magnevist), the structure of which is shown in Figure 4.35.

Signal is not detected directly from the contrast agent per se, but rather the biodistribution of the agent is visualized as a result of its effect on the relaxation times of

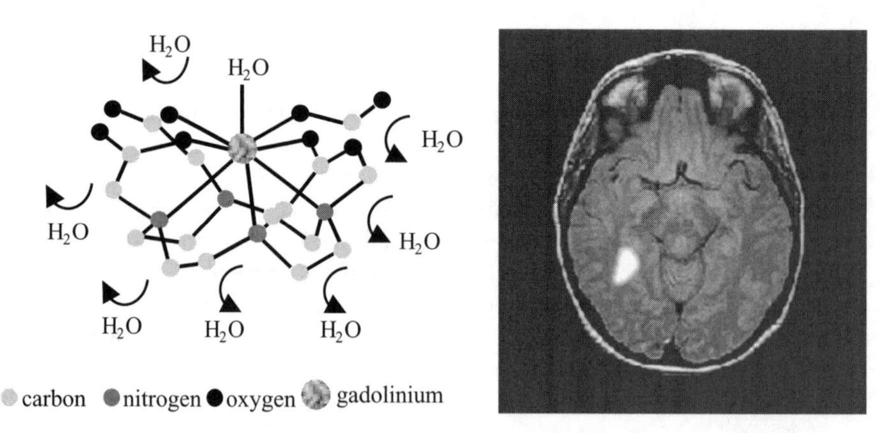

FIGURE 4.35. *(Left) The chemical structure and mode of operation of Gd-DTPA. Water molecules that diffuse close to the contrast agent, but do not bind to it, have a relatively small reduction in their T_1 value (outer-sphere relaxation). Water molecules that occupy the one free binding site are relaxed very efficiently (inner-sphere relaxation), and have a large reduction in their T_1 value. (Right) A brain scan taken after administration of Gd-DTPA showing enhancement of a tumor.*

neighboring water molecules. The interactions between the unpaired electrons of the metal ion and the water molecules cause the proton T_1 and T_2 relaxation times to be shortened, the effect being quantified by the relaxivity of the agent:

$$\frac{1}{T_{1,C}} = \frac{1}{T_{1,0}} + \alpha_1 C \tag{4.60}$$

where $T_{1,C}$ is the T_1 of water containing a concentration C of the contrast agent, $T_{1,0}$ is the corresponding value without contrast agent, and α_1 is the T_1 relaxivity of the contrast agent. For Gd-DTPA the value of α_1 is approximately 5 mM^{-1} s^{-1}.

There are two mechanisms which result in enhanced relaxation efficiency. These are termed "inner-sphere" and "outer-sphere" relaxation. Figure 4.35 shows that the metal ion in Gd-DTPA has one binding site that is not occupied by the chelate. A water molecule can temporarily bind at this position, and will be relaxed very efficiently due to its proximity to the unpaired electrons on the metal ion. This process is called inner-sphere relaxation. On the time scale of the imaging sequence, many thousands of water molecules are bound, relaxed, and released via this chemical coordination. Water molecules that diffuse close to the agent, but are not bound, undergo a process called outer-sphere relaxation, which is not as efficient as inner-sphere relaxation, but still results in shortened relaxation times.

Typical doses of Gd-DTPA administered to patients are 10 ml at a concentration of 0.5 M, which results in a concentration in the body of ~0.1 mmol/kg. At this concentration, the shortening of the water T_1 relaxation time is much greater than that of the T_2 value. The DTPA chelate is ionic and highly hydrophilic and does not bind to the proteins in blood, ensuring very rapid distribution throughout the bloodstream and fast clearance through the kidneys. There are a number of other gadolinium chelates, with very similar chemical structures, but which are nonionic in nature, including Gd-1,4,7,10-tetraazacyclododecane-1,4,7,10-tetraacetic acid (Gd-DOTA; trade name Dotarem), Gd-DTPA-bis(methylamide) (Gd-DTPA-BMA; trade name Omniscan), and (±)-10-(2-hydroxypropyl)-1,4,7,10-tetraazacyclodecane-1,4,7-triacetatogadolinium[III] (Gd-HP-DO3A; tradename Prohance).

Gd-DTPA is most often used in the diagnosis of brain disorders, such as the presence of gliomas, meningiomas, and various other types of tumors, as described further in Section 4.12.1. Disruption of the blood brain barrier allows the agent to enter into the brain and T_1-weighted images show the tumor as an area of increased brightness, as seen on the right of Figure 4.35. Gd-DTPA is also used in magnetic resonance angiography, covered in Section 4.8, where it is used to reduce the T_1 value of the blood.

4.7.2. Superparamagnetic Agents

Superparamagnetic MRI contrast agents consist of small magnetic particles containing iron. If these particles are very small, 30 nm or less in diameter, then they possess extremely high magnetic moments, which arise from the cooperative alignment of the electron spins within the particle. These contrast agents work by causing inhomogeneities in the local magnetic field. Water molecules diffusing through these local gradients undergo fast T_2 and T_2^* relaxation via an outer-sphere mechanism. Superparamagnetic particles are therefore negative contrast agents, causing a reduction in signal intensity in the tissues in which they accumulate on T_2^*-weighted gradient-echo or T_2-weighted spin-echo sequences. These particles usually consist of a crystalline core comprising a mixture of Fe_2O_3 and Fe_3O_4, coated in a polymer matrix such as dextran, and are referred to as superparamagnetic iron oxides (SPIOs).

In the body, small particles are taken up primarily by Kuppfer cells in the liver, but also accumulate in the lymph nodes, spleen, and bone marrow. The particles only enter the healthy Kuppfer cells in the liver and do not accumulate in tumors or other pathological tissue. Therefore, these particles reduce the signal intensity from the healthy tissue, with the tumor intensity remaining unaffected as a relatively bright area.

4.8. MAGNETIC RESONANCE ANGIOGRAPHY

Unlike X-ray angiographic techniques, magnetic resonance angiography (MRA) does not require the use of a contrast agent, although Gd-DTPA is often used to increase the signal difference between flowing blood and tissue. Due to the health risks of X-ray contrast agents, the ability of MRA to visualize vessels without a contrast agent is a major advantage, although very fine vessels are visualized more clearly using X-ray techniques. There are two major techniques for obtaining MRAs: time-of-flight and phase contrast angiography methods.

4.8.1. Time-of-Flight Methods

Time-of-flight (TOF) methods are based on the shortening of the effective T_1, $T_{1(\mathrm{eff})}$, of blood as it flows into and through the imaging slice (or volume) during data acquisition. The actual T_1 value of blood at 1.5 T is $\sim$1.2 s, which is not dissimilar to the value for many tissues. The reason for the effective shortening of the T_1 of blood is that, at each incremental value of phase-encoding gradient, protons in blood that have not experienced the previous RF pulse enter the slice with full magnetization ($M_z = M_0$). For a given slice thickness S_{th} and blood velocity v, the value of $T_{1(\mathrm{eff})}$ is given by

$$\frac{1}{T_{1(\mathrm{eff})}} = \frac{1}{T_1} + \frac{v}{S_{\mathrm{th}}} \tag{4.61}$$

For example, if the slice thickness is 5 mm and a value of TR of 50 ms is used, blood flowing at speeds greater than 10 cm/s will flow completely out of the slice in the time between successive phase-encoding steps. The value of $T_{1(\mathrm{eff})}$ is therefore zero.

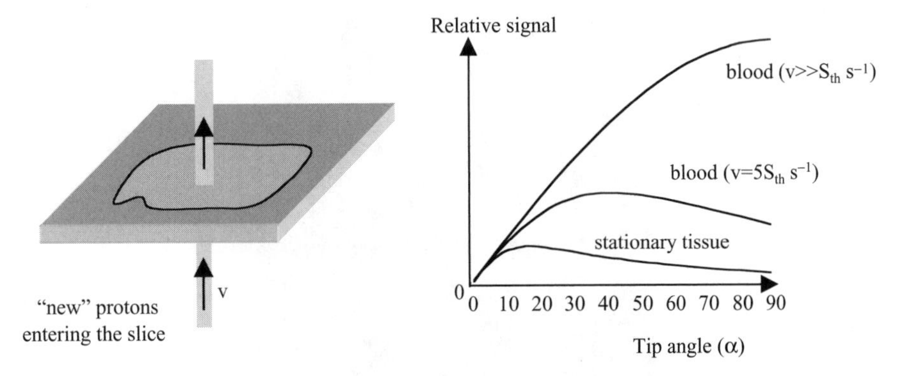

FIGURE 4.36. *(Left) A schematic of blood flow perpendicular to the imaging slice. (Right) A graph of signal intensity versus tip angle for tissue and blood flowing at two different rates with a TR set to 50 ms. The T_1 value of blood is 1.2 s and that of tissue is 1 s. A short value of TE is used so that the blood does not travel a substantial distance through the slice during the TE interval. If a tip angle of 18° (the Ernst angle for tissue at this TR) is used in the gradient-echo sequence, relatively little difference in SNR is seen between tissue and blood. If the tip angle is increased to 60°, then a large difference can be seen.*

The simplest implementation of the TOF principle uses a rapid gradient-echo sequence with a tip angle that is large compared to the Ernst angle for the tissue. This means that the sequence is heavily T_1-weighted, with the signal intensity from tissue being very small, and that from flowing blood much larger, due to its shorter effective T_1 value. Figure 4.36 shows the behavior of the signal intensities from flowing blood and stationary tissue.

There are many other imaging sequences based on the TOF, or inflow, principle. One such sequence excites the protons in a blood vessel at a particular position using a large-volume RF coil. A specific time delay is inserted into the imaging sequence to allow the blood to flow into the sensitive region of a surface coil, which is positioned above the area where the angiogram is to be recorded. Because protons in the static tissue below the surface coil have not experienced the RF pulse from the volume coil, signal is only detected from protons in the blood.

Multislice or three-dimensional angiography is normally performed to obtain flow images throughout a given volume of the brain, for example. The data are then processed and displayed using a maximum intensity projection (MIP) algorithm, as shown in Figure 4.37. For the observation of very small vessels, contrast agents such as Gd-DTPA can be used in order to reduce further the effective T_1 of blood and increase the contrast between flowing spins and stationary tissue.

4.8.2. Phase-Contrast Methods

Phase-contrast (PC) angiographic techniques are based on inducing phase shifts in the precessing magnetization of flowing blood by means of flow-sensitive "bipolar" gradient pulses, as shown in Figure 4.38.

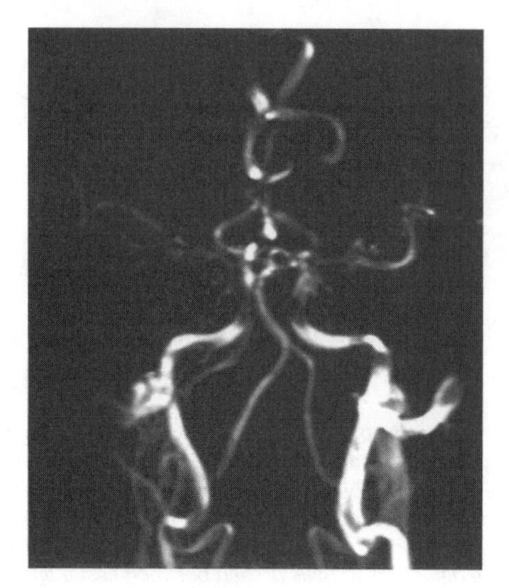

FIGURE 4.37. *A time-of-flight angiogram obtained from the brain. The image represents a maximum intensity projection of a three-dimensional dataset.*

The effect of applying a bipolar gradient pulse pair is to introduce a velocity-dependent phase into the signal. For the gradient waveform shown on the left of Figure 4.38, this phase ϕ is given by

$$\phi = \int_{t=0}^{\tau/2} \gamma G_x x(t)\, dt + \int_{t=\tau/2}^{\tau} \gamma(-G_x)x(t)\, dt \tag{4.62}$$

For stationary protons, $x(t) = x = \text{const}$, and the value of ϕ is zero. However, for protons in blood flowing at constant velocity v_x in the x direction, the value of ϕ is

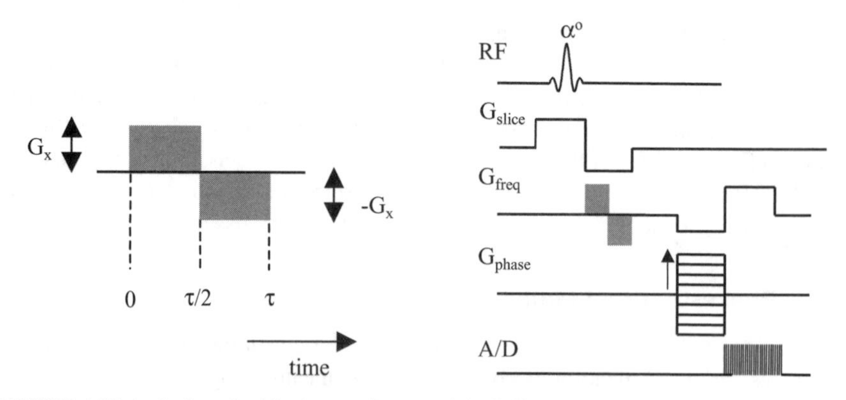

FIGURE 4.38. *Inclusion of a bipolar gradient module (left) into a two-dimensional imaging sequence (right) can be used to produce phase contrast angiograms.*

given by

$$\phi = \gamma v_x \tau^2 G_x \tag{4.63}$$

Bipolar gradients can be inserted into a gradient-echo or spin-echo imaging sequence. The phase of a single image cannot be used directly to measure the velocity. Instead, a second image must be acquired, in which the polarity of the bipolar gradients are reversed, that is, the negative waveform is applied first, followed by the positive one. The phase of the precessing protons in static tissue remains the same in both images, whereas the phase of protons in blood flowing at a constant velocity is reversed in sign from that in equation (4.63). Subtraction of the phase images therefore gives a net phase shift $\Delta\phi$ given by

$$\Delta\phi = 2\gamma v_x \tau^2 G_x \tag{4.64}$$

The PC method potentially allows not only the selective visualization of flowing blood, but also the quantitation of the flow velocities via the measured phase shifts in the image. An additional advantage is that flow in any direction, x, y, or z, can be measured simply by changing the particular gradient used in the bipolar waveform.

4.9. DIFFUSION-WEIGHTED IMAGING

One very important physical parameter that MRI can measure is the diffusion coefficient of water. The rate of water diffusion is often indicative of the health of tissues. For example, it is well known that in conditions such as stroke, cells swell and cell membranes can rupture. This means that water in these tissues can diffuse much faster because there are fewer physical barriers. The simplest pulse sequence used to measure diffusion is based on a spin-echo sequence, with symmetric "diffusion-encoding" gradients applied either side of the 180° refocusing pulse, as shown in Figure 4.39.

The effect of the first diffusion gradient is to encode each proton with a certain phase, in exactly the same mechanism as in phase-encoding. If the proton does not move position, that is, if it does not diffuse, then the second diffusion-encoding gradient will impose an equal and opposite phase on the proton, and therefore there is no net dephasing of the magnetization. If, however, the proton diffuses to a different position in the time between the two encoding gradient pulses, then the proton magnetization is only partially rephased, and there is a loss in signal intensity. The faster the proton diffuses, the greater is the loss in signal. In order to obtain a quantitative measurement of the diffusion coefficient, more accurately termed the apparent diffusion coefficient, of water, the imaging sequence is repeated a number of times with different values of the diffusion-encoding gradient. The signal intensities are then fitted, on a pixel-by-pixel basis, to the basic equation describing diffusive signal loss:

$$I(G_n) = I_0 e^{-D\gamma^2 G_n^2 \delta^2 (\Delta - \delta/3)} \tag{4.65}$$

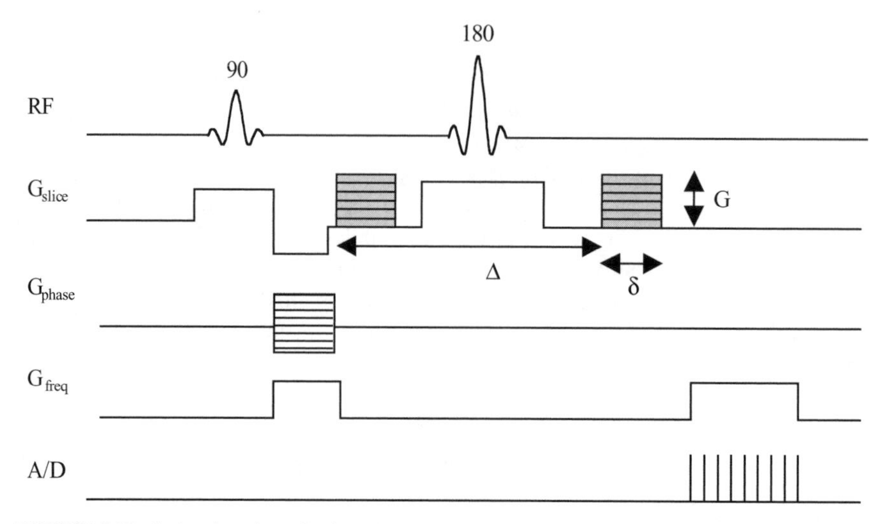

__FIGURE 4.39.__ A simple spin-echo imaging sequence used to measure the diffusion coefficient of water for each pixel in an image. The diffusion-encoding gradients are shown as shaded areas. If only one value of the gradient G is used, then a diffusion-weighted image is produced. The gradient can be applied along any of the three axes, depending upon the particular diffusion coefficient to be measured.

where I_0 is the signal intensity with no diffusion-encoding gradients applied, D is the apparent diffusion coefficient of water, G_n represents the n different values of encoding gradients, and the variables δ and Δ are shown in Figure 4.39. Diffusion coefficients are often not uniform in all directions of the tissue. For example, in muscle fibers, water diffusion along the length of the fiber is much faster than in a direction across the fiber. By applying diffusion-encoding gradients separately in three different directions, the water diffusion coefficients in the x, y, and z directions can be measured. In fact, water diffusion is technically characterized by a second-order tensor, and so-called diffusion tensor imaging is a technique which can measure this tensor for each pixel in an image. This allows, for example, maps of diffusion anisotropy to be produced, and has recently enabled the technique of fiber tracking to be implemented *in vivo*.

4.10. *IN VIVO* LOCALIZED SPECTROSCOPY

The hardware and pulse sequences used in MRI can be adapted very simply to the acquisition of *in vivo* localized NMR spectra. In these measurements, an FID is acquired from a defined volume within the body. The FID is then Fourier-transformed to give an NMR spectrum. In proton spectroscopy, the major signals come from water and lipid, and in order to see the signals from much more dilute metabolites, these signals must be suppressed. This is usually carried out by means of frequency-selective irradiation techniques. The proton spectrum of brain, for example, includes

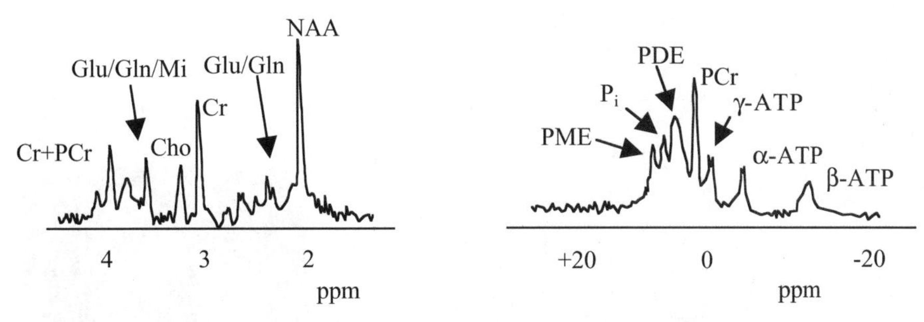

FIGURE 4.40. *(left) A localized proton spectrum obtained from the brain at 3 T. The peaks correspond to Cr (creatine), Glu (glutamate), Gln (glutamine), Cho (choline), Mi (myo-inositol), and NAA (n-acetylaspartate). (Right) A corresponding localized phosphorus spectrum from the brain. The peaks shown are PME (phosphomonoester), P_i (inorganic phosphate), PDE (phosphodiester), PCr (phosphocreatine), and ATP (adenosine triphosphate), which gives three peaks.*

peaks from creatine, choline, *N*-acetylaspartate, lactate, and myo-inositol. The relative levels of these proton metabolites can reflect the cellular status and health of the tissue. Many tumors, for example, are characterized by increased levels of lactate. Spectral linewidths *in vivo* are quite broad, as shown in Figure 4.40, due to the presence of tissue inhomogeneities. Phosphorus spectra are also often acquired. As can be seen from Table 4.1, the phosphorus resonance frequency is approximately 40% that of protons, and therefore the Larmor frequency is correspondingly lower. This means that the RF coils used to transmit the RF pulses and receive the signal must be designed to operate at this lower frequency. The spin-active ^{31}P isotope is almost 100% naturally abundant, and so sufficient SNR can be acquired in a time scale

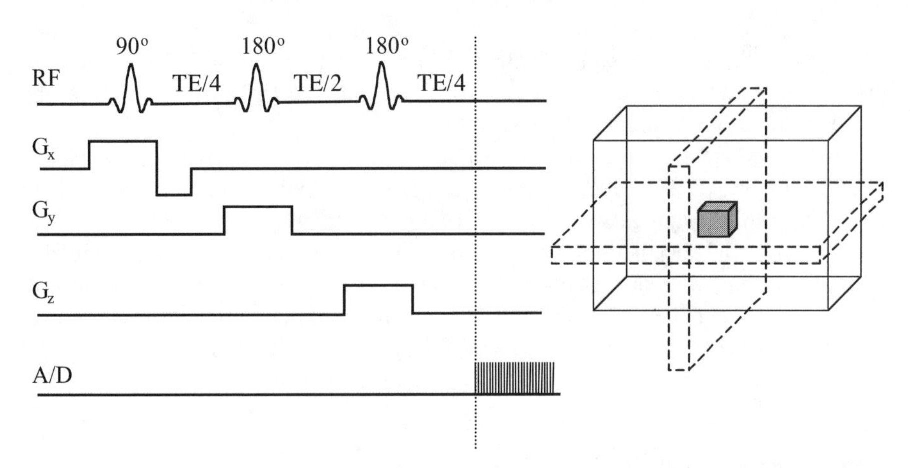

FIGURE 4.41. *(Left) A PRESS pulse sequence used to acquire an NMR spectrum from a single voxel. (Right) the voxel (shaded) is defined by the intersection of the three slices in the sequence. Only nuclei within this voxel will experience all three RF pulses and therefore be refocused to give an NMR signal. In practice, extra RF pulses and gradients are used for water suppression.*

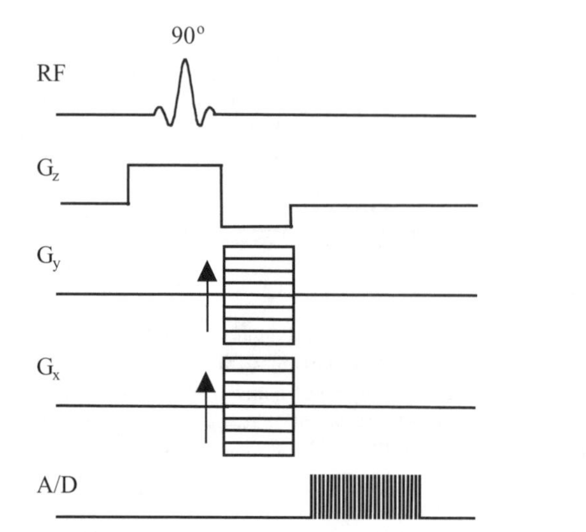

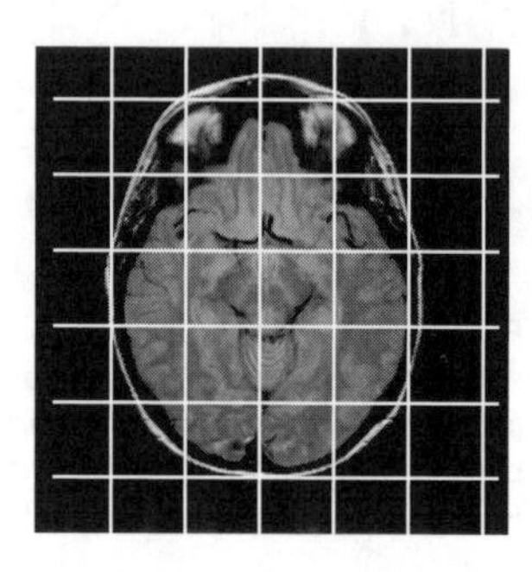

FIGURE 4.42. *(Left) A two-dimensional CSI sequence that produces NMR spectra from a range of voxels in the xy plane (right). The voxels are often overlaid on the axial image for correlating the anatomical structure with the biochemical information.*

commensurate with clinical scanning. The major phosphorus-containing metabolites are phosphomonoesters and phosphodiesters, phosphocreatine, inorganic phosphate, and adenosine triphosphate. Once again, the relative amounts of these metabolites are, in many cases, indicative of the health of the tissue. A typical *in vivo* phosphorus spectrum is also shown in Figure 4.40.

There are two basic classes of methods used to obtain localized spectra. The first one localizes the acquired FID to a single, defined voxel. One of the most commonly used sequences is shown in Figure 4.41, and is called point-resolved spectroscopy (PRESS). A single voxel is localized using three frequency-selective RF pulses, and gradients are applied in all three directions. The acquired FID arises only from the voxel representing the intersection of all three slices.

The second class of methods is based on one-, two-, or three-dimensional phase-encoding of the FID to produce separate spectra from multiple voxels, and is referred to as chemical shift imaging (CSI). A sequence for two-dimensional CSI is shown in Figure 4.41. An axial slice is first selected in the z dimension. The FID is phase-encoded in the x and the y dimensions. Two-dimensional inverse Fourier transformation with respect to the x and the y spatial dimensions and forward Fourier transformation with respect to the time dimension gives a series of spectra from each of the voxels shown on the right of Figure 4.42.

4.11. FUNCTIONAL MRI

Functional MRI (fMRI) is a relatively new technique, developed in the early 1990s, which can be used to determine which areas of the brain are involved in specific cognitive tasks. The basis for the technique is the sensitivity of the MRI signal intensity to the level of oxygen in the blood in the brain, a phenomenon termed the blood-oxygen-level-dependent (BOLD) effect.

In gray matter in the brain, a modest increase in the cerebral metabolic rate of oxygen ($CMRO_2$) and of glucose occurs in areas involved in neural activation. As a result of the release of vasodilatory compounds at an increased rate within the active tissue, local blood flow in the capillary bed is increased significantly. This increased blood flow leads to decreased oxygen extraction by the tissue due to the decreased capillary transit times. The overall effect is that the rate of delivery of oxygen to neurally "activated" tissue increases to a much lesser extent than the increase in blood flow, resulting in an increase in the oxygenation state of blood. In turn, this increase corresponds to an increase in the concentration of oxyhemoglobin and a decrease in that of deoxyhemoglobin. Deoxyhemoglobin has a magnetic susceptibility which is more paramagnetic than that of tissue, whereas oxyhemoglobin has a diamagnetic susceptibility very similar to that of tissue. The decrease in the deoxyhemoglobin concentration, therefore, reduces the local magnetic field gradients between the blood in the capillary bed and tissue. As a result, the values of T_2 and T_2^* increase locally in areas of the brain associated with neuronal activation, the value of T_2^* increasing by a greater amount than that of T_2.

fMRI studies are usually carried out using imaging sequences sensitive to changes in tissue T_2^* values. The most commonly used sequence is multislice echo-planar imaging because data acquisition is fast enough to obtain whole-brain coverage in a few seconds. The changes in image intensity in activated areas are very small, typically only 0.1–1% using a 1.5-T scanner, and so the experiments are repeated a number of times, and the data are then subjected to statistical analysis. Data processing involves correlation, on a pixel-by-pixel basis, of the change in MRI signal intensity with the time course of the presented stimulus, as shown in Figure 4.43. The spatial resolution of most fMRI studies is approximately $7 \times 7 \times 7$ mm due to the small data matrix collected (64×64), the inherent PSF of the EPI sequence, and the widespread use of postacquisition spatial filtering of the data. It should be noted, however, that very high resolution fMRI can also be performed, particularly at high magnetic fields, and reports with in-plane resolution of 1×1 mm have been published.

The change in MRI signal intensity at sites associated with neuronal activation has three components, shown schematically in Figure 4.43. The first component is a small signal decrease immediately after the onset of the stimulation. This corresponds to the total deoxyhemoglobin increasing for the first 3 s or so due to an initial increase in oxygen extraction before the large increase in blood flow. The second feature is an increase in signal intensity, which reaches a maximum at about 7 s after the onset of the stimulus. This time lag is referred to as the hemodynamic response time. The final stage is a signal undershoot, which can last up to 1 min poststimulation, and corresponds to the blood volume in the venules, which drain the activated areas, remaining elevated after blood flow has reequilibrated.

Although neuronal activation is itself highly localized, the BOLD fMRI signal contains contributions not only from the capillary bed close to the area of activation, but also from venules and veins that are connected to the capillary bed. Because roughly 75% of the blood in the brain is contained in venous vessels, whereas only 5% of the blood is contained in capillaries, a significant part of the

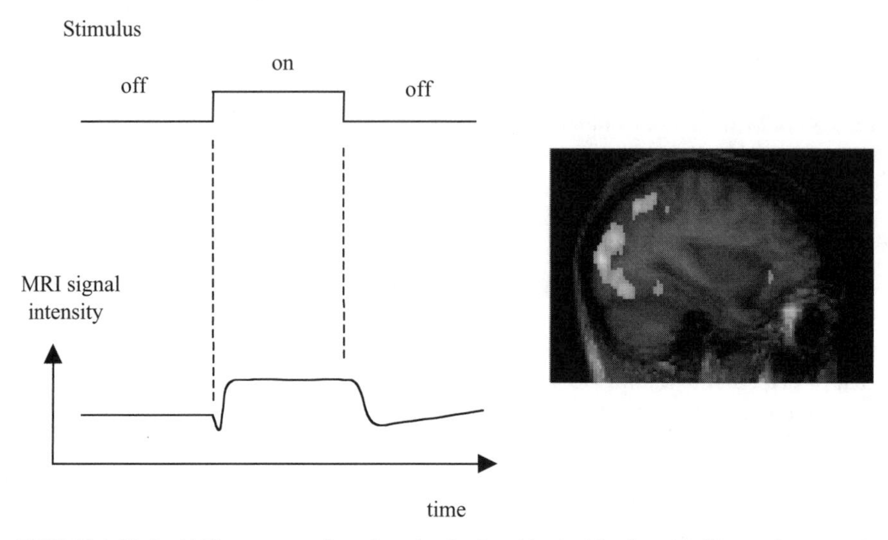

FIGURE 4.43. *(Left) The presentation of a stimulus in a blocked "on" and "off" paradigm results in an idealized waveform of the MRI signal intensity shown below. After an initial undershoot, the signal increases to a maximum approximately 7 s after the onset of stimulation and then undershoots for 30–60 s after stimulation has ceased. (Right) An "activation map" produced by correlating the pixel-by-pixel MRI signal with the waveform shown on the left. Pixels that show statistically significant correlation are shown as areas of high signal intensity overlaid on one of the EPI scans used to acquire the raw data.*

stimulus-induced signal change results from oxygenation changes in veins, which may be up to 1 cm from the actual area of activation. One of the advantages of operating at higher field strengths, apart from the intrinsic increase in image SNR, is the increased contribution of the component of the BOLD signal from the capillary bed.

Although fMRI is currently used more for academic research than routine clinical use, it is being used in a number of presurgical planning studies. Here, the exact procedure for removing, for example, a tumor from the brain is planned around knowing the location of areas that control tasks such as language recognition and motor processes.

4.12. CLINICAL APPLICATIONS OF MRI

The majority of clinical diagnoses using MRI rely on the intrinsic contrast between pathological and healthy tissue. Based on patient history, and coupled with the results of other types of imaging such as ultrasound and CT, the appropriate scanning protocol (T_1-weighted, T_2-weighted, or proton density-weighted) is performed. Very often a contrast agent such as Gd-DTPA is used to increase the image contrast. The MRI signal is also sensitive to a number of other parameters. For example, the diffusion coefficient of water has been found to be an extremely sensitive parameter related to the extent of stroke in the very early stages after the episode. Diffusion-weighted sequences show areas of tissue damaged by stroke much earlier than relaxation time-weighted sequences. Images can also be acquired in which the signal intensity is related to the amount of blood perfusion in tissue. This section outlines a few of the basic clinical applications of MRI.

4.12.1. Brain

The detection of brain disease depends mainly on the changes in relaxation times associated with cellular damage. In brain tumors, there is an increase in the water concentration, as well as an increase in the T_1 and T_2 relaxation times. T_2-weighted sequences, for example, show the tumor as an area of higher signal intensity than the surrounding tissue, as shown in Figure 4.44.

Other conditions which can be diagnosed by MRI are Parkinson's disease and Alzheimer's disease. These both lead to the deposition of iron in the putamen. The effect of the iron is to reduce the T_2 and T_2^* of the surrounding water molecules, and so there is a reduction in signal intensity on T_2-weighted sequences. Hemorrage and hematomas are also associated with increased levels of iron in the brain. Hydrocephalus is particularly easy to diagnose, given the distinct signal from water in its free state, with very long T_1 and T_2 values. Multiple sclerosis produces many lesions in the brain by the process of demyelination. Plaques typically vary in size between 1 and 10 mm and have prolonged T_1 and T_2 relaxation times with respect to the white matter in brain where most occur.

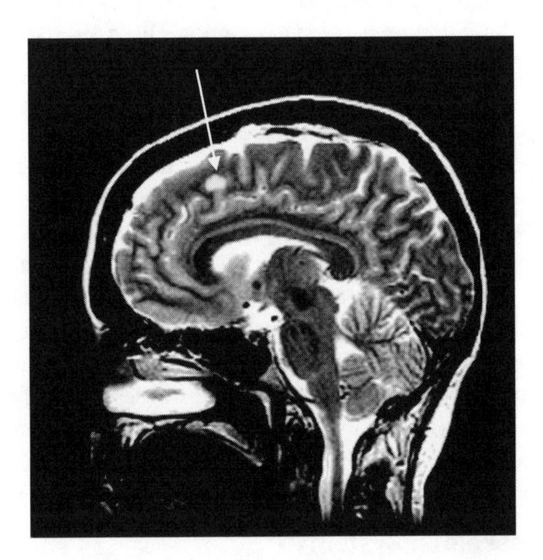

FIGURE 4.44. A T_2-weighted image of a brain tumor, which shows up as a hyperintense region because its T_2 value is longer than that of the surrounding healthy tissue.

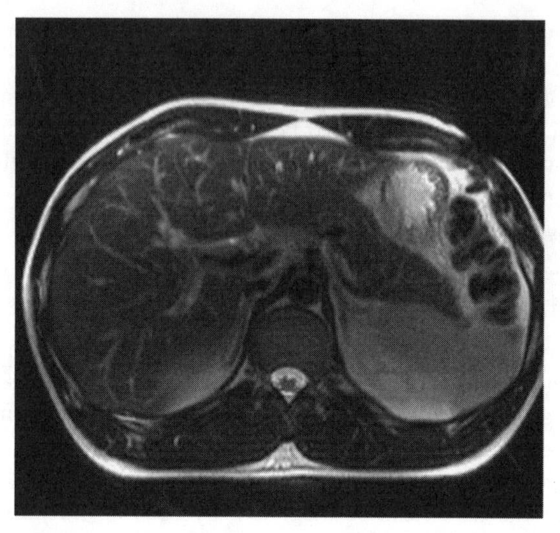

FIGURE 4.45. A FLASH image of the liver acquired in a single breath-hold.

4.12.2. Liver and the Reticuloendothelial System

Imaging of the liver requires rapid imaging sequences so that the entire image can be acquired within a single breath-hold: an example of a rapid hepatic scan is shown in Figure 4.45. Diseases such as hemosiderosis and hemochromatosis cause iron to be deposited in the parenchyma of the liver, reducing both the T_1 and T_2 relaxation times. In hemosiderosis, iron is also deposited in the spleen. Cirrhosis of the liver is often characterized by fatty infiltrations into the tissue, and is relatively easy to diagnose using MRI. MRA techniques can be used to diagnose diseases associated with reduced flow through the portal vein of the liver. Tumors within the liver can be delineated on the basis of their differences in relaxation times with respect to healthy tissue. For example, hepatocellular carcinomas are normally hyperintense on T_2-weighted scans. If it is not possible to differentiate the tumor, then a superparamagnetic contrast agent can be administered, as covered in Section 4.7.2. Paramagnetic contrast agents can also be used in detecting hepatic tumors. The distribution of the paramagnetic agent in tumor and healthy liver parenchyma occurs at different rates. More rapid uptake in normal parenchyma means that the tumor is visible as a region of lower signal intensity. Recently, paramagnetic contrast agents have been designed specifically for liver imaging, with the aim of increasing the time during which the signal from the normal parenchyma is higher than that of the tumor. Two such agents are Gd-ethoxybenzyl-DTPA (trade name Eovist) and Gd-benzyloxypropionictetraacetate (Gd-BOPTA; trade name MultiHance).

4.12.3. Musculoskeletal System

MRI is particularly useful in high-resolution imaging of the musculoskeletal system. Developmental abnormalities or degenerative diseases of the spinal cord are

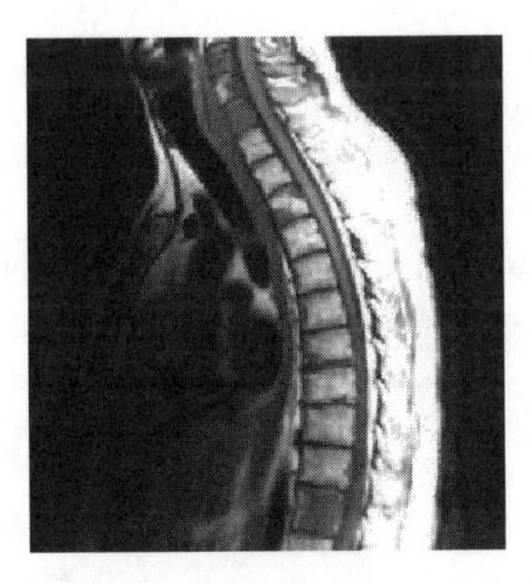
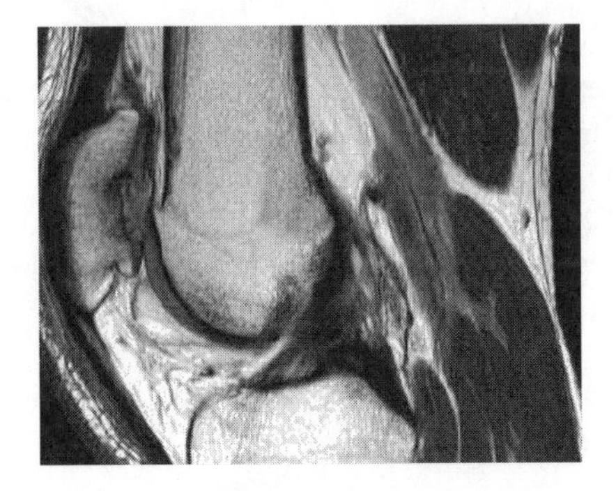

FIGURE 4.46. *(Left) An image of the spinal cord, showing the individual disks and a slight curvature of the spine. (Right) One image from a three-dimensional dataset of the knee.*

very commonly diagnosed using MRI. Traumatic injury such as disk herniation, disk compression, or epidural hematoma similarly show up well on images. Spinal cord tumors and plaques associated with multiple sclerosis can also be detected using high-resolution imaging of the spinal cord. A typical image is shown on the left of Figure 4.46, demonstrating the excellent delineation of cord morphology. In terms of other tissues, imaging of the shoulder is very common for sports injuries. Imaging of the knee is also used to diagnose degenerative cartilage waste and the state of connective tissue, as shown on the right of Figure 4.46.

4.12.4. Cardiac System

The detection of cardiovascular disease is based mainly on anatomical changes. There is excellent intrinsic contrast between flowing blood and the walls of vessels and the cardiac chambers, as shown in Figure 4.47. The left ventricular volume and ejection fraction are very important measures of heart function, and both can be measured using MRI. In addition, using spin-tagging techniques, the complex motion of the heart wall during systole and diastole can be investigated for abnormalities. Ischemic heart disease is characterized by a decrease in the wall thickness of the left ventricle, which can be seen directly on the images. Hypertrophy leads to the opposite effect, a thickening of the myocardial wall. Tumors are detected by an increased signal intensity on T_2-weighted images. Cardiomyopathy produces enlargement of the left ventricular chamber. Congenital heart disease can involve cardiac valve stenosis, valve

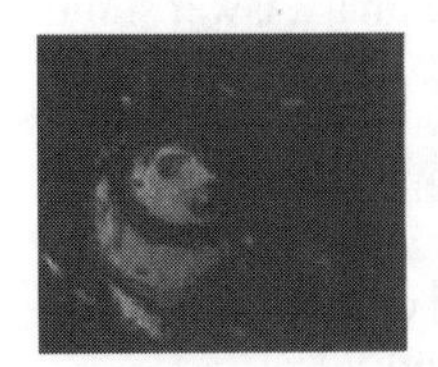
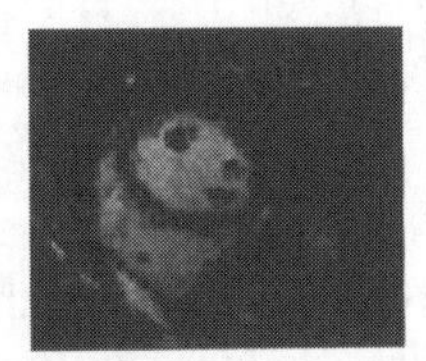
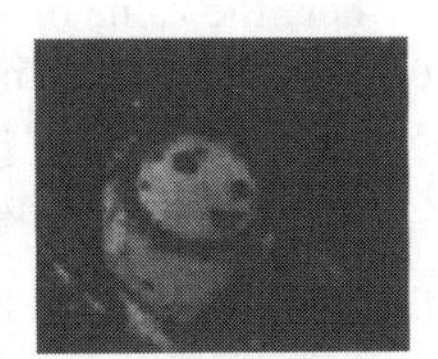
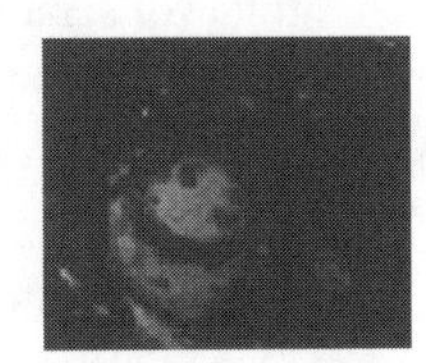

FIGURE 4.47. *A series of cardiac images taken at various times throughout the cardiac cycle.*

deficiencies, or abnormal connections between the individual components of the heart. In heart transplants, rejection is often associated with an increased concentration of water in the tissue and a higher T_2 value, and therefore T_2-weighted imaging is used as a test for the rejection process.

Electronic gating of the MRI data acquisition to the cardiac cycle, via electrocardiogram measurements, is necessary to reduce the motion artifacts associated with heart motion.

EXERCISES

4.1. Assuming that there are 6.7×10^{22} protons in 1 cm^3 of water, what is the magnetization contained within this volume at a magnetic field strength of 1.5 T?

4.2. Show schematically the effects of a 90°, a 180°, a 270°, and a 360° pulse on thermal equilibrium magnetization, using the vector model.

4.3. Calculate the effects of the following pulse sequences on thermal equilibrium magnetization. The final answer should include x, y, and z components of magnetization.

- **(a)** 90_x (a pulse with tip angle 90°, applied about the x axis).
- **(b)** 80_x.
- **(c)** 90_x 90_y (the second 90° pulse is applied immediately after the first).
- **(d)** 80_x 80_y.

4.4. Answer true or false with one or two sentences of explanation:

- **(a)** Recovery of magnetization along the z axis after a 90° pulse does not necessarily result in loss of magnetization from the xy plane.
- **(b)** A static magnetic field $\mathbf{B}_0$ that is homogeneous results in a free induction decay that persists for a long time.
- **(c)** When the magnetization relaxes from the xy plane back to the z axis, it absorbs energy from the lattice.
- **(d)** A short tissue T_1 indicates a slow spin–lattice relaxation process.

4.5. Using the vector model, show the effects of the pulse sequence given below on thermal equilibrium magnetization for two cases. First, for a water proton exactly on resonance, that is, stationary in the rotating reference frame. Second, for a fat proton, which has a precessional frequency in the rotating reference frame of ω rad/s, where the value of ω is given by π/τ. The final answer should include x, y, and z components of magnetization:

$$12.5^{\circ}_{x} - \tau - 37.5^{\circ}_{-x} - \tau - 37.5^{\circ}_{x} - \tau - 12.5^{\circ}_{-x}$$

4.6. **(a)** Plot qualitatively the dependence of T_1 on the strength of the applied magnetic field for a mobile, intermediate, and viscous liquids.

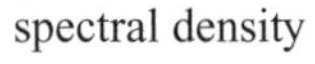

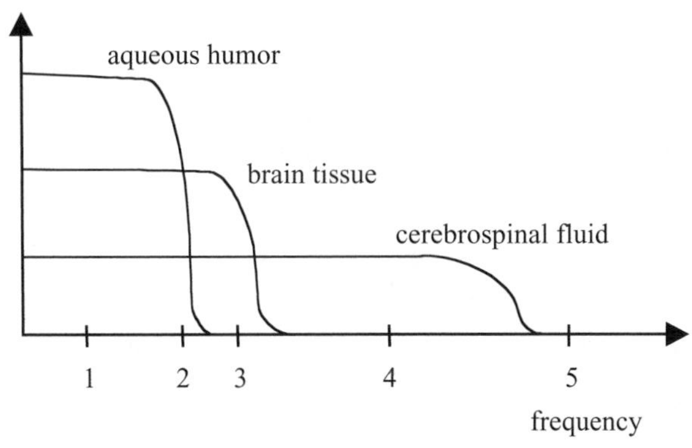

FIGURE 4.48. Illustration for Exercise 4.7.

(b) Plot qualitatively the variation in T_1 as a function of the mobility of a liquids.

4.7. For the five frequencies (1–5) shown in Figure 4.48, state the order of the T_1 and T_2 values, for example, $T_1(\text{brain}) > T_1(\text{CSF}) > T_1(\text{aqueous humor})$.

4.8. The hydrogen nuclei in the body are found mainly in fat and water. The T_2 value of fat was measured to be 100 ms and that of water to be 500 ms. In a spin-echo experiment, calculate the delay between the 90° pulse and the 180° pulse that maximizes the difference in signal intensities between the fat and the water.

4.9. Write an expression for the M_z magnetization as a function of time after a 180° pulse. After what time is the M_z component zero? Plot the magnetization after instead applying a 135° pulse.

4.10. Explain why a three-dimensional image cannot be obtained by applying all three gradients simultaneously during data acquisition.

4.11. Derive the value of the Ernst angle given in equation (4.54).

4.12. What is the form of the PSF in the phase-encoding direction of an EPI sequence?

4.13. Suggest an imaging sequence that could be used for "black-blood imaging," that is, where flowing blood appears with very low signal intensity in the image.

4.14. A brain tumor has a lower concentration of water than surrounding healthy tissue. The T_1 value of the protons in the tumor is shorter than that of the protons in healthy tissue, but the T_2 value of the tumor protons is longer. Which kind of weighting should be introduced into the imaging sequence in order to ensure that there is contrast between the tumor and healthy tissue? If a large concentration of superparamagnetic contrast agent is injected and accumulates in the tumor only, which kind of weighting would now be optimal?

FURTHER READING

Original Papers

The Basics of NMR and Data Acquisition

F. Bloch, Nuclear induction, *Phys. Rev.* **70,** 460–474 (1946).

N. Bloembergen, E. M. Purcell, and R. V. Pound, Relaxation effects in nuclear magnetic resonance absorption, *Phys. Rev.* **73,** 679–712 (1948).

E. L. Hahn, Spin-echoes, *Phys. Rev.* **80,** 580–594 (1950).

Signal Detection

R. R. Ernst and W. A. Anderson, Application of Fourier transform spectroscopy to magnetic resonance, *Rev. Sci. Instrum.* **37,** 93–102 (1966).

D. I. Hoult, The NMR receiver, *Progr. NMR. Spectr.* **12,** 41–77 (1978).

Magnetic Resonance Imaging

P. C. Lauterbur, Image formation by induced local interactions: Examples employing nuclear magnetic resonance, *Nature* (London) **242,** 190–191 (1973).

P. Mansfield and P. K. Grannell, NMR diffraction in solids, *J. Phys. C Solid State Phys.* **6,** L422–L426 (1973).

A. Kumar, D. Welti, and R. R. Ernst, NMR Fourier zeugmatography, *J. Magn. Reson.* **18,** 69–83 (1975).

W. A. Edelstein, J. Hutchinson, G. Johnson, and T. W. Redpath, Spin warp NMR imaging and applications to human whole-body imaging, *Phys. Med. Biol.* **25,** 751–756 (1980).

k-Space

S. Ljunggren, A simple graphical representation of Fourier-based imaging methods, *J. Magn. Reson.* **54,** 338–343 (1983).

D. B. Twieg, The *k*-trajectory formulation of the NMR imaging process with applications in analysis and synthesis of imaging methods, *Med. Phys.* **10,** 610–621 (1983).

Radiofrequency Coils and Magnetic Field Gradients

J. E. Tanner, Pulsed field gradients for NMR spin-echo diffusion measurements, *Rev. Sci. Instrum.* **36,** 1086–1090 (1965).

D. I. Hoult and R. E. Richards, The Signal-to-noise ratio of the nuclear magnetic resonance experiment, *J. Magn. Reson.* **24,** 71–85 (1976).

C. E. Hayes, W. A. Edelstein, J. F. Schenck, O. M. Mueller, and M. Eash, An efficient, highly homogeneous radiofrequency coil for whole-body NMR imaging at 1.5 T, *J. Magn. Reson.* **63,** 622–628 (1985).

Fast Imaging Techniques.

P. Mansfield, Multi-planar image formation using NMR spin echoes, *J. Phys. C Solid State Phys.* **10,** L55–L58 (1977).

A. Haase, J. Frahm, D. Matthaei, W. H¨anicke, and K. D. Merboldt, FLASH imaging. Rapid NMR imaging using low flip-angle pulses, *J. Magn. Reson.* **67,** 258–266 (1986).

J. Hennig, A. Naureth, and H. Friedburg, RARE imaging: A fast imaging method for clinical MR, *Magn. Reson. Imag.* **3,** 823–833 (1986).

A. B. Ahn, J. H. Kim, and Z. H. Cho, High-speed spiral-scan echo planar NMR imaging—I, *IEEE Trans. Med. Imag.* **MI-5,** 1–6 (1986).

Magnetic Resonance Angiography

L. E. Crooks, C. M. Mills, P. L. Davis, *et al.,* Visualization of cerebral and vascular abnormalities by NMR imaging: The effects of imaging parameters on contrast, *Radiology* **144,** 843–852 (1982).

D. J. Bryant, J. A. Payn, D. N. Firmin, and D. B. Longmore, Measurement of flow with NMR imaging using a gradient pulse and phase difference technique, *J. Comput. Assist. Tomogr.* **8,** 588–593 (1984).

In Vivo Localized Spectroscopy

T. R. Brown, B. M. Kincaid, and K. Ugurbil, NMR chemical shift imaging in three dimensions, *Proc. Natl. Acad. Sci. USA* **79,** 3523–3526 (1982).

A. Haase, J. Frahm, W. Hanicke, and D. Matthei, ^{1}H NMR chemical shift selective (CHESS) imaging, *Phys. Med. Biol.* **30,** 341–344 (1985).

J. Frahm, K. D. Merboldt, and W. Hanicke, Localized proton spectroscopy using stimulated echoes, *J. Magn. Reson.* **72,** 502–508 (1987).

P. A. Bottomley, Spatial localization in NMR spectroscopy *in vivo, Ann. N. Y. Acad. Sci.* **508,** 333–348 (1987).

Functional MRI.

S. Ogawa, T. M. Lee, A. R. Kay, and D. W. Tank, Brain magnetic resonance imaging with contrast dependent on blood oxygenation, *Proc. Natl. Acad. Sci. USA* **87,** 9868–9872 (1990).

R. Turner, D. Le Bihan, C. T. Moonen, D. Despres, and J. Frank, Echo-planar time course MRI of cat brain oxygenation changes, *Magn. Reson. Med.* **22,** 159–166 (1991).

Books

Nuclear Magnetic Resonance

R. R. Ernst, G. Bodenhausen, and A. Wokaun, *Principles of Nuclear Magnetic Resonance in One and Two Dimensions,* Clarendon, Oxford (1987).

C. P. Slichter, *Principles of Magnetic Resonance,* Springer-Verlag, Berlin (1990).

P. T. Callaghan, *Principles of nuclear magnetic resonance microscopy,* Clarendon, Oxford (1991).

Instrumentation

E. Fukushima and S. B. W. Roeder, *Experimental Pulse NMR: A Nuts and Bolts Approach,* Addison-Wesley, Reading, Massachusetts (1981).

C.-N. Chen and D. I. Hoult, *Biomedical Magnetic Resonance Technology,* Adam Hilger, Bristol, England (1989).

J.-M. Jin, *Electromagnetic Analysis and Design in Magnetic Resonance Imaging,* CRC Press, Boca Raton, Florida (1998).

Magnetic Resonance Imaging

P. G. Morris, *Nuclear Magnetic Resonance Imaging in Medicine and Biology,* Oxford University Press, Oxford (1990).

D. D. Stark and W. G. Bradley, Jr., *Magnetic Resonance Imaging,* 2nd ed., Mosby-Year Books, St. Louis (1992).

R. H. Hashemi and W. G. Bradley, Jr., *MRI: The Basics,* Lippincott, Williams and Wilkins, Philadelphia (1997).

M. A. Brown and R. C. Semelka, *MRI: Basic Principles and Applications,* 2nd ed., Wiley-Liss, New York (1999).

E. M. Haake, R. W. Brown, M. R. Thompson, and R. Venkatesan, *Magnetic Resonance Imaging: Physical Principles and Sequence Design,* Wiley-Liss, New York (2000).

Magnetic Resonance Angiography

E. J. Potchen, E. M. Haake, J. E. Siebert, and A. Gottschalk, eds., *Magnetic Resonance Angiography: Concepts and Applications,* Mosby-Year Book, St. Louis (1993).

M. R. Prince, T. M. Grist, and J. F. Debatin, *3D Contrast MR Angiography,* Springer, Berlin, (1998).

Functional MRI

C. T. W. Moonen and P. A. Bandettini, *Functional MRI (Medical Radiology),* Springer-Verlag, Berlin (2000).

R. B. Buxton, *An Introduction to Functional Magnetic Resonance Imaging: Principles and Techniques,* Cambridge University Press, Cambridge (2001).

P. Jezzard, P. M. Matthews, and S. M. Smith, eds., *Functional Magnetic Resonance Imaging: An Introduction to Methods,* Oxford University Press, Oxford (2001).

Contrast Agents

A. E. Merbach and E. Toth, eds., *The Chemistry of Contrast Agents in Medical Magnetic Resonance Imaging,* Wiley, New York (2001).

W. Krause, ed., *Magnetic Resonance Contrast Agents,* Springer-Verlag, Berlin (2002).

Rapid Imaging

F. W. Wehrli, *Fast Scan Magnetic Resonance: Principles and Applications,* Raven Press, New York (1991).

F. Schmitt, M. K. Stehling, and R. Turner, eds., *Echo-Planar Imaging: Theory, Technique and Application,* Springer-Verlag, Berlin (1998).

Signal Processing

Z.-P. Liang and P. C. Lauterbur, *Principles of Magnetic Resonance Imaging. A Signal Processing Perspective,* IEEE Press, New York (2000).

Review Articles

J. Link, The design of resonator probes with homogeneous radiofrequency fields, in *NMR:Basic Principles and Progress* (P. Diehl, E. Fluck, H. Guenther, R. Kosfeld, and J. Seelig, eds.), pp. 1–32 Springer-Verlag, Berlin (1992).

R. Turner, Gradient coil design: A review of methods, *Magn. Reson. Imag.* **11,** 903 (1993).

B. L. Chapman, Shielded gradients. And the general solution to the near field problem of electromagnet design. *MAGMA* **9,** 146 (1999).

R. Turner and R. J. Ordidge, Technical challenges of functional magnetic resonance imaging, *IEEE Trans. Biomed. Imag.* **19,** 42–54 (2000).

R. C. Semelka and T. Helmberger, New contrast agents for imaging the liver, *Magn. Reson. Imag. Clin. N. Am.* **9,** 745 (2001).

Specialized Journals

Concepts in Magnetic Resonance

Journal of Magnetic Resonance

Journal of Magnetic Resonance Imaging

MAGMA: Magnetic Resonance Materials in Physics, Biology and Medicine

Magnetic Resonance Engineering

Magnetic Resonance in Chemistry

Magnetic Resonance in Medicine

NMR in Biomedicine

5

General Image Characteristics

5.1. INTRODUCTION

Irrespective of the method used to acquire medical images, whether it be X-ray, nuclear medicine, ultrasound, or MRI, there are a number of criteria by which the image characteristics can be evaluated and compared. The most important of these criteria are the spatial resolution, the signal-to-noise ratio, and the contrast-to-noise ratio. In addition to measurements made on humans, new acquisition and processing techniques are often tested on "phantoms," examples of which are shown in Figure 5.1. This chapter covers a number of general concepts applicable to all of the modalities in this book.

5.2. SPATIAL RESOLUTION

There are a number of measures used to describe the spatial resolution of an imaging modality: the three most common in the spatial domain are the point spread function (PSF), the line spread function (LSF), and the edge spread function (ESF). These measures correspond to a modulation transfer function (MTF) in the spatial frequency domain.

5.2.1. The Point Spread Function

The concept of the PSF is most easily explained by considering a very small "point source" positioned within the imaging FOV, as shown in Figure 5.2. This point source could be a small sphere of water for MRI, a small reflector for ultrasound, a sphere

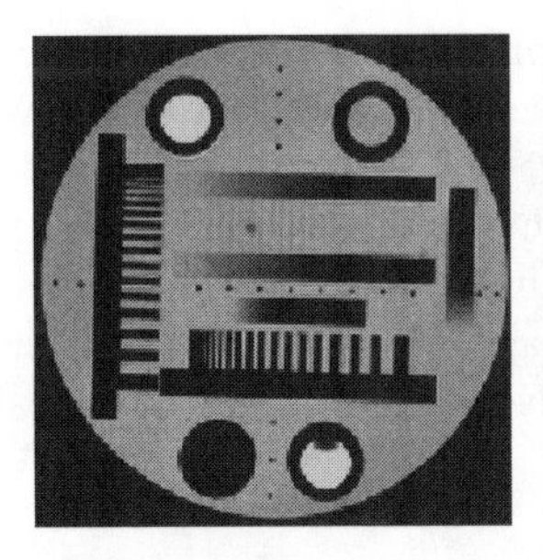

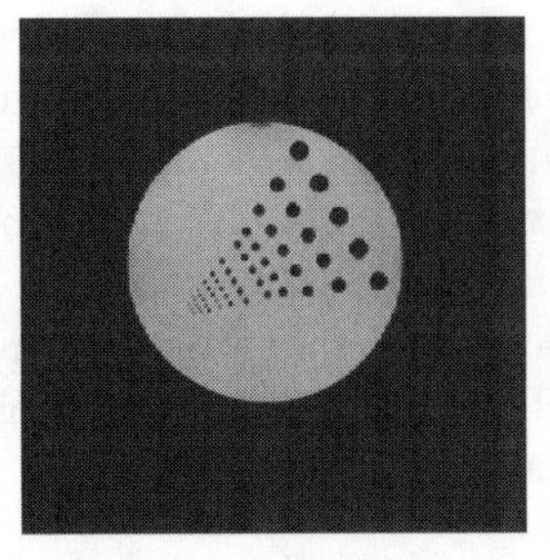

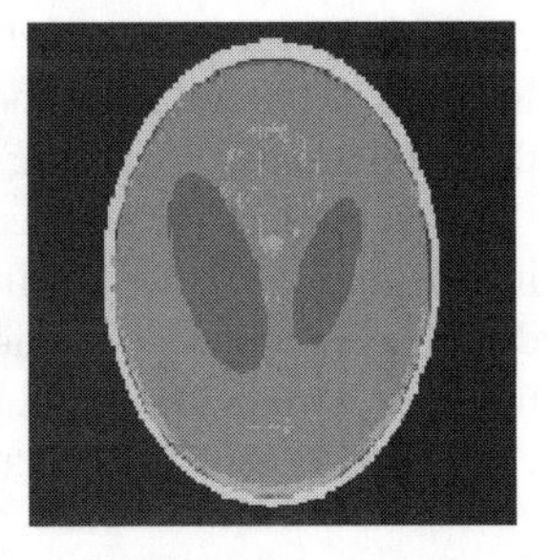

FIGURE 5.1. *Images of various phantoms used for the measurement of image characteristics. (Left, center) MRI phantoms used for spatial-resolution, signal-to-noise, and contrast-to-noise measurements. (Right) A Shepp–Logan phantom often used to compare the results from different image processing methods.*

filled with a γ-ray emitter for nuclear medicine, or a lead sheet with a pinhole for X-ray imaging. The mathematical relationship between the reconstructed image $I(x, y, z)$ and the object $O(x, y, z)$ being imaged can be represented by

$$I(x, y, z) = O(x, y, z) * h(x, y, z) \tag{5.1}$$

where $*$ represents a convolution, and $h(x, y, z)$ is the three-dimensional PSF. In a perfect imaging system, the PSF would be a delta function in all three dimensions, and in this case the image would be a perfect representation of the object. In practice, as has been described for each imaging modality, the PSF has a finite width, which may be different in the x, y, and z directions, and can also contain side lobes if, for

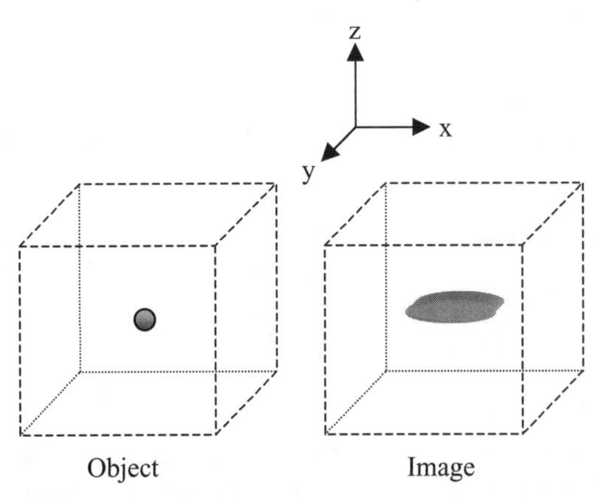

FIGURE 5.2. *(Left) The object to be imaged consists of a small point source. (Right) The image obtained is larger than the actual object, and may be blurred asymmetrically in the x, y, and z dimensions. In this illustrative case the PSF is broad in the x dimension and relatively narrow in the y and the z dimensions.*

example, image reconstruction involves Fourier transformation of a truncated dataset. In terms of the imaging modalities covered, nuclear medicine and ultrasound have the strongest asymmetry in the three-dimensional PSF.

In addition to the PSF associated with the intrinsic physics of the particular imaging method, each stage of image formation, such as the individual components of the detection system, the method of data sampling, and image reconstruction and filtering has an associated PSF. The total system PSF involves a series of mathematical convolutions of the individual PSFs for each stage:

$$\begin{aligned} h_{\text{total}}(x, y, z) \\ = h_{\text{detector}}(x, y, z) * h_{\text{sampling}}(x, y, z) * h_{\text{reconstruction}}(x, y, z) * h_{\text{filter}}(x, y, z) \end{aligned} \quad (5.2)$$

The degree to which a particular PSF blurs the image depends upon the nature of the object being imaged, as shown in Figure 5.3.

5.2.2. Resolution Criteria

The spatial resolution of an image is defined as the smallest separation of two point sources necessary for the sources to be resolved. The spatial resolution is clearly related to the PSF, which can have many different mathematical forms depending upon the particular imaging modality. There are many different criteria for describing

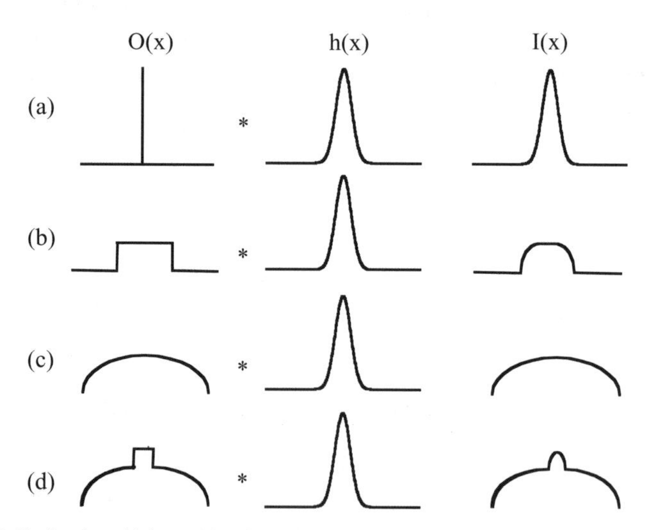

FIGURE 5.3. Projections I (x) resulting from the convolution of different one-dimensional objects O(x) with a one-dimensional Gaussian PSF, h(x). (a) If O(x) is a delta function I (x) and h(x) are identical, and thus the acquired image can be used to estimate h(x). (b) Sharp edges and boundaries in the object are blurred in the image I (x). (c) If the image is very smooth, then the overall effect of h(x) is small, but if, within the smooth structure, there are sharp boundaries, as in (d), then these boundaries appear blurred in the image.

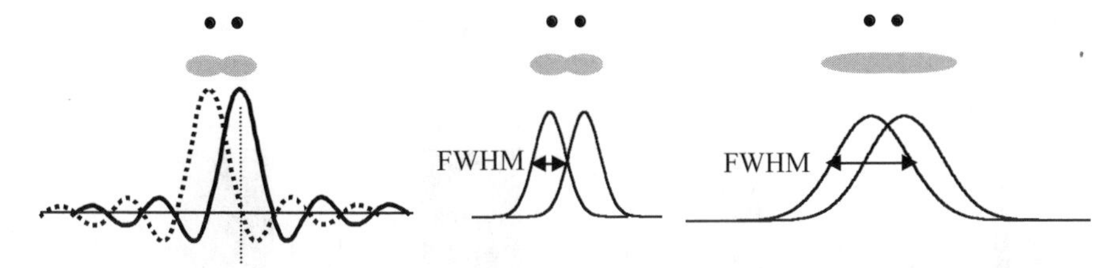

FIGURE 5.4. *(Left) For a sinc PSF, the signals from the two point sources can be resolved when the separation between them is less than half the width of the main lobe of the sinc function. (Center) For an arbitrary form of the PSF, the two point sources can be resolved when their separation is less than the FWHM of the function. (Right) The two point sources can no longer be resolved due to the broad FWHM of the PSF.*

the spatial resolution in terms of the PSF. If the PSF is a sinc function, then the Rayleigh criterion can be applied, which states that the two point sources can be resolved if the peak intensity of the PSF from one source coincides with the first zero-crossing point of the PSF of the other, as shown in Figure 5.4. In this case the spatial resolution is defined as one-half the width of the central lobe of the sinc function.

If the form of the PSF is arbitrary, then it can be characterized in terms of its FWHM. Then the criterion for resolution can be stated such that, if the two points sources are separated by a distance greater than the FWHM, then they can be resolved, as shown in Figure 5.4.

The PSF for many imaging techniques is well-approximated by a Gaussian function. The one-dimensional PSF, $h(x)$, can be written as

$$h(x) = \frac{1}{\sqrt{2\pi\sigma^2}} \exp\left(-\frac{(x-x_0)^2}{\sigma^2}\right) \tag{5.3}$$

where σ is the standard deviation of the distribution and x_0 is the center of the function. The FWHM of a Gaussian function is given by

$$\text{FWHM} = 2\sqrt{2\ln 2}\sigma \cong 2.36\sigma \tag{5.4}$$

5.2.3. The Line Spread Function and Edge Spread Function

A second commonly used function to characterize spatial resolution is the line-spread function (LSF), which is illustrated in Figure 5.5. The LSF is defined in terms of the PSF by

$$\text{LSF}(y) = \int \text{PSF}(x, y)\, dx \tag{5.5}$$

The LSF is most often used in X-ray imaging, where a line phantom is easy to construct, and usually consists of a grid of thin lead septa placed between the X-ray source and the detector.

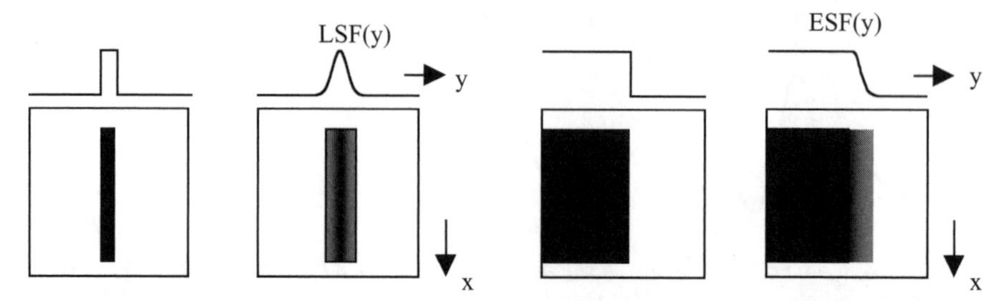

FIGURE 5.5. Illustration of the concept of (left) the line spread function (LSF) and (right) the edge spread function (ESF). For measuring the LSF, the object consists of a thin line, with the one-dimensional projection of the object in the y dimension shown above. The actual image is broadened, with the LSF defined by the one-dimensional y projection of the image. (Right) For measurement of the ESF, a wide object with a sharp edge is used.

The edge spread function (ESF) can be defined as the convolution of the LSF with a step function. It is measured experimentally using a block of material with a sharp edge, as shown in Figure 5.5.

5.2.4. The Modulation Transfer Function

As outlined in Section 5.2.1, calculation of the overall PSF of an imaging system requires the convolution of the PSFs from each of the individual components of that system. This process can be mathematically extremely complicated. It is much easier to consider the situation in the spatial frequency domain, where the equivalent of the PSF is termed the modulation transfer function (MTF). Because the the spatial frequency domain and the spatial domain are related by the Fourier transform, as decribed by equations (A3) and (A4) in Appendix A, the MTF and the PSF are related similarly:

$$\mathrm{MTF}(k_x, k_y, k_z) = \iiint \mathrm{PSF}(x, y, z) e^{-j2\pi k_x x} e^{-j2\pi k_y y} e^{-j2\pi k_z z}\, dx\, dy\, dz \qquad (5.6)$$

where k_x, k_y, and k_z are the spatial frequencies, measured in cycles/millimeter or line pairs/millimeter. Features within the image that are large and contain many pixels of very similar signal intensity correspond to low spatial frequencies. Very small objects, and the edges of image features, represent high spatial frequencies, with the maximum spatial frequency corresponding to large changes in image intensity from one pixel to the next. Randomly distributed noise corresponds to high spatial frequencies because its value changes from pixel to pixel.

The relationship between a one-dimensional MTF and image spatial resolution is shown in Figure 5.6. The ideal MTF, which is independent of spatial frequency, is the Fourier transform of the ideal LSF, which is a delta function.

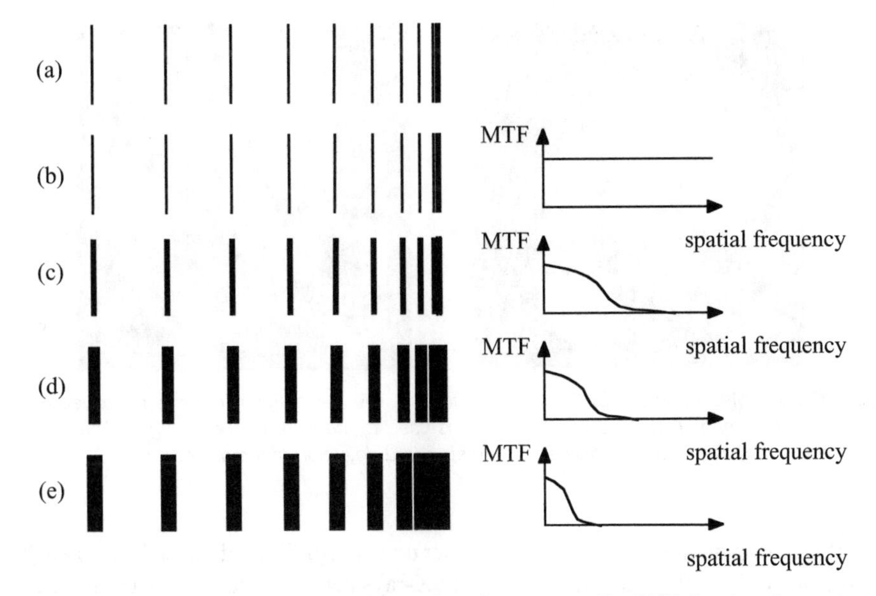

FIGURE 5.6. *(a) A schematic of a line phantom used to measure the MTF of an imaging system. (b–e) The images produced from the phantom by imaging systems with the MTF shown on the right. As the MTF becomes progressively narrower (corresponding to a broader LSF), the image becomes more blurred.*

5.3. SIGNAL-TO-NOISE RATIO

The factors that affect the SNR for each imaging modality are described in detail in the relevant sections of each chapter. In cases, such as MRI, where the noise is distributed uniformly throughout the imaging FOV, the SNR can be measured by computing the mean signal intensity over a certain region of interest (ROI) and dividing this by the standard deviation of the signal from a region outside the image, as shown in Figure 5.7. In other imaging modalities, the noise is not distributed uniformly, and so there is no simple method of measuring the SNR.

In this section, two important concepts related to image SNR are described: Poisson statistics and signal averaging.

5.3.1. The Poisson Distribution

The Poisson distribution is most commonly used to model the number of occurrences of some random phenomenon in a specified unit of space or time. Examples encountered in medical imaging include the spatial and temporal distribution of X-rays produced from the source and the corresponding distributions of γ-rays emitted by a radioisotope. In X-ray CT and nuclear medicine, it is usually true that the image SNR is determined solely by the Poisson statistics of the X-ray beam and the radioactive source, respectively.

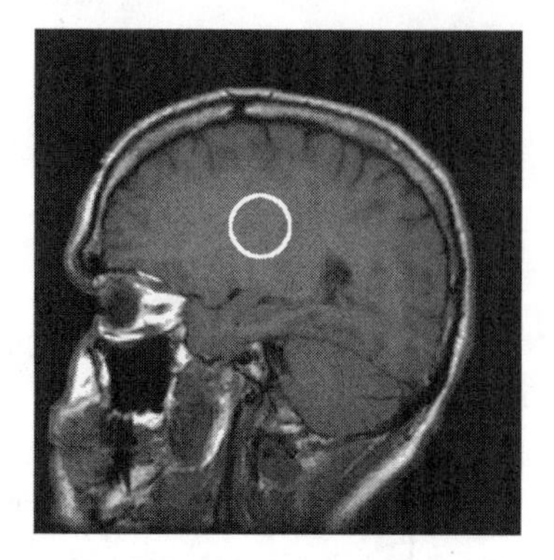

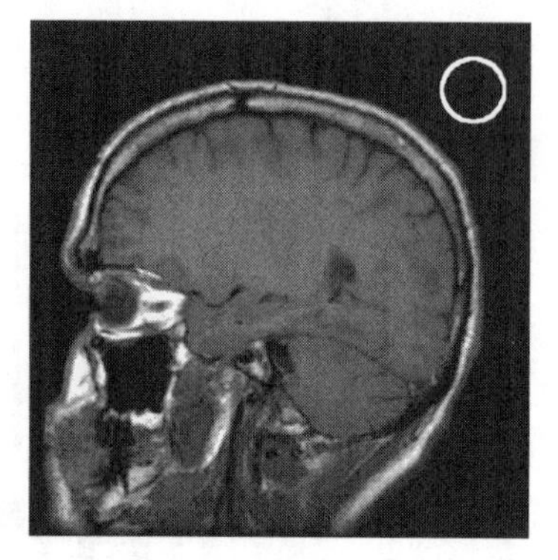

FIGURE 5.7. *Measuring the SNR for an MRI image. The mean signal intensity is derived from an ROI in the image (left), and the same area is used to measure the noise (right). The SNR is defined as the mean intensity divided by the standard deviation of the noise.*

If the mean number of incident X-rays per unit area of film is denoted by μ, then the probability $P(N)$ that there are N incident X-rays per unit area is shown graphically in Figure 5.8, and is described mathematically as

$$P(N) = \frac{\mu^N e^{-\mu}}{N!} \tag{5.7}$$

For the Poisson distribution, the standard deviation σ is defined as the difference between the values of μ and of N for which the value of $P(N)$ is one-half that of

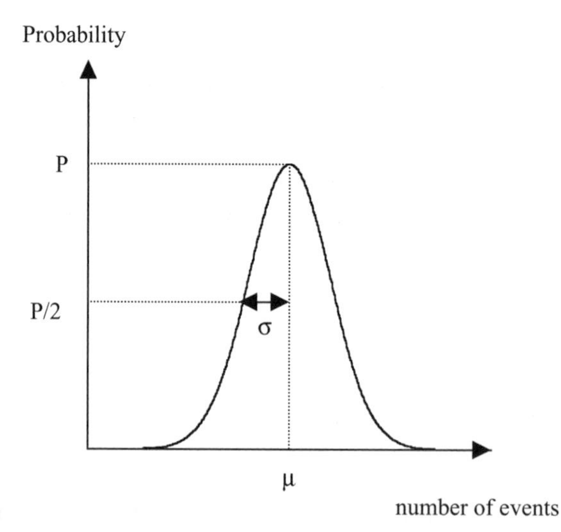

FIGURE 5.8. *The Poisson distribution describes the probability of a particular number of events happening for a random process.*

$P(\mu)$. A characteristic of the Poisson distribution is that the value of σ is related to μ by

$$\sigma = \sqrt{\mu} \tag{5.8}$$

For large values of N, μ can be well-approximated by N. The SNR, defined as N/σ, is therefore given by

$$\text{SNR} \propto \sqrt{N} \tag{5.9}$$

Equation (5.9) shows that the greater the number of X-rays or γ-rays that can be detected, the higher is the image SNR. To double the image SNR, for example, requires four times the number of counts.

5.3.2. Signal Averaging

The image SNR can be increased by averaging the signals from a number of images if the signal from successive images is coherent and the noise is at least partially incoherent. In MRI, for example, noise voltages are produced from conducting samples such as the human body and Johnson noise in the receiver electronics. This noise is, to a good approximation, random, and therefore "signal averaging" is widely used in MRI to increase the image SNR. The measured signal $\hat{x}$ can be represented as

$$\hat{x} = x + \xi \tag{5.10}$$

where x is the true signal and ξ is the noise component with a mean value of zero and a standard deviation denoted by σ_ξ. The SNR for a single measurement is given by

$$\text{SNR}_{\hat{x}} = \frac{|x|}{\sigma_\xi} \tag{5.11}$$

If N measurements are acquired, the averaged signal is given by

$$\hat{y} = x + \frac{1}{N}\sum_{n=1}^{N} \xi_n \tag{5.12}$$

Assuming that the noise for each measurement is uncorrelated, then the SNR for the averaged scans is given by

$$\text{SNR}_{\hat{y}} = \frac{|x|}{\sqrt{\text{var}\left\{(1/N)\sum_{n=1}^{N} x + \xi_n\right\}}} = \sqrt{N}\frac{|x|}{\sigma_\xi} = \text{SNR}_{\hat{x}}\sqrt{N} \tag{5.13}$$

Equation (5.13) shows that the SNR increases as the square root of the number of averaged images. The tradeoff in signal averaging is clearly the additional time required for data acquisition.

In ultrasonic imaging the noise contribution from speckle is coherent, and so simple signal averaging does not increase the SNR. However, if images are acquired with the transducer oriented at different angles with respect to the transducer, a technique known as compound imaging (Section 3.9), then the speckle in different images is only partially coherent. Averaging of the images therefore gives an increase in the SNR, but by a factor less than the square root of the number of images.

5.4. CONTRAST-TO-NOISE RATIO

Even if the image has a very high SNR, it is not useful unless there is a high enough CNR to be able to distinguish among different tissues, and in particular between healthy and pathological tissue. Various definitions of image contrast exist, the most common being

$$C_{\mathrm{AB}} = |S_{\mathrm{A}} - S_{\mathrm{B}}| \tag{5.14}$$

where C_{AB} is the contrast between tissues A and B, and S_{A} and S_{B} are the signals from tissues A and B, respectively. The CNR between tissues A and B is defined in terms of the respective SNRs of the two tissues:

$$\mathrm{CNR}_{\mathrm{AB}} = \frac{C_{\mathrm{AB}}}{\sigma_N} = \frac{|S_{\mathrm{A}} - S_{\mathrm{B}}|}{\sigma_N} = |\mathrm{SNR}_{\mathrm{A}} - \mathrm{SNR}_{\mathrm{B}}| \tag{5.15}$$

where σ_N is the standard deviation of the noise. Figure 5.9 shows the decrease in the CNR as the noise level in an image increases.

The CNR also depends upon the spatial resolution of the image. If the FWHM of the image PSF is on the order of the size of a particular image feature, then image blurring reduces the contrast significantly, as also shown in Figure 5.9.

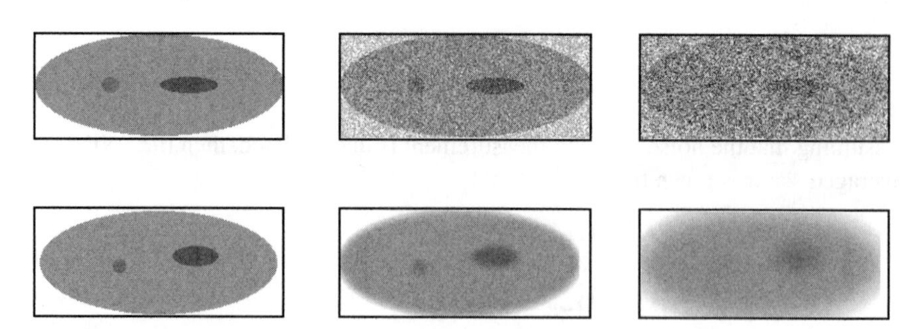

FIGURE 5.9. *(Top left-to-right) As the noise level increases in an image with high intrinsic contrast, the CNR degrades such that structures within the image can no longer be discerned. (Bottom left-to-right) As the spatial resolution of the image decreases, then the image contrast becomes worse, particularly for small objects within the body.*

5.5. IMAGE FILTERING

Postacquisition processing of images usually involves some form of filtering. Different filters can be used, for example, to improve the image SNR or spatial resolution or to highlight features such as edges and boundaries in the image. Such filtering involves tradeoffs between, in particular, image SNR and spatial resolution.

The simplest method of improving the SNR after data acquisition is to apply a low-pass filter to the image. Low-pass filtering is most commonly used in nuclear medicine scans because the intrinsic SNR is low due to the relatively small number of counts recorded per pixel. The term "low-pass" refers to the characteristics of the filter in the spatial frequency domain, that is, this type of filter amplifies the low spatial frequencies in the image with respect to the high spatial frequencies. As described earlier, low spatial frequencies are associated with areas of relatively uniform signal intensity, whereas high spatial frequencies represent the fine detail within tissue and sharp boundaries between tissues. Noise in an image, due to its random spatial distribution from pixel to pixel, corresponds to high spatial frequencies. A low-pass filter therefore improves the image SNR by attenuating the contribution from noise, but it also degrades the spatial resolution. If the imaging data are acquired in the spatial frequency domain, as in MRI, for example, then a filter can be applied directly to the data in this domain. Filters can also be applied in the spatial, that is, image, domain, in the form of convolution with a particular filter kernel. Simple examples of low-pass kernels are

$$\begin{matrix} 1 & 2 & 1 \\ 2 & 4 & 2 \\ 1 & 2 & 1 \end{matrix} \qquad \text{and} \qquad \begin{matrix} 1 & 1 & 1 \\ 1 & 4 & 1 \\ 1 & 1 & 1 \end{matrix}$$

Implementation of filtering using a 3×3 convolution kernel is shown schematically in Figure 5.10. The process involves placing the kernel over the image pixels, multiplying each pixel by the corresponding component of the kernel, and replacing the center pixel by the average of these values. The kernel is then displaced by one pixel in the horizontal dimension, for example, and the process repeated until the kernel has been applied to all the pixels in this horizontal dimension. This process is repeated for the next row of pixels until the whole image has been covered. An example of low-pass filtering of an MRI brain scan is shown in Figure 5.11(b).

Improvements in spatial resolution, a process often called resolution enhancement, can be achieved by using a high-pass filter, which uses convolution kernels such as

$$\begin{matrix} -1 & -1 & -1 \\ -1 & 9 & -1 \\ -1 & -1 & -1 \end{matrix} \qquad \text{or} \qquad \begin{matrix} -1 & -1 & -1 \\ -1 & 12 & -1 \\ -1 & -1 & -1 \end{matrix}$$

The SNR of the image is reduced using this type of filter because it amplifies the high spatial frequency noise, as shown in Figure 5.11(c).

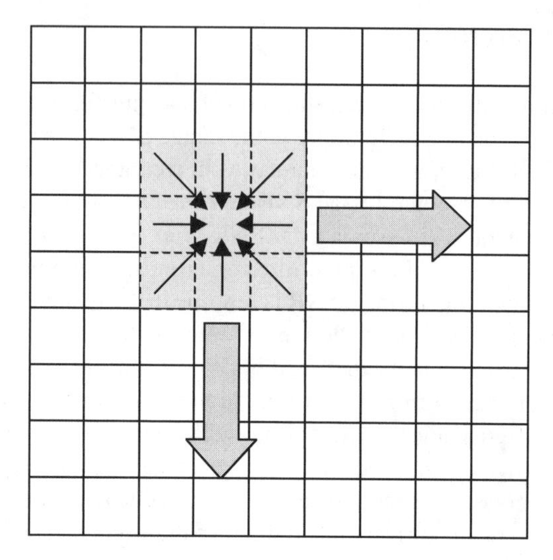

FIGURE 5.10. *Implementation of image filtering in two-dimensions using a 3 × 3 convolution kernel.*

Edge detection in nuclear medicine images is important for implementation of attenuation correction algorithms. This process is difficult because of the low SNR and the relatively poor spatial resolution of the raw image. Simple high-pass filtering results in too high a noise level, and so edge detection involves applying a smoothing function first, followed by a second convolution kernel to emphasize

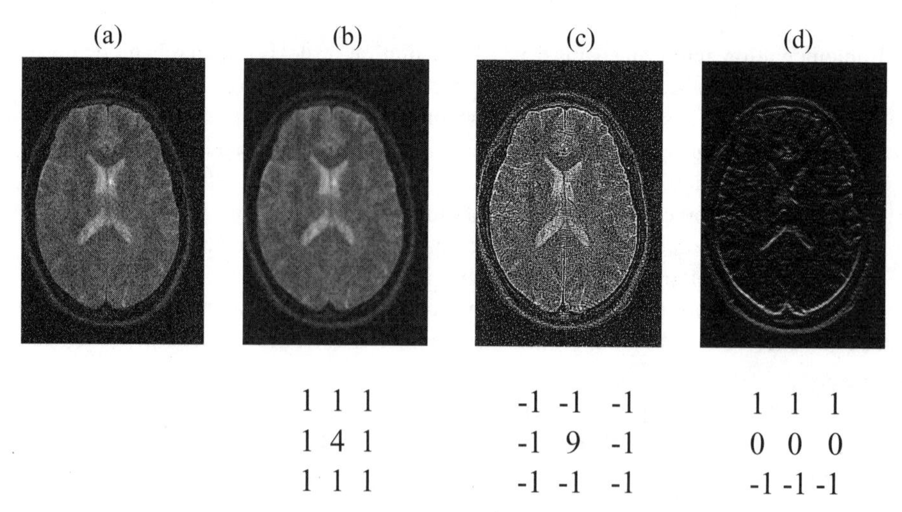

FIGURE 5.11. *Effects of different types of image filtering. (a) The original MRI image of the brain. (b) Low-pass filtering. (c) High-pass filtering. (d) Edge detection.*

the image edges. An example of an edge detection filtered image is shown in Figure 5.11(d).

More sophisticated filtering is often performed on medical images, in which the filter applied has different characteristics for different parts of the image. One common procedure is to apply a Wiener, or minimum mean-square estimation (MSE), filter, which provides the optimum tradeoff between improved SNR and minimal degradation of the spatial resolution.

5.6. THE RECEIVER OPERATING CURVE

As discussed in this chapter, several instrumental and patient-related characteristics affect the SNR, the spatial resolution, and the CNR of an image. The inherent tradeoffs among these parameters are case- and disease-specific, and methods of assessing the relative importance of each parameter for a particular application are very useful. One such method uses the so-called receiver operating curve (ROC). As an example, consider the situation in which a patient is suspected of having a tumor. There are four possibilities for a radiologist making the diagnosis: a true positive (where true refers to the correct diagnosis and positive to the tumor being present), a true negative, a false positive, and a false negative, as shown in Figure 5.12. Three measures are commonly used in ROC analysis: the accuracy is the number of correct diagnoses divided by the total number of diagnoses, the sensitivity is the number of true positives divided by the sum of the true positives and the false negatives, and the specificity is the number of true negatives divided by the sum of the number of true negatives and false positives.

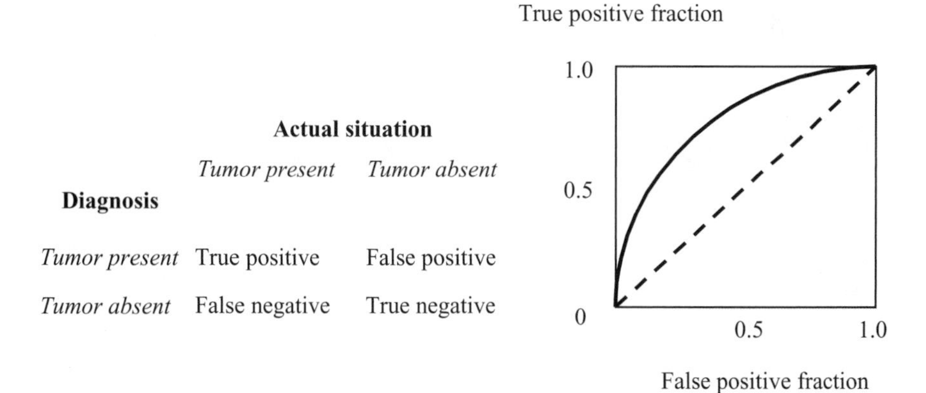

Diagnosis	**Actual situation** *Tumor present*	*Tumor absent*
Tumor present	True positive	False positive
Tumor absent	False negative	True negative

FIGURE 5.12. *(Left) A table showing the four possible outcomes of a tumor diagnosis. (Right) The ROC represented by the dashed line represents a random diagnosis. The upper curve represents an improved diagnosis. The better the diagnosis, the larger is the integrated area under the ROC.*

The ROC plots the fraction of true positives versus the fraction of false positives for a series of images acquired under different conditions, or with different values of the image spatial resolution and SNR, for example. The area under the ROC is a measure of the effectiveness of the imaging system and/or the radiologist: the greater the area under the curve, the more effective is the diagnosis.

Appendix A

The Fourier Transform

A.1. INTRODUCTION

The Fourier transform is an integral part of data processing in each of the image modalities studied. In X-ray CT, SPECT, and PET, filtered backprojection reconstruction is implemented using a Fourier transform. In ultrasonic imaging, spectral Doppler graphs are produced by Fourier transformation of the acquired time-domain signals. In MRI, the acquired spatial frequency-domain signals are inverse-Fourier-transformed to give the image. This Appendix summarizes the basis mathematics and properties of the Fourier transform.

A.2. FOURIER TRANSFORMATION OF TIME-DOMAIN AND SPATIAL FREQUENCY-DOMAIN SIGNALS

The forward Fourier transform of a time-domain signal $s(t)$ is given by

$$S(f) = \int_{-\infty}^{\infty} s(t)e^{-j2\pi ft}dt \tag{A.1}$$

The inverse Fourier transform of a frequency-domain signal $S(f)$ is represented by

$$s(t) = \frac{1}{2\pi}\int_{-\infty}^{\infty} S(f)e^{+j2\pi ft}df \tag{A.2}$$

Similarly, the forward Fourier transform of a spatial-domain signal $\rho(x)$ has the form

$$S(k) = \int_{-\infty}^{\infty} \rho(x) e^{-j2\pi kx} dx \tag{A.3}$$

The corresponding inverse Fourier transform of a spatial frequency-domain signal $S(k)$ can be expressed as

$$\rho(x) = \int_{-\infty}^{\infty} S(k) e^{+j2\pi kx} dk \tag{A.4}$$

Some useful Fourier pairs are shown in Figure A.1.

Signals are often acquired in more than one dimension, and image reconstruction then requires multidimensional Fourier transformation:

$$S(k_x, k_y) = \int_{-\infty}^{\infty} \int_{-\infty}^{\infty} \rho(x, y) e^{-j2\pi(k_x x + k_y y)} dx\, dy \tag{A.5}$$

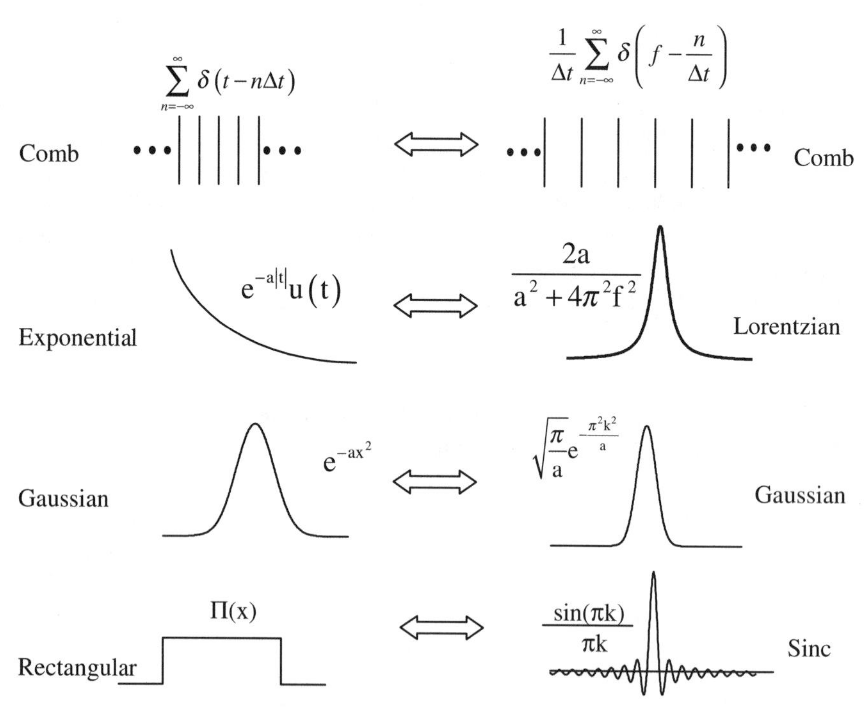

FIGURE A.1. *Some Fourier transform pairs commonly encountered in imaging methods. For example, the comb function represents the process of the discrete sampling of a continuous signal. A negative exponential characterizes spin–spin relaxation of MRI signals, as well as radioactive decay. The beam profile in ultrasound is often Gaussian, as is the line spread function in many imaging modalities. Finally, the rectangular function describes truncation effects in the total number of time-domain data points acquired in MRI, for example.*

$$\rho(x, y) = \int_{-\infty}^{\infty}\int_{-\infty}^{\infty} S(k_x, k_y)e^{+j2\pi(k_x x + k_y y)}dk_x dk_y \tag{A.6}$$

$$S(k_x, k_y, k_z) = \int_{-\infty}^{\infty}\int_{-\infty}^{\infty}\int_{-\infty}^{\infty} \rho(x, y, z)e^{-j2\pi(k_x x + k_y y + k_z z)}dx\, dy\, dz \tag{A.7}$$

$$\rho(x, y, z) = \int_{-\infty}^{\infty}\int_{-\infty}^{\infty}\int_{-\infty}^{\infty} S(k_x, k_y, k_z)e^{+j2\pi(k_x x + k_y y + k_z z)}dk_x\, dk_y\, dk_z \tag{A.8}$$

These higher-dimension Fourier transforms can be expressed, and implemented, as sequential one-dimensional transforms along the respective dimensions. For example, this means that a two-dimensional Fourier transform of a function $f(x, y)$ can be implemented by first carrying out a one-dimensional Fourier transform along the x axis and then the second Fourier transform along the y axis.

A.2.1. Useful Properties of the Fourier Transform

There are a number of mathematical properties of the Fourier transform that are extremely useful in analyzing the signals acquired using different imaging techniques. The following list is not exhaustive, but highlights relevant properties for the imaging systems covered in this book.

1. Linearity. The Fourier transform of two additive functions is also additive:

$$\begin{aligned} as_1(t) + bs_2(t) &\Leftrightarrow aS_1(f) + bS_2(f) \\ a\rho_1(x) + b\rho_2(x) &\Leftrightarrow aS_1(k) + bS_2(k) \end{aligned} \tag{A.9}$$

where $\Leftrightarrow$ represents the Fourier transform This theorem is useful in considering, for example, time-domain Doppler ultrasound signals, which consist of many frequency components, each frequency component having a different amplitude. The linearity property means that the relative amplitudes of these components are maintained when the data are Fourier-transformed into the frequency domain.

2. Convolution. If two time-domain signals are multiplied together, then the frequency-domain signal is the convolution of the two individual Fourier-transformed components:

$$s_1(t)s_2(t) \Leftrightarrow S_1(f) * S_2(f) \tag{A.10}$$

where $*$ represents a convolution. The convolution $f(x)$ of two functions $p(x)$ and $q(x)$ is defined as

$$f(x) = p(x) * q(x) = \int_{-\infty}^{\infty} p(x - \tau)q(\tau)\, d\tau \tag{A.11}$$

One example is the real component of the time-domain NMR signal, which can be represented by a cosine function multiplied by a negative exponential due to T_2^* relaxation. The frequency-domain signal is given by the convolution of a delta function (the Fourier transform of a cosine function) with a Lorentzian function (the Fourier transform of an exponential function).

3. Parseval's theorem: The total energy of a function in the time domain/spatial domain is the same as the total energy of the Fourier transform of that function in the frequency domain/spatial frequency domain:

$$\int_{-\infty}^{\infty} |s(t)|^2 \, dt = \int_{-\infty}^{\infty} |S(f)|^2 \, df$$
$$\int_{-\infty}^{\infty} |\rho(x)|^2 \, dx = \int_{-\infty}^{\infty} |S(k)|^2 \, dk \tag{A.12}$$

An example of Parseval's theorem can also be found in NMR, in which the amplitude of the signal directly after an RF pulse is proportional to the integrated area of the NMR spectrum after Fourier transformation.

4. Scaling law. If a time-domain signal is expanded by some factor, then its Fourier transform is compressed by the same factor:

$$s(at) \Leftrightarrow \frac{1}{|a|} S\left(\frac{f}{a}\right) \tag{A.13}$$

For example, in MRI, if the T_2^* value of tissue is increased through better shimming, the time-domain signal decays to zero more slowly, and the corresponding frequency-domain spectrum is narrower.

Appendix B

Backprojection and Filtered Backprojection

B.1. INTRODUCTION

The problem of reconstructing a two-dimensional image from a series of one-dimensional projections is common to a number of imaging modalities. Of those covered in this book, CT, SPECT, and PET produce data exclusively as a series of projections, and, less commonly, MRI projection reconstruction sequences are used, typically for imaging samples with very short T_2 values. In each of these methods a number of one-dimensional projections, $p_1, p_2, \ldots, p_n$, are acquired with the detector oriented at different angles with respect to the object, as shown in Figure B.1. In the following analyses, the object is represented as a function $f(x, y)$, in which the spatially dependent values of f correspond to the distribution of radiopharmaceutical in SPECT or PET or attenuation coefficients in X-ray CT.

The coordinate system in the measurement frame is represented by (r, s), where r is the direction parallel to the detector and s is the direction along the ray sum at 90° to the r dimension. The angle between the x and r axes is denoted as ϕ, and so by simple trigonometry

$$\begin{aligned} r &= x\cos\phi + y\sin\phi \\ s &= -x\sin\phi + y\cos\phi \end{aligned} \tag{B.1}$$

The measured projection is denoted by $p(r, \phi)$. Projections are acquired at different values of ϕ until coverage over a range of 180° or 360°, depending upon the particular application, has been reached. A number of schemes exist for the reconstruction of the image, covered in the following sections.

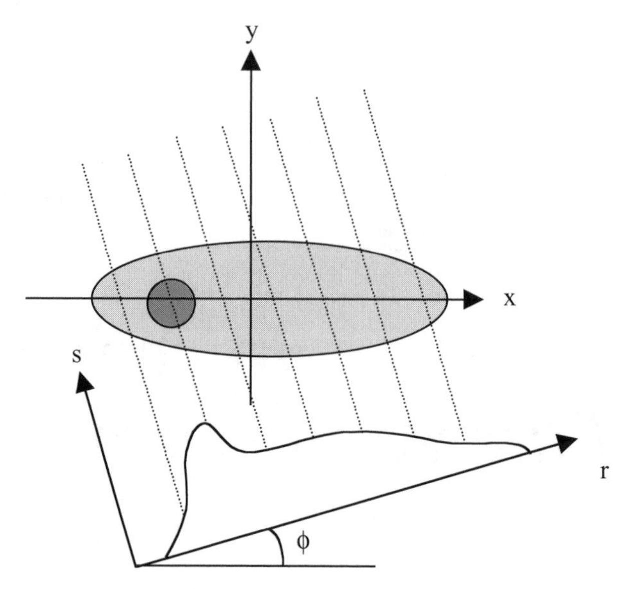

FIGURE B.1. *The coordinate system used for analyzing backprojection algorithms. The object can be represented as f(x, y), where x and y represent the image coordinates. Successive projections of the object are obtained with the detector aligned at different values of the angle ϕ.*

B.2. BACKPROJECTION

Simple backprojection of the acquired projections corresponds to direct implementation of the inverse Radon transform. Backprojection assigns an equal weighting to the pixels contributing to each point in a particular projection. This process is repeated for all of the projections, and the pixel intensities are summed to give the reconstructed image $\hat{f}(x, y)$. Mathematically, $\hat{f}(x, y)$ can be represented as

$$\hat{f}(x, y) = \sum_{j=1}^{n} p(r, \phi_j)\, d\phi \tag{B.2}$$

where n is the number of projections. Figure B.2 shows the typical artifacts associated with simple backprojection.

The backprojected image of a well-known model of the head, the Shepp–Logan phantom, is shown in Figure B.3. This phantom is often used to assess the effect of newly developed reconstruction algorithms and consists of a set of ellipses: the largest outer ellipse represents the head, with smaller ellipses representing features within the head. Notice that, in addition to blurring the edges of the image, the contrast within the phantom is also greatly reduced by simple backprojection.

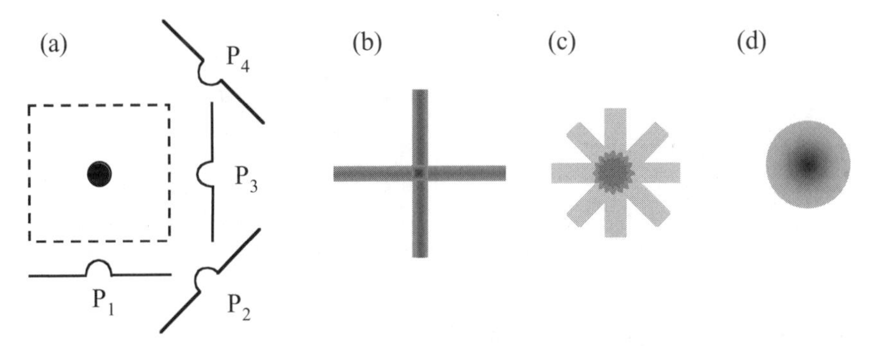

FIGURE B.2. (a) A series of projections P_1–P_4 acquired for a simple circular object. The dashed lines represent the FOV of the image. (b) A simple backprojection reconstruction using only projections P_1 and P_3. (c) The "star artifact" produced by the reconstruction of a moderate number of projections. (d) The radial blurring produced using simple backprojection of an infinite number of projections.

B.3. FILTERED BACKPROJECTION

The widely implemented method of filtered backprojection consists in applying a filter to each projection before backprojection in order to reduce the artifacts associated with simple backprojection. One of the most common implementations uses the Ramachandran–Lakshminarayanan (Ram–Lak) filter. If the filter is applied in the spatial domain, then the filtered projection $p'(r, \phi)$ can be represented as

$$p'(r, \phi) = p(r, \phi) * h(r) \tag{B.3}$$

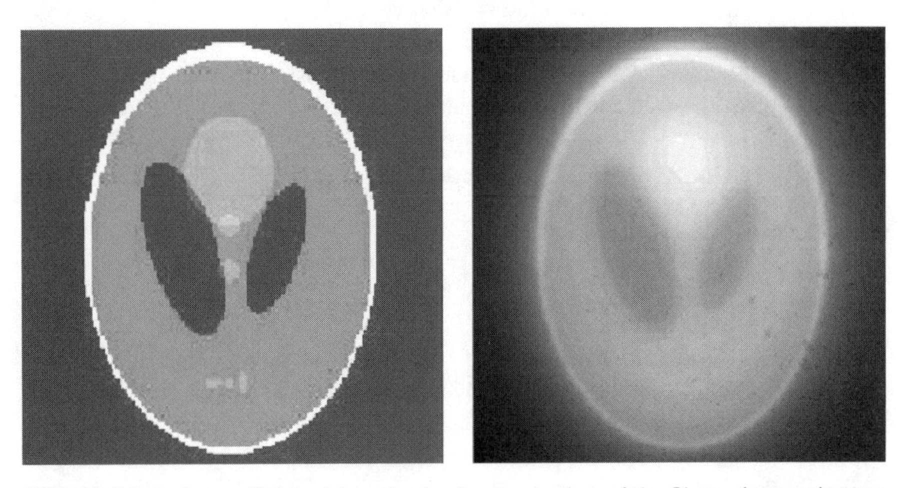

FIGURE B.3. An image (right), obtained using backprojection, of the Shepp–Logan phantom (left) shows considerable blurring and contrast loss.

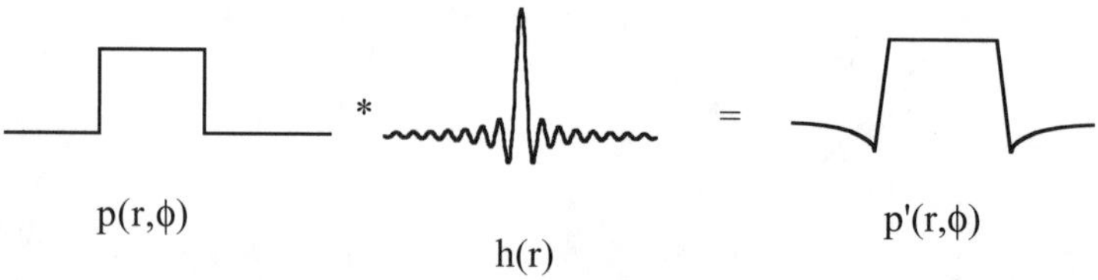

p(r,ϕ)
h(r)
p'(r,ϕ)

FIGURE B.4. *The effect of convolving a projection $p(r, \phi)$ with the spatial filter function $h(r)$. The negative lobe in the filtered projection minimizes the "star artifact" in the reconstructed image.*

The expression for $h(r)$, the Ram–Lak filter, is given by

$$h(r) = \frac{1}{2(dr)^2}\left[\text{sinc}\left(\frac{r}{dr}\right)\right] - \frac{1}{4(dr)^2}\left[\text{sinc}^2\left(\frac{r}{2dr}\right)\right] \tag{B.4}$$

where dr is the sampling interval along the r axis. The form of $h(r)$ is shown in Figure B.4. After filtering, the projections are then backprojected as described previously. The major effect of the convolution of $p(r, \phi)$ with $h(r)$ is to decrease the intensity of the "star artifact" produced by simple backprojection.

Because the mathematical process of convolution is computationally intensive, in practice filtered backprojection is carried out in the spatial frequency domain using fast Fourier transform methods. Convolution in the spatial domain is equivalent to multiplication in the spatial frequency domain, and multiplication can be performed much faster computationally than convolution. Each projection $p(r, \phi)$ is Fourier-transformed along the r dimension to give $P(k, \phi)$, and then $P(k, \phi)$ is multiplied by $H(k)$, the Fourier transform of $h(r)$, to give $P'(k, \phi)$:

$$P'(k, \phi) = P(k, \phi)H(k) \tag{B.5}$$

The filtered projections $P'(k, \phi)$, are inverse-Fourier-transformed back into the spatial domain and backprojected to give the final image $\hat{f}(x, y)$:

$$\hat{f}(x, y) = \sum_{j=1}^{n} \mathbb{F}^{-1}\{P'(k, \phi_j)\}\, d\varphi \tag{B.6}$$

where $\mathbb{F}^{-1}$ represents an inverse Fourier transform. The expression for H(k) in equation (B.5) is given by

$$H(k) = |k| \text{ rect}(k) \tag{B.7}$$

where:

$$\begin{aligned} \text{rect}(k) &= 1 \qquad \text{if} \quad |k| \leq 0.5 \\ &= -1 \qquad \text{if} \quad |k| \geq 0.5 \end{aligned} \tag{B.8}$$

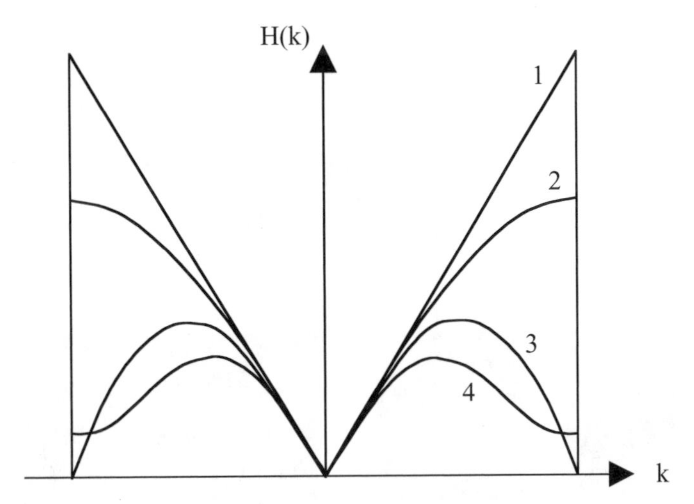

FIGURE B.5. *Some common filter functions used for backprojection. 1, Ram–Lak; 2, Shepp–Logan; 3, low-pass cosine; and 4, generalized Hamming.*

The form of $H(k)$ in the spatial frequency domain is shown in Figure B.5. As can be appreciated, this filter does not have very desirable noise characteristics because it amplifies high spatial frequencies. In order to improve the noise performance of the filter, the amplification of high spatial frequencies can be reduced, resulting in commonly used functions such as Shepp–Logan, low-pass cosine, or generalized Hamming filters, which are also shown in Figure B.5.

Figure B.6 compares the results of filtered backprojection of the Shepp–Logan phantom with a Ram–Lak and a Hamming filter.

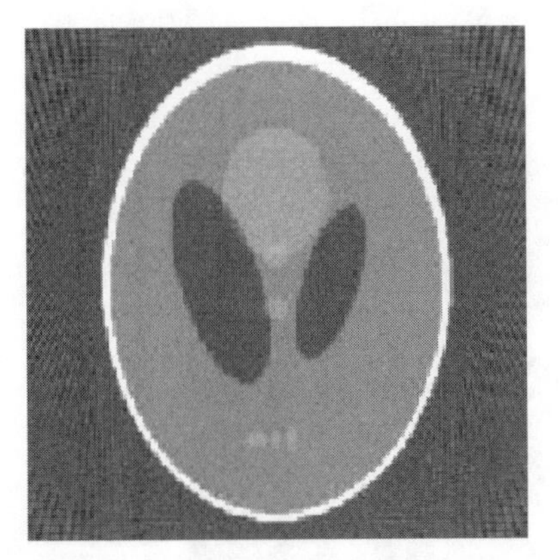

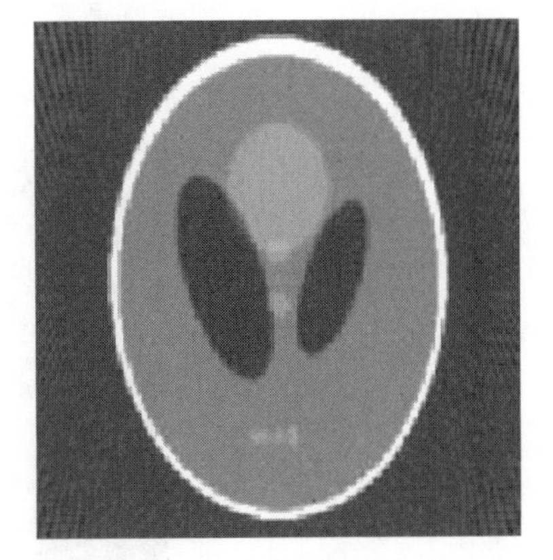

FIGURE B.6. *Filtered backprojections of the Shepp–Logan phantom using (left) the Ram–Lak filter and (right) a generalized Hamming filter. Results using the Hamming filter give a higher SNR image, but one which is also more blurred.*

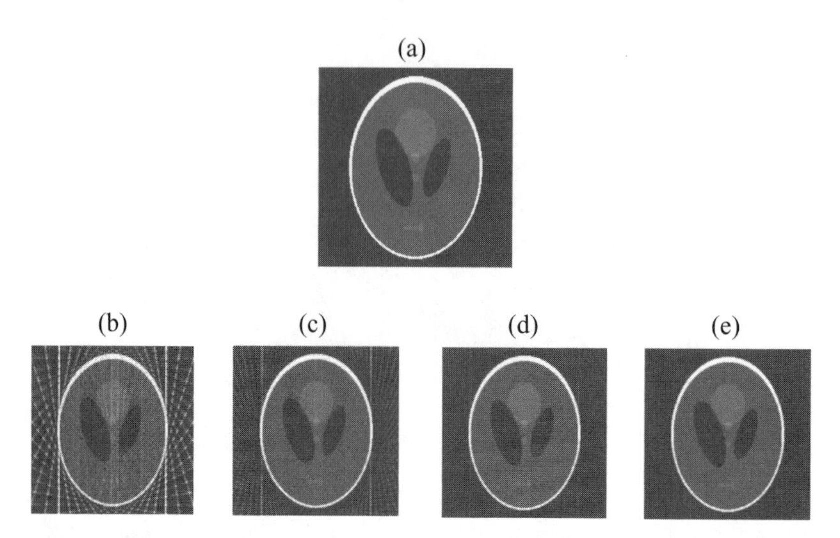

FIGURE B.7. *The effect of the number of projections on the final image using filtered backprojection with a Shepp–Logan filter. (a) The original Shepp–Logan phantom. (b–e) The effect of increasing the number of projections for reconstruction: (b) 20 projections, (c) 45 projections, (d) 90 projections, and (e) 180 projections.*

An important data acquisition parameter is the number of projections required to produce a high-quality image. If too few projections are acquired, then significant image artifacts occur in data reconstruction. Figure B.7 shows examples of these so-called "streak" artifacts.

A common method of displaying projection data is called a sinogram, in which the projections are plotted as a function of the angle ϕ. In order to reduce the

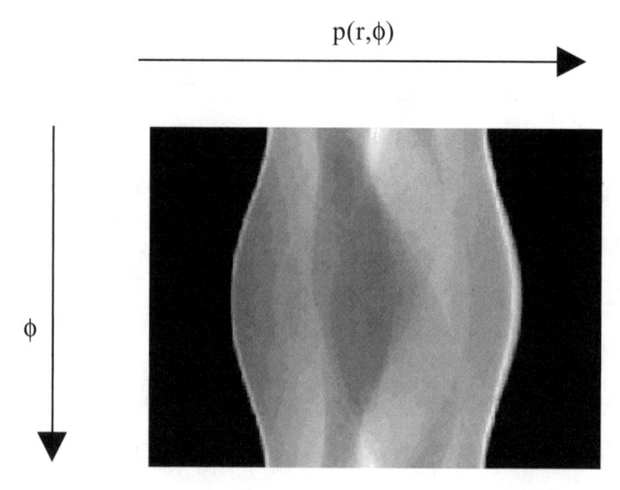

FIGURE B.8. *Sinogram from a Shepp–Logan phantom.*

dimensionality of the plot, the projections are plotted with the signal amplitude represented by the brightness of the sinogram, with a high amplitude corresponding to a bright pixel and a low amplitude to a dark pixel. Figure B.8 shows a sinogram from the Shepp–Logan phantom used in the previous examples. Sinograms can be used to detect the presence of patient motion, which is visible as a signal discontinuity. Such motions can cause severe artifacts in the reconstructed images.

ABBREVIATIONS

A/D	analog-to-digital
ACD	annihilation coincidence detection
AEC	automatic exposure control
BBB	blood brain barrier
BGO	bismuth germanate
BOLD	blood oxygen level dependent
CBF	cerebral blood flow
CCD	charge coupled device
$CMRO_2$	cerebral metabolic rate of oxygen
CNR	contrast-to-noise ratio
CR	computed radiography
CSF	cerebrospinal fluid
CSI	chemical shift imaging
CT	computed tomography
CTDI	computed tomography dose index
CW	continuous wave
CZT	cadmium lead telluride
DNA	deoxyribonucleic acid
DOF	depth-of-focus
DQE	detective quantum efficiency
DR	digital radiography
DSA	digital subtraction angiography
DTPA	diethylenetriaminepentaacetic acid
EPI	echo planar imaging
ESF	edge spread function
FDG	fluorodeoxyglucose
FID	free induction decay
FLASH	fast low angle shot
fMRI	functional magnetic resonance imaging
FOV	field-of-view
FPD	flat-panel detector
FWHM	full-width-at-half-maximum
GI	gastrointestinal

HSA	human serum albumin
HOCM	high osmolarity contrast media
HVL	half value layer
IVP	Intravenous pyelogram
kV_p	accelerating voltage
LED	Light-emitting diode
LOCM	low osmolarity contrast media
LSF	line spread function
MAA	macroaggregated albumin
MIP	maximum intensity projection
MRA	magnetic resonance angiography
MRI	magnetic resonance imaging
MSE	mean squared error
MTF	modulation transfer function
NEX	number of excitations
NFB	near-field boundary
NMR	nuclear magnetic resonance
OD	optical density
PC	phase contrast
PET	positron emission tomography
PHA	pulse height analyzer
PMT	photomultiplier tube
PRESS	point resolved spectroscopy
PRR	pulse repetition rate
PSF	point spread function
PSPMT	position sensitive photomultiplier tube
PVDF	polyvinylidine difluoride
PZT	lead zirconate titanate
QF	quality factor
RBC	red blood cell
RES	reticuloendothelial system
RF	radiofrequency
ROC	receiver operating curve
ROI	region-of-interest
SATA	spatial average temporal average
SD	standard deviation
SNR	signal-to-noise ratio
SPECT	single photon emission computed tomography
SPIO	superparamagnetic iron oxide
SPTA	spatial peak temporal average
TDC	time-domain correlation
TFT	thin-film transistor
TGC	time-gain compensation
TOF	time-of-flight

INDEX